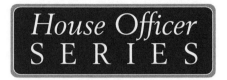

House Officer
S E R I E S

Psychiatry

SEVENTH EDITION

The House Officer Series is based on Weiner and Levitt's *Neurology for the House Officer*, first published in 1973.

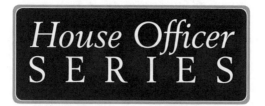

House Officer SERIES

Psychiatry

SEVENTH EDITION

David A. Tomb, M.D.

Associate Professor
Department of Psychiatry
University of Utah School of Medicine
Salt Lake City, Utah

 Wolters Kluwer | Lippincott Williams & Wilkins
Health

Philadelphia · Baltimore · New York · London
Buenos Aires · Hong Kong · Sydney · Tokyo

Acquisitions Editor: Charles W. Mitchell
Managing Editor: Sirkka Howes Bertling
Associate Director of Marketing:
    Adam Glazer
Production Manager: Bridgett Dougherty

Senior Manufacturing Manager:
    Benjamin Rivera
Creative Director: Doug Smock
Production Services: Nesbitt Graphics, Inc.

© 2008 by LIPPINCOTT WILLIAMS & WILKINS- a Wolters Kluwer business
530 Walnut Street
Philadelphia, PA 19106 USA
LWW.com

Printed in the USA

Library of Congress Cataloging-in-Publication Data

Tomb, David A.
    Psychiatry / David A. Tomb. — 7th ed.
      p. ; cm. — (House officer series)
    Includes bibliographical references and index.
    ISBN-13: 978-0-7817-7452-9
    ISBN-10: 0-7817-7452-7
    1. Psychiatry—Handbooks, manuals, etc. 2. Mental illness—Handbooks, manuals, etc. 3. Psychological manifestations of general diseases—Handbooks, manuals, etc. I. Title. II. Series.
    [DNLM: 1. Mental Disorders—Handbooks. WM 34 T656pa 2007]
RC456.T64 2007
616.89—dc22

                              2007014411

                    10 9 8 7 6 5 4 3 2 1

Contents

Preface ix

1 Psychiatric Classification 1
   A description of psychiatric classification and DSM-IV
   is presented.

2 Assessment 4
   DSM-IV has clarified the procedure of diagnosis, yet
   there is still need for a good history and mental status
   examination. Additional useful information may be
   obtained from psychological testing, EEG, brain
   imaging, and the Amytal interview.

3 Psychotic Disorders 20
   Schizophrenia, the major psychotic disorder, is a
   chronic disorder. There are several other psychoses
   that mimic schizophrenia but that appear to have
   different etiologies.

4 Mood Disorders 40
   Mood disorders include both depression and mania.
   They can be major or minor and primary or due to
   medical causes. Treatment is often quite specific and
   successful.

5 Delirium and Amnestic and Other
   Cognitive Disorders 56
   The unique syndromes produced by compromised brain
   function must be considered prominently in the differential diagnosis of almost all other psychiatric disorders.

6 Dementia 62
   Dementia is defined and clues for making the diagnosis are given. Treatable and untreatable types are
   listed along with general treatment principles.

7 **Suicidal and Assaultive Behaviors** 72
Suicidal patients are common and diagnostically diverse. They need to be identified and vigorously treated. Violent patients require special handling and a careful workup.

8 **Anxiety Disorders** 81
Anxiety disorders include not just patients with anxiety but also patients with phobias, unfortunate reactions to severe stress, and obsessive compulsive disorders.

9 **Dissociative Disorders** 93
These dramatic conditions include amnesias, fugues, dissociative identity disorder, and depersonalized states. All are uncommon but striking when encountered.

10 **Grief and the Dying Patient** 98
A description of normal grief and unresolved grief, with treatment principles. Clinical presentation and treatment of the response to chronic illness and dying are described.

11 **Conditions which Mimic Physical Disease** 105
Some medical patients may really have a psychiatric illness. Possibilities include conversion disorder, somatization disorder, hypochondriasis, and pain disorder.

12 **Psychosomatic Disorders** 116
The general characteristics of psychophysiologic illness are described and the psychological and physiological mechanisms are detailed. Specific psychosomatic disorders are listed.

13 **Psychiatric Symptoms of Nonpsychiatric Medication** 126
The medications most likely to cause psychiatric symptoms are presented along with the clinical pictures they produce.

14 Psychiatric Presentations of Medical Disease 131
*Anxiety, depression, and confusion may all have a
purely medical cause. The physical disorders which
most commonly present with psychiatric symptoms
are described.*

**15 Psychiatric Presentations of
Neurological Disease** 137
*Neurological disease produces psychiatric symptoms
partially based on the location of the CNS pathology.
Specific diseases are described.*

16 Psychiatry of Alcohol 142
*Alcohol-related conditions are common and include
intoxication, abuse, withdrawal, DTs, and hallucinosis. Treatments are described.*

17 Psychiatry of Drug Abuse 154
*Drugs covered include opioids, sedative-hypnotics,
hallucinogens, stimulants, and inhalants.*

18 Psychosexual Disorders 176
*Disorders of normal sexual performances are
covered, as are sexual deviations, and disorders of
gender identity. Available treatments are presented.*

19 Sleep Disturbances 186
*An understanding of normal sleep and a careful
history are key to a good evaluation of the
two common sleep disturbances, insomnia and
hypersomnia.*

20 Personality Disorders 195
*Several different personality disorders are recognized.
Although all of them produce dysfunction, in each
case the personality characteristics seem "natural" to
the patient.*

21 Mental Retardation 203
*Mental retardation is common and due to a variety
of causes. It is not necessarily an irreversible
condition.*

22 The Psychotherapies 207
*There are numerous different psychotherapies in use
but the major ones include psychoanalysis, supportive
psychotherapy, group therapy, cognitive-behavior
therapy, and family therapy.*

23 Biological Therapy 215
*The major drugs in adult psychiatry are the antide-
pressants, the major and minor tranquilizers, and
lithium. ECT plays a major role, and psychosurgery a
minor role in modern treatment.*

24 The Elderly Patient 260
*The elderly patient has some unique sensitivities.
Knowledge of special psychopharmacologic and psychotherapeutic principles is needed to treat these
patients satisfactorily.*

25 Legal Issues 267
*Legal matters are assuming ever greater importance
in psychiatry. Particularly complex are involuntary
commitment and treatment issues as well as the
interface between psychiatry and the criminal
courts.*

26 Impulse-Control Disorders 274
*This grouping constitutes an odd collection of condi-
tions which have just enough in common to be placed
together. However, specific disorders from this group
could just as easily be placed elsewhere in DSM-IV-TR.
Moreover, a number of other disorders are discussed
which could as easily (and perhaps will) be placed
here as well.*

Index 279

Preface

Who would have thought when I wrote the first edition of this book that psychiatry would advance at a rate requiring seven editions in my lifetime? But advance it has. New and useful information and explanations continue to tumble over one another in an effort to squeeze their way into these pages. They show no signs of slowing. This makes the field exciting and has given me an embarrassing plenitude of riches from which to construct the latest edition. I hope I have chosen well.

Among the many individuals who have helped this book appear in its numerous editions over 2 ½ decades, I would like specially to thank the residents and students with whom I have worked. It would be an impossible task to list the colleagues and trainees who have shared their knowledge with me over the years but I can take comfort in the fact that "you know who you are." Once again I wish to thank Bernie Grosser, MD, Department Chairman, for his support and Gloria J. Tong, MD, a fine young colleague, for sharing both her enthusiasm and innumerable cases with me, providing a diversity which has kept me honest. Perhaps the best concealed secret in education, but well known by "educators," is that as much learning flows from students to teachers as the reverse.

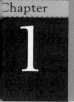

1 Psychiatric Classification

DSM-IV

Psychiatric diagnosis has long been criticized as ambiguous and unreliable. Some diagnoses have been based on subjective, unverifiable, intrapsychic phenomena, whereas others have been heterogeneously broad.

Modern diagnosis attempts to avoid these pitfalls through the use of the 4th edition of the *Diagnostic and Statistical Manual of Mental Disorders* (DSM-IV-TR) (1), which identifies each disorder by a unique specific collection of symptoms. (Note: throughout this text, the term "DSM" will be used to represent the most recent edition, DSM-IV-TR.) It defines a limited number of identifiable (although possibly overlapping) psychiatric disorders and contains specific diagnostic criteria for each diagnosis. One matches facts from a particular patient's history and clinical presentation with criteria from a likely diagnosis, and if an adequate number are met (a **polythetic** diagnosis; not all the criteria are needed to make the diagnosis), that diagnosis should be made. Each disorder has a unique set of these "operationally defined" diagnostic criteria. Multiple diagnoses are permitted, and each general group of disorders has one disorder, "Not Otherwise Specified" (NOS), that allows placement of the (often many) patients who have unusual presentations. In addition, some disorders have **subtypes,** which are mutually exclusive (e.g., *paranoid* schizophrenia) or **specifiers** that are not (may change with time; e.g., mild, moderate, and severe, or in full remission) or both. Finally, it is okay to make a **provisional** (you are not sure) or a **deferred** (not enough information) diagnosis.

For example, a patient who (a) has been having delusions and auditory hallucinations that (b) have impaired social relations and functioning at work (c) for at least 6 months and who is without evidence of (d) a general medical condition or (e) prominent symptoms of a major mood disorder must be given the diagnosis of schizophrenia. If the patient also has (f) a flat, inappropriate, or silly affect and (g) disorganized speech and behavior, an additional diagnosis of "disorganized" subtype should be made.

DSM-IV has improved diagnostic **reliability** (the likelihood that different professionals would make the same diagnosis on the same patient) but has had only a modest impact on **validity** (the certainty that the diagnoses identify unique meaningful conditions). It may well be that DSM-IV has broken psychiatric conditions into too many pieces and that each piece does not represent a "valid" condition (2,3). A common criticism is that the criteria allow too many minor human behaviors to be classed as disorders (false positives), a problem partially corrected by insisting that each set of behaviors has serious clinical significance (4).

Note also that DSM-IV makes no assumptions about what causes these disorders (it just describes and categorizes them), and in most cases, the etiology is unknown. Although DSM-IV holds up well across cultures, its use in those settings requires special care in the interpretation of symptoms. DSM-IV is far from perfect (5) and thus allows the use of "clinical judgment" as well as strict application of the criteria in making a final diagnosis. Remember, ultimately it is the patient and the patient's narrative/life story that we are treating, not the diagnosis.

MULTIAXIAL CLASSIFICATION

In addition to operationally defined criteria, DSM-IV also uses a multiaxial system of classification to capture other important information. A patient is not fully classified until coded on each of five axes (although only the first three axes are needed for an official diagnosis):

- **Axis I:** The clinical disorder(s) described earlier.
- **Axis II:** Personality disorders or mental retardation (none may be present) or both.
- **Axis III:** Physical disorders relevant to the mental disorder.
- **Axis IV:** A listing of psychosocial and environmental *problems*, usually but not always during the preceding year, such as unemployment, divorce, financial problems, victim of child neglect, and so on.
- **Axis V:** The Global Assessment of Functioning Scale (GAF) (DSM, p. 34), which is a measure, typically, of *current* general functioning but at times of the highest functioning over the preceding year (scale range is 1 to 100) and which is used in treatment planning and predicting outcome.

REFERENCES

1. American Psychiatric Association. *Diagnostic and Statistical Manual of Mental Disorders*, 4th ed., Text Revision. Washington, DC: American Psychiatric Association, 2000.
2. Phillips KA, First MB, Pincus HA. *Advancing DSM*. Washington, DC. American Psychiatric Association, 2003.
3. Sullivan PF, Kendler KS. Typology of common psychiatric syndromes. *Br J Psychiatry* 1998;173:312–319.
4. Spitzer RL, Wakefield JC. DSM-IV diagnostic criterion for clinical significance: does it help solve the false positives problem? *Am J Psychiatry* 1999;156:1856–1864.
5. Tucker GJ. Putting DSM-IV in perspective. *Am J Psychiatry* 1998;155:159–161.

Assessment

A psychiatric evaluation helps to (a) make a diagnosis, (b) estimate the severity of the patient's condition, (c) decide on an initial course of action, (d) develop a relationship with the patient (therapeutic alliance), (e) assemble a dynamic understanding of the patient, and (f) engage the patient in psychotherapy. Some (primarily analytically oriented) psychiatrists argue that the most reliable understanding of a patient results from an open-ended interview in which the course of the interview is directed by the patient's conscious and unconscious concerns. An alternate form of interview, and one encouraged by the requirements of *Diagnostic and Statistical Manual of Mental Disorders* (DSM), uses a structured format that demands precise historic and descriptive information and the answers to specific questions (1–4). Which technique produces a more accurate and useful understanding of the patient remains unresolved, yet modern diagnosis requires the structured form described later.

A thorough evaluation of a psychiatric patient consists of a psychiatric history, mental status examination, complete physical examination, laboratory screening evaluation, and, when indicated, specific psychological and biologic tests. The history and mental status are usually obtained during the initial interview.

More is required than merely collecting facts. The interviewer seeks useful information not only from the history and mental status examination but also from the patient's interpersonal style and nonverbal communications and from the sequence and choice of issues raised by the patient. Because so much information is available from the patient outside the formal part of the interview, it is essential to avoid structuring the interview too early. Initially, allow the patient to express concerns and find out the reason for coming for help (*Why now?*). Be supportive, attentive, nonjudgmental, and encouraging—develop a rapport with the patient and try to get an empathic understanding of his or her distress. Develop a qualitative sense for the patient's impairment. Help allay anxiety, if present. Be patient, friendly, and receptive if the patient is quiet. If the patient rambles, you may have to impose a structure early. If the patient is paranoid, progress slowly. Decide early if he or she is likely to be aggressive, suicidal, or in need of hospitalization.

If the interview is skillfully conducted, much of the information required by the history and mental status examination may be obtained unobtrusively. As the interview proceeds, you usually can identify and narrow missing data so that more formal questions are minimal. However, certain information is almost always required (e.g., data to satisfy DSM diagnostic criteria, family psychiatric history, or mental status responses to rule out organicity or loss of abstracting ability). At times during the interview, mentally review what is missing, and save time toward the end to pursue it by direct questioning. The transition to a more formal style of interviewing can be smooth if rapport has been developed beforehand ("Now I need to ask you some very specific questions").

PSYCHIATRIC HISTORY

Identification of the Patient

1. Name, age, birth date, marital status and children, ethnic status, religion, occupation, education, social class, handicaps, and so on;
2. Identification of informants (if not the patient), as well as mood and apparent biases of informants;
3. Estimate of the reliability of the information.

Chief Complaint

Usually a verbatim statement of "the problem." Does it differ significantly from the reports of those who accompany the patient?

Present Illness

Usually the focus of the interview. Get the patient's description of and feelings about the illness (problem) and need for care ("why now," if ever). Establish the chronologic order of recent *symptoms* and *treatments* from an appropriate historic reference point (varies but often weeks). Has the patient noticed any other changes in him or herself? Have there been major life changes during this time or particular stresses and conflicts? Is any secondary gain identifiable? What is the patient's legal status? *Is the patient suicidal* or homicidal?

Past Psychiatric Illness

Backtrack any current psychiatric problems to their inception. Ask about the other most common psychiatric disorders; their diagnoses, and severity of illnesses. Get a chronologic history of symptoms, associated life problems, past psychopharmacology and its usefulness, psychotherapy, and hospitalizations. Get a detailed history of alcohol and drug use/abuse and history of past suicidal or homicidal behavior. Determine reliability of this history (attempt to obtain past records).

Personal History

- **Birth and early development:** Mother's pregnancy and delivery: Prematurity? Planned pregnancy? Get estimate of temperament and behavior problems. Are there any psychophysiologic problems? (Relatives may be a source of information.)
- **Childhood:** Personality traits, behavior problems, social relationships, school adjustment, family relationships, and family stability. Any personal abuse (physical, sexual, neglect) or family violence?
- **Social history:** What kind of interpersonal relationships can the patient make? Has he or she been a loner? Follower? Leader? What kind of group activities has he or she had in the past and in the present? Who are the people important to the patient now and in the past? What was the patient's *premorbid personality?* Does the patient have any military history?
- **Marriage:** At what age? How many times? Relationship patterns within the marriage? Number of children and attitude toward them?
- **Education:** Highest grade attained? Specific academic difficulties? Behavior problems? Social problems?
- **Occupational history:** Concentrate on job changes, length of time jobs have been held, best job obtained and when—get details. Social relations on job; with boss? With workers? How does job compare with ambition? With family expectations?
- **Sexual history:** Sexual orientation? Psychosexual problems or deviant behavior? Feelings about sex?

- **Current social situation:** Personal living situation, income? Social environment? Estimated current marital and family stability and happiness?

Family History

Who lives in the home? The patient should describe them and the relationship with them. Get description of patient's family of origin and his or her role in it. Upwardly mobile family? Get a detailed description of psychiatric (and medical) illnesses in family members (**family psychiatric history**).

Medical History

Obtain current and past medical problems and treatments (medications, etc.). Ask about the most common or serious "likely suspects" (see Chapters 13–15), [e.g., HIV/AIDS (risk of?), thyroid, cardiac, steroid use, head injury].

MENTAL STATUS EXAMINATION

A mental status examination (5) is a systematic documentation of the quality of mental functioning *at the time of interview*. It helps both with current diagnosis and treatment planning, and it serves as a baseline for future reference. Although much of the information sought in a mental status examination is obtained informally during other parts of the interview, it is usually necessary for the patient to answer a few formal questions if the interviewer is to learn the patient's abilities in each category of mental functioning listed below. After concluding the mental status examination, estimate its reliability. (Note: do not "over-read" mistakes on the MSE; we all make errors.)

General Presentation

- **Appearance:** Overall impression of the patient: attractive, unattractive, posture, clothes, grooming, healthy versus sickly, old looking (vs.) young looking, angry, puzzled, frightened, ill

at ease, apathetic, contemptuous, effeminate, masculine, and so on.
- **General behavior:** Mannerisms, gestures, combative, psychomotor retardation, rigid, twitches, picking, clumsy, hand wringing, and so forth.
- **Attitude toward the examiner:** Cooperative, hostile, defensive, seductive, evasive, ingratiating, and so on.

The psychotic patient may appear disheveled and bizarre with odd posturing (particularly catatonics) and grimacing. Some schizophrenics may stare, and others look "blank." Paranoid patients may be hostile and suspicious; borderline patients, hostile and angry; whereas histrionic patients often are seductive in manner and dress. Depressed patients may be nearly mute and display psychomotor retardation. Restlessness may suggest anxiety, withdrawal, mania, etc.

State of Consciousness

Is the patient *alert* (e.g., normally aware of both internal and external stimuli) or *hyperalert*? Is the patient *lethargic* (e.g., does he "drift off," or do his thoughts wander)? The patient must be reasonably alert for the remainder of the examination to be reliable. The causes for decreased alertness are usually organic.

Attention

Can the patient pay attention for short periods (*attend*) without being distracted by minor stimuli? Can the patient attend for lengths of time (*concentrate*)? This ability is necessary if you are to assess higher-level functions (i.e., they may be intact, but the patient cannot demonstrate them because of lack of attention). Test attention level with digit recall (digit span) (e.g., speak a series of numbers in a monotone and ask the patient to repeat them; begin with three numbers and increase by one with each successful trial; a normal maximum is seven numbers repeated). Have them repeat numbers backward; the norm is five. Test concentration by the Random Letter Test [e.g., tell the patient to note (by raising a finger) each time a certain letter is mentioned, and then read a long string of letters; most people make very few errors]. Defects in attention usually are due to organic causes but may be caused by marked anxiety or psychotic interruption of thoughts. Ask patient to spell "watch" forward, then backward (also involves intelligence).

Speech

Listen to the patient's speech. Is it loud, soft, fast, slow, pressured, mute, etc? Does the patient speak spontaneously? With good vocabulary? Does the patient articulate with difficulty (dysarthria)?

Is there a deficiency in *language* (e.g., aphasia)? This speech is usually identifiable by the experienced listener (e.g., patient tries to communicate, but incorrect words are chosen and grammatical errors made) but may be confused with rambling psychotic speech. Manic patients often speak loudly and rapidly; depressed patients are soft and slow. Bizarre speech usually suggests a psychotic or organic state or both.

Orientation

Check for *person* (name? age? when born?), *place* (what place is this? what is your home address?), *time* (today's date? day of the week? time? season?), and *situation* (why are you here?). Sense of time is usually the first thing lost. Major disorientation suggests organicity. Minor loss may reflect temporary stress. If without problems, they are "oriented × 4."

Mood and Affect

Mood is a sustained emotional state (e.g., depressed, euphoric, elevated, anxious, angry, irritable). *Affect* is the patient's current emotional state—it is the state the interviewer can *observe*. Common abnormal affects include flat, blunted, restricted, and inappropriate.

Note whether the affect you observe is consistent with the patient's expressed mood and congruent with thought content. Distinguish a depressed mood from an organically caused apathy. The affective disorders most commonly display alterations in mood, but so do psychotic, anxiety (e.g., panic), and organic (e.g., drug use) disorders.

Form of Thought

Does the patient's thinking make sense? Does one thought follow another logically, or does the patient display *circumstantiality* (take forever to make a point; many irrelevant details—overinclusiveness), *flight of ideas* (rapidly jumping from idea to idea; usually stimulated by a previous word or thought but with understandable associations), *evasiveness*, *loosening of associations* (tangentiality or derailment—thoughts are unrelated, but the patient seems unaware of this), *perseveration* (needless repetition of the same thought or phrase), or *blocking* (speech and train of thought is interrupted and picked up again a few moments or minutes later). Are answers to questions relevant? Ask the patient for impressions of his or her own thoughts. Record quotes of abnormal speech—it adds clarity.

These abnormalities in thought processes are most commonly associated with schizophrenic or affective disorders. None is pathognomonic, but any major abnormality suggests a psychotic process.

Thought Content

Check for abnormal preoccupations and obsessions, excessive suspiciousness, phobias, rituals, hypochondriacal symptoms, *déjà vu* experiences, depersonalization, *delusions* (fixed false beliefs—characterize them as persecutory, of grandeur, of reference, of influence, unsystematized, etc.). *Always* check for preoccupations about suicide or homicide.

Get at the presence of delusions with questions like "Do you have any strong ideas other people don't share?" or "Are there things you think about a lot?"

Delusions usually suggest a psychotic disorder (most commonly schizophrenia), but other conditions may display them (e.g., poorly systematized delusions in delirium). Obsessions may occur with psychosis but also are typical of obsessive compulsive disorder (OCD). Phobias characterize phobic disorders.

Is the patient unaware that he or she is ill or has abnormal thinking (lacks *insight*)? Does the patient have a generalized loss of ability for *abstractive* thinking (i.e., concreteness)? Test for abstractive ability by

1. **Similarities:** "What do these things have in common?"
   baseball—orange
   car—train
   desk—bookcase
   happy—sad
   horse—apple
2. **Proverbs:** "What do people mean when they say . . . ?"
   When the cat's away, the mice will play.
   The proof of the pudding is in the eating.
   A golden hammer breaks an iron door.
   The tongue is the enemy of the neck.
   The hot coal burns, the cold one blackens.

Always correlate abstractive thinking with intelligence. Concreteness in the face of normal intelligence "suggests" a psychotic thought disorder. Note any bizarre responses to similarities or proverbs—are the answers personalized? Are the answers vague because the patient is aware of failing (e.g., delirium, early dementia) and is obfuscating?

Perceptions

Does the patient display *misperceptions* (draw wrong conclusions from self-evident information)? Are there *illusions* (misinterpretations of sensory stimuli; e.g., a shadow becomes a person) or *hallucinations* (totally imagined sensory perceptions: note whether auditory, visual, tactile, olfactory, etc.)? *Always* determine whether hallucinations are accusatory, threatening, or commanding. If not volunteered, detect the presence of hallucinations by questions like "Have you had the experience of walking down the street, hearing your name called, and finding no one there?" or "Have you had any mystical or psychic experiences?"

Illusions are most common in delirium but also may occur in other psychoses. Hallucinations occur in a variety of conditions but most commonly in psychotic disorders. Schizophrenia usually has auditory hallucinations, whereas visual hallucinations are more common in organic conditions. Tactile hallucinations are frequent in sedative-hypnotic and alcohol-withdrawal states.

Judgment

An estimate of the patient's real-life problem-solving skills is often difficult to make. Judgment is a complex mental function that depends on maturation of the nervous system (poor in children). The best indicator is usually the patient's behavior, so history is very important. Some sense of the patient's judgment can be obtained through hypothetical examples: "What should you do if you find a stamped, addressed letter?" "What should you do if you lose a book belonging to a library?"

Judgment is regularly impaired in delirium, dementia, psychosis, and some retardation. Its assessment helps determine the patient's capacity for independent functioning.

Memory

Test all three types of memory: immediate (registration), short-term (recent), and remote.

■ **Immediate:**

1. Digit repetition.
2. Ask the patient immediately to repeat three to four items (e.g., mixture of physical objects and concepts).

■ **Recent:**

1. Ask questions about the past 24 hours (e.g., "How did you travel here?" "What was on the TV news last night?").
2. Ask the patient to repeat the three to four items listed earlier after 5 minutes (they should be recalled).
3. Ask the patient to count—stop at 27—(wait 1 minute)—tell him to continue counting—stop at 42—(wait 3 minutes)—and then continue counting.

■ **Remote:**

1. Get personal information such as: when were you born? School? Work?
2. Ask historic information (for example, name four presidents in this century, the dates of World War II).

Recent and remote memory usually can be tested inconspicuously during the interview. Is the patient aware of her deficit? What is her attitude toward it? Loss of memory usually indicates an organic process unless it has some of the characteristics of the dissociative disorders (see Chapter 9).

Constructional ability is a sensitive test for early diffuse cortical damage. Draw a diamond and a three-dimensional cube, and have the patient copy them. Ask the patient to draw a flowerpot with a flower or the face of a clock set at 2:45. Incomplete or very poorly done responses are suggestive of early organicity.

Intellectual Functioning

Intelligence is a global function that can be estimated from the general tone and content of the interview and by the patient's fund of information and ability to perform calculations.

Fund of knowledge:

How many weeks in a year?
Name the last six presidents.
What does the liver do?
How far is it from Chicago to Los Angeles?
Why are light-colored clothes cool?
Who wrote *Remembrances of Things Past*?

What causes rust?
How many nickels in $1.15?
Calculations:
    Serial 7s—"take 100 and subtract 7 from it, and then take 7
        from that answer, etc.";
    Serial 3s—"take 3 from 20, etc.";
    Simple calculations—2 × 3, 5 × 3, 4 × 9.

Calculation relies on functions other than intelligence, including concentration and memory. If in doubt, ask for formal IQ testing. Organic conditions may produce a loss of intellectual functioning, but psychoses seldom do (as long as the patient can concentrate on the tests).

PSYCHOLOGICAL TESTS

Psychological testing is requested for occasional psychiatric patients and may provide a useful enlargement of the understanding of those patients. Although not essential for most patients, testing may
1. Help identify organic syndromes;
2. Help localize organic pathology;
3. Contribute to the identification of borderline psychotic states;
4. Provide a baseline of general and specific functioning;
5. Generally help with differential diagnosis among psychiatric conditions.

Talk to the psychologist. Describe what you are looking for. Ask for recommendations. Although most patients receive a battery of tests, very specific questions may be answered by only one test. Carefully integrate the psychologist's report with your own evaluation, but do not allow test results to supersede clinical judgment. Commonly used tests for adults include the following:

WECHSLER ADULT INTELLIGENCE SCALE (WAIS): A very useful test. Although it does yield three separate IQ scores (full-scale, verbal, and performance), a careful evaluation of how the patient answered the 11 different subtests within the WAIS provides clues to the presence of a thought disorder, an attention or memory deficit, visual–motor impairment, and so forth.

MINNESOTA MULTIPHASIC PERSONALITY INVENTORY (MMPI): This is a true–false self-administered personality test of 567 items that takes little of the therapist's time, produces a general description of the patient's personality characteristics, and can even be computer scored. Although it provides a useful global description of the patient, do not stretch it too far diagnostically.

BENDER-GESTALT TEST: This test is easily administered—the patient draws nine specific geometric figures on a blank sheet of paper. Its greatest application is in detecting visual–motor impairment and organic deficits.

RORSCHACH TEST: This is an unstructured *projective* test that asks the patient to "describe what he sees" in a series of ten standardized ink blots. Elaborate scoring systems exist that allow a skilled examiner to infer elements of the patient's personality functioning. It is used diagnostically to help identify psychoses and personality disorders. Its diagnostic validity, although not ensured, is reasonably high by using the standardized rating system devised by Exner.

THEMATIC APPERCEPTION TEST (TAT): This projective test, similar to the Rorschach, draws conclusions from stories a patient generates in response to a series of suggestive but ambiguous human figure drawings.

DRAW-A-PERSON TEST: The patient is asked to draw a picture of a "person" and then a picture of a person of the opposite sex. The results are then interpreted by the examiner, usually as a screen for brain damage.

MINI-MENTAL STATE EXAMINATION (MMSE): A brief, formal, mental status screening examination devised by Folstein (6) for a "bedside" assessment of dementia. It tests orientation to time and place, immediate and short-term memory, calculation, language, and constructive ability. Although (too) widely used because of its simplicity, it is flawed (7), and improved versions exist.

Psychiatric rating scales are a class of measures that rate emotional symptoms or disorders. They usually consist of lists of short questions that require brief numeric answers and typically are filled out by the patient or the therapist. They serve several purposes: provide a baseline measure of a set of symptoms or diagnoses, allow the severity of psychopathology to be followed up longitudinally, complement clinical judgment with an objective measure, evaluate the effectiveness of treatment, provide a uniform standard across evaluators, help determine disposition, and function as a standard measure of patients' symptoms in research trials. They assess differing psychopathology, including general emotional problems [Global Assessment Scale (GAS); Brief Psychiatric Rating Scale (BPRS)], organicity (such as the Folstein MMSE, mentioned earlier), the diagnosis of mood and psychotic disorders (Schedule for Affective Disorders and Schizophrenia; SADS), depression (Beck Depression Inventory; Hamilton Depression Rating Scale), and anxiety (Hamilton Anxiety Rating Scale; State–Trait Anxiety Scale). Dozens of rating scales are available, and their use is growing rapidly both because they give the advantage/illusion of objectivity and because managed-care agencies increasingly demand objective measures of the severity and course of a patient's illness. Moreover, they are philosophically consistent with the concepts of psychiatric disorder underlying the DSM, yet may be misleading in some situations because of their very simplicity.

ELECTROENCEPHALOGRAM (EEG)

The EEG plays a useful, but only supportive, role in psychiatry. It is suggestive but not definitive in any psychiatric condition, but it does help rule in or out a diversity of conditions. Its primary use is in the differentiation between organic and functional conditions.

1. Patients with epilepsy (particularly temporal lobe epilepsy) often mimic "pseudoseizure" psychiatric patients—the EEG helps differentiate (although 30% of those with epilepsy have a normal tracing between attacks).
2. The patient who is confused and disoriented (delirium) due to organic factors usually has diffuse EEG slowing. A major exception is alcohol-withdrawal delirium (delirium tremens), which shows increased fast activity, as does confusion due to sedative–hypnotics. Major tranquilizers increase slow-wave activity.
3. The patient who has dementia of the Alzheimer type (50% of demented patients) usually has a normal EEG early on, with abnormalities later (a help in staging). Most reversible forms of dementia produce abnormal tracings. The EEG of a person with pseudodementia (e.g., depression that mimics dementia) is usually normal.
4. A variety of organic causes can produce bizarre behavior (e.g., brain tumor, cerebral infarcts, cerebral trauma). A normal EEG does not rule out organic pathology, but an abnormal tracing is suggestive.

Several populations of psychiatric patients have a slightly increased frequency of nonspecific abnormalities on the EEG (e.g., schizophrenics, particularly catatonics, and those with dementia or panic disorder). Patients with antisocial personality disorder have perhaps the highest frequency of abnormal tracings; look for but do not over-read organic pathology in these patients.

Brain electrical activity topographic mapping (quantitative EEG or QEEG) groups each wavelength type and plots their positions over a map of the head. This new technology may extract more information from EEG data and increase its usefulness, although it is plagued by misreading artifacts. Its real value remains uncertain. A related EEG technique, visual and/or auditory evoked potentials (EPs), remains a (actively investigated) research tool in psychiatry.

BRAIN IMAGING

Structural Techniques

Both computed tomography (CT) and magnetic resonance imaging (MRI; sMRI) supply brain *structure* information primarily useful in identifying brain lesions but not particularly helpful for diagnosing psychiatric conditions. Even though it is more expensive, MRI has become the standard because it gives a better image and is much more capable of differentiating between gray and white matter; thus it is more effective at identifying subtle shape and size differences in CNS structures, as well as detailing demyelinating disorders, dementia, infarctions, and neoplasms. MRI can produce a good picture of the demented brain, and early *suggestions* exist that (a) enlarged lateral ventricles or decreased medial temporal lobe volume on MRI or both are associated with negative symptoms in schizophrenia, (b) decreased superior temporal lobe size is linked to positive symptoms, (c) hippocampal atrophy is associated with major depression and posttraumatic stress disorder (PTSD), and (d) serious depression in the elderly is associated with large lateral and third ventricles as well as general cerebral atrophy. Because it is relatively inexpensive, CT is used to screen for organic brain disease, particularly in older patients with sudden psychiatric symptoms. Moreover, it is superior to MRI at investigating bone injury (e.g., trauma), calcification, and acute hemorrhage. A CT scan or MRI may be combined with neuropsychological testing or functional imaging like functional MRI (*f*MRI) or both, or single-photon emission CT (SPECT) for more information.

Functional Techniques

Two principle ways exist of measuring the brain as it *functions* (i.e., "in action"): (a) inject (IV) molecular radioisotopes (e.g., oxygen [^{15}O], nitrogen [^{13}N], carbon [^{11}C], fluorine [^{18}F]) attached to molecules that are metabolized in some way by the brain (e.g., glucose, water) or attached to neurotransmitters, their receptors, or a few drugs, and then measure location and intensity as the brain deals with them [in positron emission tomography or PET scanning, the isotopes emit short-lived positrons, which requires the presence of a nearby cyclotron to make the isotope (very expensive)] or apply a similar method that uses isotopes that release photons, which are then measured (single-photon emission computed tomography or SPECT uses tracers that last longer and so can be used in most major hospitals but measure fewer items [e.g., blood flow (an indirect measure of metabolism) and several receptors]); or (b) use the very safe, noninvasive, and increasingly available method of functional MRI (fMRI), which measures increased (or decreased) levels of deoxyhemoglobin, which generates an indirect map of neural activity.

All these functional methods remain primarily research techniques, even though they have provided many fascinating, but unproven, insights into psychiatric disorders [e.g., various semireproducible abnormalities in CNS regions such as the orbitofrontal gyri, hippocampal regions, caudate nuclei, various parts of the limbic system, and the frontal lobes as a whole in conditions such as unipolar and bipolar mood disorders, panic disorder, OCD, and different presentations of schizophrenia (8)]. SPECT now has clinical utility in the differential diagnosis of stroke, dementia, and epilepsy. In the near future, it is likely that PET will teach us much more about the psychobiologic functioning of the brain, and SPECT and fMRI will become useful diagnostic tools for specific psychiatric conditions.

THE AMYTAL INTERVIEW

The administration of amobarbital (Amytal), thiopental (Pentothal), or pentobarbital (Nembutal) during an interview to produce a sedated state has been used for many years both diagnostically (Amytal interview) and therapeutically (narcoanalysis). Despite a long history of use, the indications for and value of this technique are unclear, and it is currently out of favor.

The technique usually consists of administering 200–500 mg (occasionally more) of sodium amobarbital IV at a rate of 25–50 mg/min. The interviewer talks with the patient throughout administration and halts the drug temporarily when the desired level of sedation is attained (e.g., appearance of lateral nystagmus for light sedation; development of slurred speech for a deeper state). Additional Amytal may be given if the interview is lengthy.

In this sedated state, some patients demonstrate a markedly altered clinical picture that may be of diagnostic value. Although opinion varies, diagnostic uses for the Amytal interview may include the following:

1. Evaluation of mute patients: Patients with *catatonic schizophrenia* often recover dramatically when sedated (although a thought disorder usually remains) but return to the full catatonic state when the Amytal wears off. This helps differentiate catatonia from marked psychomotor retardation in the depressed patient (they show little improvement). Patients mute for other reasons (e.g., hysterical, acute stress) may begin to talk under sedation.
2. *Acute panic states:* Patients immobilized by severe stress may talk about their concerns when sedated and find some relief.
3. *Organic versus functional differentiation:* Patients who are confused, disoriented, or demented due to organic factors usually worsen with Amytal, whereas clinically similar functional patients often clear temporarily.
4. Hysterical phenomena: *Amnesias, fugues,* and *conversion disorders* often are temporarily relieved by Amytal. Useful information may be obtained during this time (e.g., the patient's name and address; the cause of the patient's anger).
5. The interview is less reliably useful with psychotic states (except for catatonic schizophrenia), although some patients may contribute information they would not have otherwise.

Although helpful in confirming some diagnoses, the Amytal interview also may contribute to the treatment of a few patients by allowing them to confront and deal with stressful or troubling experiences that they previously had been reluctant or unable to face. However, the validity of old memories in patients with a presumed history of child abuse or a current dissociative disorder (or both) recalled under the Amytal interview is uncertain (the "false memory" vs. "repressed memory" controversy).

REFERENCES

1. Carlat DJ. *The Psychiatric Interview.* 2nd ed. Philadelphia: Lippincott Williams & Wilkins, 2005.
2. Morrison J. *The First Interview.* New York: Guilford Press, 1993.
3. Othmer E, Othmer SC. *The Clinical Interview Using SDM-IV.* Vol. 1. Washington, DC: American Psychiatric Press, 1994.

4. Shea SC. *Psychiatric Interviewing: the Art of Understanding.* Philadelphia: WB Saunders, 1998.
5. Strub RL, Black FW. *The Mental Status Examination in Neurology.* 3rd ed. Philadelphia: PA Davis, 1993.
6. Folstein MF, Folstein SE, McHugh PR. "Mini-mental state:" a practical method for grading the mental state of patients for the clinician. *J Am Geriatr Soc* 1975;12:189–198.
7. Wind AW, Schellevis FG, van Staveren G, et al. Limitations of the mini-mental state examination. *Int J Geriatr Psychiatry* 1997;12:101–108.
8. Sukhwinder SS, Brammer MJ, Williams SCR, et al. Mapping auditory hallucinations in schizophrenia using functional magnetic resonance imaging. *Arch Gen Psychiatry* 2000;57:1033–1038.

Chapter 3

Psychotic Disorders

Psychosis describes a degree of severity, not a specific disorder. A psychotic patient has a grossly impaired sense of reality, often coupled with emotional and cognitive disabilities, which severely compromise the ability to function. The patient is likely to talk and act in a bizarre fashion, have hallucinations, or have strongly held ideas that are contrary to fact (delusions). He or she may be confused and disoriented and typically is not aware of the impairment (lacks insight).

This chapter covers the major psychotic disorders [i.e., conditions that present with some combination of psychotic symptoms at some time during their course (although the patients may be nonpsychotic most of the time)]. Recognize that these are descriptive groupings of clinical syndromes, *not* discrete diseases.

Schizophrenia
  Disorganized type
  Catatonic type
  Paranoid type
  Undifferentiated type
  Residual type
Schizophreniform disorder
Brief psychotic disorder
Schizoaffective disorder
Shared psychotic disorder
Delusional (paranoid) disorder
Psychotic disorder due to a general medical condition
Substance-induced psychotic disorder
Psychotic disorder not otherwise specified (NOS)

DIFFERENTIAL DIAGNOSIS

Most psychotic disorders have an organic base, although poorly understood. Start by identifying any underlying medical and neurologic causes or psychoses due to substance intoxication or withdrawal. Obtain a complete history and physical on all psychotic patients. Most psychotic disorders present with emotion and thinking disturbances in a patient with a clear sensorium, whereas obviously organic psychoses usually have a degree of delirium (e.g., clouding of consciousness, confusion, disorientation). Unfortunately, exceptions to either pattern are frequent. Possible organic causes of psychosis include almost any type of serious medical illness or drug abuse (see Chapters 5, 6, 14, and 15). Suspect an organic etiology if

- The patient has significant memory loss, confusion, disorientation, or clouding of consciousness;
- No personal or family history of serious psychiatric illness is known;
- The patient has a serious medical illness or a chronic medical condition with periodic relapses;
- The psychosis has developed rapidly (e.g., days) in a patient who previously had been functioning well.

Psychiatric conditions that *may* (but do not necessarily) reach psychotic proportions (addressed in other chapters) include the following:

1. Major depressive disorder or bipolar disorder (see Chapter 4): Look for the psychosis to coexist with and be dominated by an affective component (either manic or depressed) that preceded the development of the psychosis.
2. Brief psychotic disorders may occur from stress in patients with personality disorders of the histrionic, borderline, paranoid, and schizotypal types. In some obsessive–compulsive persons, a psychosis may at times develop if they fail to control their environment.
3. Some acute panic or rage attacks may be of psychotic intensity [e.g., rage in the patient with an explosive disorder (see Chapter 7)].
4. A few psychotic conditions develop in childhood and continue into the adult years [e.g., **AUTISTIC DISORDER** (DSM, p. 70, 299.00) and **PERVASIVE DEVELOPMENTAL DISORDER NOS** (DSM, p. 84, 299.80)].
5. Psychotic states occasionally may be mimicked unconsciously or even "faked": Factitious Disorder with Predominantly Psychological Signs and Symptoms; Malingering.

SCHIZOPHRENIA

Schizophrenia is the most common psychotic disorder; almost 1% of people worldwide develop it during their lifetime; more than 2 million persons are affected in the United States. It occurs more frequently in urban populations and in lower socioeconomic groups, probably because of a "downward drift" (i.e., poorly functional unemployable persons end up in marginal settings). Poor environments do not "cause" the disorder, although they make it more intractable.

The diagnosis of schizophrenia has had a checkered history. Many different ways have been used to make the diagnosis, which have thus represented different populations of patients. The current diagnostic scheme (DSM-IV) uses specific objective criteria to define several forms of schizophrenia. Because no pathognomonic findings exist, "schizophrenia" is a *clinical* diagnosis that may represent a nonspecific syndrome of heterogeneous etiologies. However, biologic, genetic, and phenomenologic information suggest that it is a valid disorder(s). The five identified subtypes also are based on clinical variables.

Clinical Presentation

Although the nature of schizophrenia is uncertain, the current clinical description and method of making the diagnosis are more clear (DSM-IV).

Most schizophrenics are psychotic for only a small part of their lives. Typically they spend many years in a **residual phase**, during which time they display minor features of their illness. During these residual periods, patients may be withdrawn, isolated, and "peculiar." They usually are noticeable to others and may lose their jobs or friends, both because of their own lack of interest and ability to perform and because they behave oddly. Their thinking and speech are vague and are believed by others to be odd and to "not quite make sense." They may be convinced that they are different from others, believe that they have special powers and sensitivities, and have "mystical" or "psychic" experiences. Their personal appearance and manners deteriorate, and they may display affect that is blunted, flat, or inappropriate. Although they may maintain close to normal intelligence, they display significant cognitive deficits in memory, attention, frontal lobe function, etc., most of which can be demonstrated on neuropsychological testing. They are frequently anhedonic (unable to experience pleasure). Often this deterioration merely represents a gradual worsening of a condition the patient has displayed for many years—the first psychotic episode may have been preceded by a similar period of eccentric thinking and behavior (**prodromal phase**).

A **prepsychotic personality** is seen in some chronic schizophrenics and is characterized by social withdrawal, social awkwardness, and marked shyness in a youth who has difficulty in school despite a normal IQ. An equally common pattern is involvement in minor antisocial activities in the year or two before the initial psychotic episode. Many of these patients have previously received the diagnosis of schizoid, borderline, antisocial, or schizotypal personality disorder. It is only when the first psychotic episode develops [normally in their teens or early 20s (men) or 20s and early 30s (women); a first "breakdown" after age 40 is unusual] that the diagnosis is changed to schizophrenia. Often a presumed precipitating stress can be identified. The typical **acute psychosis** displays a variable mixture of several of the following symptoms.

■ Disturbance of Thought Form

These patients usually have a **formal thought disorder** (i.e., their thinking is frequently incomprehensible to others and appears illogical). Characteristics include

- **Loosening of associations** (derailment or tangential associations): Patients' ideas are disconnected. They may jump obliviously from topic to unconnected topic, confusing the listener. When this occurs frequently (e.g., in mid-sentence), the speech is often incoherent.
- **Overinclusiveness:** Patients continually may disrupt the flow of their thoughts by including irrelevant information.
- **Neologisms:** Patients coin new words (which may have a symbolic meaning for them).
- **Blocking:** Speech is halted (often in mid-sentence) and then picked up a moment (or minutes) later, usually at another place. This may represent the patients' ideas being interrupted by intrusive thoughts (e.g., hallucinations). These patients are often very distractible and have a short attention span.
- **Clanging:** Patients choose their next words and themes based on the sound of the words they have just used rather than the thought content (e.g., "Yesterday I went to the store." The patient looks around and then says, "I guess I'd better clean the floor.").
- **Echolalia:** Patients repeat words or phrases just spoken by another person, but without an apparent effort to communicate.
- **Concreteness:** Patients of normal or above-average IQ think in abstract terms poorly.

- **Alogia:** Patients may speak very little (but without being intentionally resistant; *poverty of speech*) or may speak a normal amount but say very little (*poverty of speech content*).

■ Disturbance of Thought Content

Delusions are fixed false beliefs far beyond credibility that may be "bizarre" (e.g., "my right eye is a computer that controls the world") or "nonbizarre" (just very unlikely; "the FBI follows me") and remain unmodified despite clear evidence to the contrary. They are common in most serious mental disorders, but some specific forms of delusional thought are particularly frequent in schizophrenia. The more acute the psychosis, the more likely the delusion is to be disorganized and nonsystematized:

- *Bizarre confused delusions;*
- *Persecutory delusions,* particularly nonsystematic types;
- *Grandiose delusions;*
- *Delusions of influence:* Patients believe they can control events through telepathy;
- *Delusions of reference:* Patients are convinced of "meanings" behind events and people's actions that are directed specifically toward themselves;
- *Delusions of thought broadcasting:* The belief that others can hear the patients' thoughts;
- *Delusions of thought insertion:* The belief that someone else's thoughts have been inserted into the patients' minds.

Many schizophrenic patients display *lack of insight* (1), that is, the patient is unaware of his or her own illness or of his or her need for treatment, even though the disorder is evident to others.

■ Disturbance of Perception

Most common are **hallucinations**, usually auditory but also visual, olfactory, and tactile. Auditory hallucinations (most often voices—one or several) may include a running commentary about the patient and events, derogatory or threatening comments made to the patient, or direct orders to the patient (command hallucinations). The voices often (but not necessarily) are perceived as coming from outside the patient's head, and occasionally the patient may hear his or her own thoughts spoken aloud (often to his or her shame or embarrassment). The voices are quite real to the patient, except in the early phases of the psychosis.

These patients may also have illusions, depersonalizations (feels as if they are observing themselves from the outside), derealizations (the world seems unreal), and a hallucinatory sense of bodily change.

■ **Disturbance of Emotions**

Acutely psychotic patients may display various emotions and may switch from one to another in a surprisingly short time. Three frequent (but not pathognomonic) underlying affects are

- **Blunted or flat affect:** The patient expresses very little emotion, even when it is appropriate to do so. He may appear to be without warmth.
- **Inappropriate affect:** The affect may be intense, but it is inconsistent with the patient's thoughts or speech.
- **Labile affect:** Marked changes in affect over a short time.

■ **Disturbance of Behavior**

Many different bizarre and inappropriate behaviors may be seen, including strange grimacing and posturing, ritual behavior, excessive silliness, aggressiveness, and some sexual inappropriateness. An acute psychotic attack can last weeks or months (occasionally years). Many patients have recurrences of the active phase periodically throughout their lives, typically separated by months or years. During the intervening periods, patients usually have residual symptoms (often with the degree of impairment gradually increasing over the years); however, a few patients are symptom free between acute episodes. Many schizophrenic patients in remission display early signs of a developing relapse—always look for them. These early signs include increasing restlessness and nervousness, loss of appetite, mild depression and anhedonia, insomnia, and trouble concentrating.

Classification

To be considered schizophrenic, a patient must (DSM, p. 312)
1. have had at least 6 *months* of
2. sufficiently *deteriorated* occupational, interpersonal, and self-supportive functioning;
3. have been *actively psychotic* in a characteristic fashion for at least 1 month of that period; and
4. must not be able to account for the symptoms by the presence of a schizoaffective or major mood disorder, autism, or an organic condition.

The *course* of the illness should be classed as continuous, episodic with or without interepisode residual symptoms, or single episode in partial or full remission. Moreover, all schizophrenic patients should be classed as one of five recognized subtypes that describes the most frequently occurring behavioral manifestations of the illness. Numerous subclassifications of schizophrenia have been used in the past, all unsatisfactory, and the current divisions share some of those deficiencies. Although genetic data suggest that schizophrenia is a fairly stable diagnosis (2), no comparable information exists for the subtypes. Symptomatically, they tend to overlap, and the diagnosis can shift from one to another with time (either during one episode or in a subsequent episode). Finally, over the years, the clinical presentations of many patients tend to converge toward a common picture of interpersonal withdrawal, flattened affect, idiosyncratic thinking, and impaired social and personal functioning. (At the same time, the course becomes more stable, with fewer acute symptoms or episodes.)

■ Disorganized Type (DSM, p. 314, 295.10)

The patient has (a) blunted, silly, or inappropriate affect; (b) frequent incoherence; and (c) no systematized delusions. Grimacing and bizarre mannerisms are common. This is the most severe subtype of schizophrenia.

■ Catatonic Type (DSM, p. 315, 295.20)

The patient may have any one (or a combination) of several forms of catatonia:

1. **Catatonic stupor or mutism:** Patient does not appreciably respond to the environment or to the people in it. Despite appearances, these patients are often thoroughly aware of what is going on around them.
2. **Catatonic negativism:** Patient resists all directions or physical attempts to move him or her.
3. **Catatonic rigidity:** Patient is physically rigid.
4. **Catatonic posturing:** Patient assumes bizarre or unusual postures.
5. **Catatonic excitement:** Patient is extremely (e.g., wildly) active and excited. May be life-threatening (e.g., because of exhaustion).

■ Paranoid Type (DSM, p. 313, 295.30)

This is the most stable, least severe, and most common (3) subtype over time and usually develops later than other forms of schizophrenia. The patient must display consistent, often paranoid, delusions that he or she may or may not act on. These patients are often uncooperative and difficult to deal with and may be aggressive, angry, or fearful, but they are less likely to display disorganized incoherent behavior.

■ **Undifferentiated Type (DSM, p. 316, 295.90)**

The patient has prominent hallucinations, delusions, and other evidence of active psychosis (e.g., confusion, incoherence) but without the more specific features of the preceding three categories.

■ **Residual Type (DSM, p. 316, 295.60)**

The patient is in remission from active psychosis but displays symptoms of the residual phase (e.g., social withdrawal, flat or inappropriate affect, eccentric behavior, loosening of associations, and illogical thinking).

Prognosis

Schizophrenia is a chronic disorder. A person gradually may become more withdrawn, "eccentric," and nonfunctional over many years. Some patients may experience low-level delusions and hallucinations indefinitely. Many of the more dramatic and acute symptoms disappear with time, but the patient may eventually need long-term sheltered living or may spend years in mental hospitals. Involvement with the law for misdemeanors is common (e.g., vagrancy, disturbing the peace), as is associated mixed drug abuse. A few patients become somewhat demented. Overall life expectancy is shortened, primarily due to accidents, suicide, and an inability of the patients to care for themselves.

This pattern has exceptions. Psychiatrists have long distinguished between *process* schizophrenia (slowly developing; chronic deteriorating course) and *reactive* schizophrenia (rapid onset; somewhat better prognosis). Likewise, they have differentiated between **positive symptoms** (hallucinations, delusions, bizarre behavior, etc.), which frequently respond to usual antipsychotic medications, and the more impairing **negative symptoms** (flattened affect, poverty of speech, anhedonia, social withdrawal, etc.), which do not (although the newer antipsychotics may produce moderate improvement). Clinical characteristics associated with an improved prognosis include (4)

1. A rapid onset of the active psychotic symptoms;
2. An onset after age 30, particularly in women;
3. Good premorbid social and occupational functioning. Past performance remains the best predictor of future performance;
4. Marked confusion and emotional features during the acute episode (positive symptoms); some question this;
5. A probable precipitating stress to the acute psychosis and no evidence of CNS abnormalities;
6. No family history of schizophrenia.

Process and reactive forms of schizophrenia may be etiologically (and biologically?) distinct. Although great variability exists, Disorganized type generally has the worst prognosis, whereas Paranoid type (and some catatonics) have the best. The prognosis is worsened if the patient abuses drugs (5) or lives in a dysfunctional family setting.

About 25% to 50% of patients recovering from an acute episode develop a major depression during the months after improvement (*postpsychotic depression*). Although treatment resistant, psychotherapy and antidepressant medication may be useful (lithium or anticonvulsants or both may also help). Watch for it—the suicide rate is increased in this population [particularly in patients aware of the seriousness of their illness (6)]—but do not overdiagnose because some of these patients may have a medication-induced akinesia, mimicking depression.

Biology

No pathognomonic structural or functional abnormality has been found in schizophrenics; however, numerous intriguing abnormalities exist (and have been replicated, as well as contested) in subpopulations of patients. The most generally accepted abnormalities include stable *lateral and third ventricular enlargements* (7) that seem to precede the onset of the illness; *bilateral atrophy of the medial temporal lobes* (8) and specifically of the amygdala and the hippocampal and parahippocampal gyri; *spacial disorientation of the hippocampal pyramidal cells* (9); and *decreased volume of the dorsolateral prefrontal cortex*. These changes all appear static and seem to have been present from about the time of birth (no gliosis) in some studies (10) but show progression in others. Their locations are suggestive of the behavioral disturbances found in schizophrenia (e.g., hippocampal abnormalities may be associated with memory impairment, and frontal lobe atrophy may account for the negative symptoms of schizophrenia). In addition, functional imaging studies have consistently found decreased frontal lobe blood flow (hypofrontality) and glucose metabolism [by positron emission tomography (PET)]. Other less well-confirmed findings include cerebrospinal fluid (CSF) cytomegalovirus antibodies, P-type (stimulated) atypical lymphocytes, abnormal left hemisphere function, impaired transmission in and reduced size of the corpus callosum, a small cerebellar vermis, impaired visual tracking with smooth-pursuit eye movements, EEG and auditory P300 EP abnormalities (by QEEM), difficulty focusing attention, and slowed reaction time, to name a few. Also, among individuals in whom schizophrenia develops, an increased incidence of birth complications is found (10) (prematurity, low birth weight, birth during an influenza epidemic), a greater likelihood to have been born in the late winter and early spring, and minor neurologic abnormalities. The significance of these findings is unknown. However, taken together, they underscore (a) the biologic nature and (b) the heterogeneity of schizophrenia.

Biochemistry

The biochemical etiology of schizophrenia is unknown. Most major hypotheses implicate an abnormality of central neurotransmitters. The best-researched theory postulates excessive central dopamine activity (the *dopamine hypothesis*) and is based on three key findings:

1. The antipsychotic activity of neuroleptic medications (e.g., phenothiazines) is derived in major part from their blockade of postsynaptic dopamine receptors (of the D_2 type).
2. Amphetamine psychosis often is clinically indistinguishable from an acute paranoid schizophrenic psychosis. Amphetamines release central dopamine. Amphetamines also worsen schizophrenia.
3. An increased number of D_2 receptors is found in the caudate nucleus, nucleus accumbens, and putamen in schizophrenics.

However, studies of the D_1 receptors have suggested that they are a major site of action and cause for the effectiveness of the newer antipsychotics. Other theories include elevated CNS serotonin (particularly $5\text{-}HT_{2A}$) receptors and excessive limbic forebrain norepinephrine (NE) (occurs in some schizophrenics and decreases with medication and improved clinical state). Clearly, a simple D_2 hypothesis is not sufficient.

Genetics

Schizophrenia has a significant inherited component: complex and polygenic (11). According to *consanguinity studies*, schizophrenia is a familial disorder (i.e., "runs in families"). The closer the relative, the greater the risk. In *twin studies* (12), monozygotic twins are 4 to 6 times more likely to develop illness than are dizygotes. In *adoption studies*, children of schizophrenic parents adopted away at birth into normal families have the same increased rate of illness as if they had been raised by their natural parents (Table 3.1).

Table 3.1 ■ Genetic Counseling: Lifetime Risk of Developing Schizophrenia	
General population	1%
Monozygotic twins[a]	40%–50%
Dizygotic twins	10%
Sibling of schizophrenic	10%
Parent of schizophrenic	5%
Child of one schizophrenic parent	10%–15%
Child of two schizophrenic parents	30%–40%

[a] Note that 50% of monozygotic twins do not both develop schizophrenia; thus clearly environment plays a role. Development of illness reflects nature and nurture.

Several nonpsychotic disorders occur with increased frequency in the families of schizophrenics and may be related genetically: schizotypal and borderline personality disorders (the *schizophrenia spectrum disorders*), obsessive–compulsive disorder, and possibly antisocial and paranoid personality disorders.

Modern molecular genetic research, primarily chromosomal linkage studies, has found nothing definitive. The strongest evidence points to chromosome 6, yet the expert consensus is that schizophrenia is genetically and environmentally multifactorial.

Family Processes

Family dynamics and turbulence play a major role in producing a relapse or maintaining a remission. Patients who are discharged to home are more likely to relapse over the following year than are those who are placed in a residential setting. Most at risk are patients from hostile families or families that display excessive anxiety, overconcern, or overprotectiveness toward the patient (called *expressed emotion*) (13). Schizophrenic patients often do not "emancipate" from their families.

Some researchers have identified peculiar and pathologic styles of communication in these families; typically, communications are vague and subtly illogical. In 1956, Bateson (14) described a characteristic "double bind" in which the patient is frequently required by a key family member to respond to an overt message that contradicts a covert message. However, recent work suggests that these family communication patterns are as likely to be the effect of having a schizophrenic child as the cause of schizophrenia in the child.

Differential Diagnosis

Schizophrenia must be differentiated from all those conditions that produce active psychoses (see earlier). Of all the possibilities, be particularly careful to eliminate schizoaffective disorder, the major affective disorders, and several organic conditions that may closely mimic schizophrenia [e.g., early Huntington chorea, early Wilson disease, temporal lobe epilepsy, frontal or temporal lobe tumors, early multiple sclerosis (MS), early systemic lupus erythematosus (SLE), porphyria, general paresis, chronic drug use, chronic alcoholic hallucinosis, and the adult form of meta-chromatic leukodystrophy]. Carefully evaluate catatonia for medical/neurologic conditions.

Treatment

■ *Biologic Methods* (see Chapter 23)

Treat acute psychoses with antipsychotics, preferably the new "atyp-ical" antipsychotics, although recent evidence suggests them to be little more effective than the traditional antipsychotics, only better tolerated (15). Low-dose antipsychotic drug maintenance is the norm; after the first relapse, maintenance medication usually should be continued for years. Because noncompliance is common (particu-larly among substance abusers), long-acting depot antipsychotics may be preferable for many patients. Traditional antipsychotics are useful primarily in controlling the positive symptoms, whereas several of the newer atypicals help with negative symptoms as well (16). Be aware that a protracted excessive dose may hinder patient functioning over the long term. A subgroup of schizophrenics may benefit from augmentation with either lithium or a benzodiazepine [particularly in agitated or anxious patients (e.g., diazepam, 15 to 30^+ mg/day, or clonazepam, 5 to 15 mg/day)].

The new gold standard is clozapine (Clozaril), an expensive, dangerous (unpredictable, potentially lethal agranulocytosis), effec-tive antipsychotic that clinically improves and is better received (because of fewer side effects) by one third or more of refractory chronic patients. It can be used safely with *uninterrupted* weekly monitoring of white blood cell (WBC) counts, presumably forever. Use it after other serious antipsychotic trials have failed (not a "first run" drug), but *be sure you monitor closely.*

Electroconvulsive therapy (ECT) may be useful for rapid control of a few acute psychotics. A very few chronic schizophren-ics who respond poorly to medication may improve with ECT (unpredictable).

■ *Psychosocial Methods*

The primary mode of treatment of schizophrenia is pharmacologic. Long-term insight psychotherapy has a limited place. Conversely, supportive reality-oriented psychosocial methods are particularly useful in the long-term treatment of schizophrenia.

The acutely psychotic patient should be approached cautiously, but *should* be approached. Keep a comfortable distance from the patient if he appears disturbed by your presence. It is essential to establish some communication with these patients.

1. Talk to the patient. Be relaxed, interested, and supportive. Give the impression that you believe the patient can respond appropriately to you.

2. Be specific. Ask pointed factual questions. Try to identify the patient's major current fears and concerns, but do not be led into a lengthy discussion of complex delusions and hallucinations.

3. Take your time during the interview. Do not rush the patient to respond to each question, but do maintain some control over the direction of the conversation.

4. Make some specific observations of the patient's behavior (e.g., "you look frightened"; "you look angry"), but do not become involved in lengthy "interpretations." Do not draw incorrect conclusions about the patient's emotional state from inappropriate affect.

5. Explain to the patient what is being done to him or her, and why.

6. If the conversation is going nowhere (e.g., the patient refuses to talk), break off the interview with a positive expectation (e.g., "I'll be back to see you in a little while when you are feeling better and are able to talk").

If the acutely psychotic patient is delirious, suicidal, homicidal, has no community support, or a combination of these, then hospitalize. It is usually better to avoid long-term hospitalization if alternate outpatient arrangements are possible: The deleterious effects of chronic hospitalization are real (regression and marked withdrawal, loss of skills, etc.). The recent trend has been toward short hospital stays during acute episodes, with maintenance as outpatients in between.

When the patient is hospitalized, allow as much independence as his or her behavior permits within the limits of a safe environment. *Therapeutic milieus* (e.g., therapeutic community, token economy) all depend on community support (staff *and* patients)—be aware of the patient's behavior, and provide helpful "corrective feedback." The milieu is a place for the patient to develop skills in maintaining interpersonal relationships and to learn new methods of coping. *Behavior modification* has been found clearly effective at eliminating specific unacceptable behaviors and in teaching low-level personal skills with some regressed, poorly functioning inpatients.

Most schizophrenics can be treated as outpatients. Several principles should be kept in mind.

- See the patient frequently enough to safely monitor medication and detect early deterioration (e.g., weekly, monthly, or even every several months—depending on the patient's course and reliability).

- Communicate with the patient clearly and unambiguously. Be factual and goal oriented. Avoid extensive discussion of hallucinations and delusions (although a recent study suggests that using cognitive therapy to change what the patient thinks of the voices may decrease their frequency). Help the patient with reality issues (e.g., living arrangements, work). Help the patient avoid excessive stress. Recognize that the more productive and skillful the patient, the more likely he or she is to maintain a recovery—encourage the patient to hold an *appropriate* job. Provide *social skills training* (17).

- Talk about medication (e.g., the need for it, the patient's feelings about taking it).

- Develop a consistent trusting relationship (often difficult). Be empathic over time, even when the patient is being "unreasonable," but also maintain a professional distance. Be a constant presence.

- Learn the patient's strengths and weaknesses. Teach him to identify an impending decompensation. What are the precipitants, if any? If the patient misses appointments, investigate (he may be relapsing). If the patient is decompensating, be ready to insist on hospitalization. Recognize that overstimulation and overindependence can precipitate a decompensation. These patients are at risk for suicide at times during their illnesses (particularly if they have self-destructive command hallucinations).

- Always evaluate the family. Have they contributed to the patient's decompensation? Can the members deal appropriately with the patient's illness? Are they hostile? Suspicious? Overprotective? Consider *family therapy*—reality-based, in-home, family/patient interventions may be particularly useful. Family members often need considerable support and understanding themselves. When worked with well, they can be a (the?) major help to the patient.

- Consider *group therapy*. The usual orientation is toward support and reality testing. It helps with resocialization, forces interpersonal interactions, and provides support. Several studies have shown it to be effective (in combination with medication) in preventing relapse in outpatients.

- Know and use community resources. Be alert to the devastating effect on the patient of a poor quality of life (e.g., does he live in a "psychiatric ghetto" or "on the street"?).
- Do not expect too much. Many patients have chronic disability.

SCHIZOPHRENIFORM DISORDER (DSM, P. 317, 295.40)

This disorder is clinically indistinguishable from brief psychotic disorder and schizophrenia except that the symptoms last more than 1 month but fewer than 6 months. This population of patients seems to differ from schizophrenic patients in several important ways:

1. Symptoms begin and end more abruptly;
2. Symptoms are usually more turbulent and "acute";
3. Good premorbid adjustment and higher functioning occurs after recovery;
4. Only a slightly increased prevalence of schizophrenia is found in the family. A higher prevalence of affective disorder may be present.

Thus schizophreniform disorder appears to be a separate disease from schizophrenia. Recognize, however, that many schizophrenic patients pass through a period (i.e., the first 6 months) when their diagnosis must be schizophreniform disorder. Also, do not miss an organic psychosis.

Treatment is similar to that for an acute schizophrenic episode, but the prognosis is better (18).

BRIEF PSYCHOTIC DISORDER (DSM, P. 329, 298.8)

This condition describes patients who experience an acute psychotic episode lasting longer than 1 day but less than 1 month and that may ["with marked stressor(s)"] or may not ["without marked stressor(s)"] immediately follow an important life stress or ("with postpartum onset") a pregnancy. The illness comes as a surprise—usually there is no forewarning that the person is likely to break down. This disorder is more common in people with a preexisting personality disorder (particularly histrionic and borderline types).

The psychosis is typically very turbulent and dramatic with marked emotional lability, bizarre behavior, confused and incoherent speech, transient disorientation and memory loss, or brief but striking hallucinations and delusions, or a combination of these. Thus it mimics the acute psychotic onset of a major affective disorder, schizophreniform disorder, or psychosis with delirium. *Always* carefully rule out medical conditions and particularly substance-induced problems. The validity of this diagnosis as a separate category is debated.

Treat the acutely psychotic patient with understanding, a secure environment, and antipsychotic medication, if needed. The patient usually recovers completely in several days, and the long-term prognosis is good, although the patient may be at risk for future brief episodes when equivalently stressed.

SCHIZOAFFECTIVE DISORDER (DSM, P. 319, 295.70)

This is a vague and poorly defined disorder meant for patients who have evidence of *both* schizophrenia and major affective disorder with depressed mood. These patients may have an affective disturbance that grades into a purely schizophrenic picture or may display symptoms of both conditions simultaneously, although the schizophrenic symptoms dominate. It is a genetically heterogeneous disorder—both schizophrenia and mood disorders occur with increased frequency in family members. Be cautious that you do not mistake it for a substance-induced psychosis [e.g., amphetamines, phencyclidine (PCP), or exogenous steroids]. Much work remains to be done to define these patients better.

Treat as one would the equivalent schizophrenic or affective patient. Antipsychotics are generally most useful, but lithium has benefitted some patients. These patients seem to have a better prognosis than do those with schizophrenia but a poorer outcome than do those with a mood disorder (19).

DELUSIONAL DISORDER (DSM, P. 323, 297.1)

These patients *do not* display the pervasive disturbances of mood and thought found in other psychotic conditions. They do not have flat or inappropriate affect, prominent hallucinations, or markedly bizarre delusions. They *do* have one or more delusions, often of persecution but also of infidelity, grandiosity, somatic change, or erotomania that are

1. Usually specific (e.g., involve a certain person or group, a given place or time, or a particular activity);
2. Usually well organized (e.g., the "culprits" have elaborate reasons for what they are doing, which the patient can detail);
3. Usually grandiose (e.g., a powerful group is interested just in *them*);
4. Not bizarre enough to suggest schizophrenia.

These patients (who can be any age but tend to be in their 40s) may be unrecognizable until their delusional system is pointed out by family or friends. Even then the diagnosis may be difficult because they may be too mistrustful to confide in the examiner and do not voluntarily seek treatment. They are frequently hypersensitive, argumentative, and litigious, and come to attention through ill-founded legal activities. Although they may perform well occupationally and in areas distant from their delusions, they tend to be social isolates either by preference or as a result of their interpersonal inhospitality (e.g., spouses frequently abandon them). Social and occupational dysfunction, when it occurs, usually is in direct response to their delusions. The course may wax and wane.

These conditions appear to form a clinical continuum with conditions like paranoid personality disorder and paranoid schizophrenia; delineation of the limits of each syndrome awaits further research. Rule out an affective disorder—morbid jealousy and paranoid ideas are common in depression. Paranoia is common among the elderly (20) (see Chapter 24) and among stimulant drug abusers. Acute paranoid reactions frequently are seen in patients with mild delirium and in patients who are bedridden (and sensory deprived).

Etiology is unknown. No genetic or biologic factors have been identified. A higher incidence occurs among refugee and minority groups and among those with impaired hearing. A tendency exists for their family relationships to be characterized by turbulence, callousness, and coldness, yet the significance of this pattern is unclear. Typical defense mechanisms seen in these patients include denial, projection, and regression.

Treatment

Treatment is notoriously difficult (21). Individual psychotherapy is useful. Emphasis should be on developing a trusting relationship, with the patient seeing the therapist as neutral and accepting. Interfere with the patient's freedom of choice as little as possible.

Gradually help the patient see his or her world from your perspective. These patients are *very* sensitive to criticism (overt or implied), so this kind of a relationship is extremely difficult to develop and maintain.

Antipsychotic medication may help a few—it may at least take the energy out of the delusion. Antidepressants appear promising—consider them.

SHARED PSYCHOTIC DISORDER (DSM, P. 332, 297.3)

An otherwise normal person may adopt the delusional system of someone else. Most commonly, a dependent isolated wife will accept the delusional ideas of her (dominant) spouse (e.g., both may come to believe that their children are attempting to murder them with poison gas). When *two* people share equally the same delusion, it is *folie à deux*. Separation of the partners with shared delusions often results in disappearance of the delusions in the healthier member.

PSYCHOTIC DISORDER DUE TO A GENERAL MEDICAL CONDITION (DSM, P. 334, 293.81 OR 293.82)

These patients have a medical condition that *causes* prominent delusions (293.81) or hallucinations (293.82) about which they have no insight and cannot appreciate the symptom's connection to their medical illness. Of course, a careful medical workup is in order, and even then, the relation between the psychosis and the medical condition is often uncertain. Look for medical symptoms that appear just after the onset or worsening of the medical problem, prominent visual or olfactory hallucinations, and/or the "wrong age" at onset for normal psychoses (e.g., often in the elderly). Many conditions can produce an isolated psychosis (see Chapters 14 and 15): Do not use this diagnosis if symptoms occur only in the presence of an illness-related delirium or dementia.

SUBSTANCE-INDUCED PSYCHOTIC DISORDER

Drugs of abuse, certain medications (see Chapter 13), and toxins all can occasionally produce flagrant psychoses, usually with marked organic features such as confusion and prominent visual, olfactory, or tactile hallucinations. Most drugs of abuse can produce temporary psychoses with intoxication, whereas a few (e.g., alcohol and hypnotic–sedatives) produce them on discontinuation in the dependent patient (see Chapters 16 and 17). Most intoxication psychoses resolve on discontinuing the drug but occasionally may persist if caused by heavy use of stimulants, PCP, or LSD.

PSYCHOTIC DISORDER NOS (DSM, P. 343, 298.9)

If a psychotic patient does not have an affective disorder, an organic condition, or one of the disorders in this chapter and is not malingering, he or she has psychotic disorder NOS. The most common use of this classification is for patients for whom there is insufficient information to make a more specific diagnosis.

REFERENCES

1. Young DA, Zakzanis KK, Bailey C, et al. Further parameters of insight and neuropsychological deficit in schizophrenia and other chronic mental disease. *J Nerv Ment Disord* 1998;186:44–50.
2. Chen YR, Swann AC, Burt DB. Stability of diagnosis in schizophrenia. *Am J Psychiatry* 1996;153:682–686.
3. Tateyama M, Kudo I, Hashimoto M, et al. Is paranoid schizophrenia the most common subtype? *Psychopathology* 1999;32:98–106.
4. Wieselgren IM, Lindstrom LH. A prospective 1–5 year outcome study in first-admitted and readmitted schizophrenic patients. *Acta Psychiatry Scand* 1996;93:9–19.
5. Gupta S, Hendricks S, Kenkel AM, et al. Relapse in schizophrenia: is there a relationship to substance abuse? *Schizophr Res* 1996;20:153–156.
6. Amador XF, Friedman JH, Kasapis C, et al. Suicidal behavior in schizophrenia and its relationship to awareness of illness. *Am J Psychiatry* 1996;153:1185–1188.
7. Gur RE, Cowell P, Turetsky BI, et al. A follow-up magnetic resonance imaging study of schizophrenia. *Arch Gen Psychiatry* 1998;55:145–152.
8. Nelson MD, Saykin AJ, Flashman LA, et al. Hippocampal volume reduction in schizophrenia as assessed by magnetic resonance imaging. *Arch Gen Psychiatry* 1998;55:433–440.
9. Conrad AJ, Abebe T, Austin R, et al. Hippocampal pyramidal cell disarray in schizophrenia as a bilateral phenomenon. *Arch Gen Psychiatry* 1991;48:413–417.

10. Buka SL, Goldstein JM, Seidman LJ, et al. Prenatal complications, genetic vulnerability, and schizophrenia. *Psychiatr Ann* 1999; 29: 151–156.

11. Tsuang MT, Gilbertson MW, Faraone SV. The genetics of schizophrenia: current knowledge and future research. *Schizophr Res* 1991;4:157–171.

12. Cannon TD, Kaprio J, Lönnqvist J, et al. The genetic epidemiology of schizophrenia in a Finnish twin cohort. *Arch Gen Psychiatry* 1998;55:67–74.

13. Butzlaff RL, Hooley JM. Expressed emotion and psychiatric relapse. *Arch Gen Psychiatry* 1998;55:547–552.

14. Bateson G, Jackson DD, Haley J, Weakland JH. Towards a theory of schizophrenia. *Behav Sci* 1956;1:251–256.

15. Lieberman JA, Stroup TS, McEvoy JP, et al. Effectiveness of antipsychotic drugs in patients with chronic schizophrenia. *N Engl J Med* 2005;353:1209–1223.

16. Schooler NR. Negative symptoms in schizophrenia: assessment of the effect of risperidone. *J Clin Psychiatry* 1994;55(suppl 5): 22–28.

17. Penn DL, Mueser KT. Research update on the psychosocial treatment of schizophrenia. *Am J Psychiatry* 1996;153:607–617.

18. Benazzi F. DSM-III-R schizophreniform disorder with good prognostic features: a six-year follow-up. *Can J Psychiatry* 1998; 43:180–182.

19. Strakowski SM, Keck PE, Sax KW, et al. Twelve-month outcome of patients with DSM-III-R schizoaffective disorder. *Schizophr Res* 1999;35:167–174.

20. Yassa R, Suranyi-Cadotte B. Clinical characteristics of late-onset schizophrenia and delusional disorder. *Schizophr Bull* 1993; 19:701–707.

21. Lane RD. Successful fluoxetine treatment of pathological jealousy. *J Clin Psychiatry* 1990;51:345–346.

Mood Disorders

Patients with disorders of mood are common (3% to 5% of the population at any one time) and are seen by all medical specialists. It is essential to identify them and either treat or refer appropriately.

Two basic abnormalities of mood are recognized: depression and mania. Both occur on a continuum from normal to the clearly pathologic; symptoms in a few patients reach psychotic proportions. Although minor symptoms may be an extension of normal sadness or elation, more severe symptoms are associated with discrete syndromes (mood disorders), which appear to differ qualitatively from normal processes and which require specific therapies.

CLASSIFICATION

Diagnostic and Statistical Manual of Mental Disorders (DSM-IV) has defined several different mood disorders that differ, among other things, in their clinical presentation, course, genetics, and treatment response. These conditions are distinguished from one another by (a) the presence or absence of mania (bipolar vs. unipolar), (b) the severity of the illness (major vs. minor), and (c) the role of medical or other psychiatric conditions in causing the disorder (1% vs. 2%).

MAJOR MOOD DISORDERS: *Major* depressive or manic signs and symptoms or both.

Bipolar I Disorder (Manic–Depression): Mania in past or present (with or without presence or history of depression). Major depression usually occurs sometime.

Bipolar II Disorder: *Hypomania* and major depression must be present or have been present sometime.

Major Depressive Disorder: Serious depression alone (unipolar).

OTHER SPECIFIC MOOD DISORDER: *Minor* depressive and/or manic signs and symptoms.

Dysthymic Disorder: Depression alone.

Cyclothymic Disorder: Depressive *and* hypomanic symptoms in the present or recent past (consistently over the past 2 years).

MOOD DISORDER DUE TO A GENERAL MEDICAL CON-
DITION and SUBSTANCE-INDUCED MOOD DISORDER:
May be depressed, manic, or mixed; these are the second-degree
mood disorders.
ADJUSTMENT DISORDER WITH DEPRESSED MOOD:
Depression caused by stress.

The DSM-IV classification also requires the examiner to specify
whether the current bipolar episode is manic, depressed, or mixed;
whether the unipolar or bipolar disorder is a single episode or
recurrent and/or shows psychotic features, catatonia, rapid cycling,
complete clearing between episodes, a seasonal pattern, or a postpartum onset; and whether a major depressive episode is *chronic*
(present at least 2 years), meets the criteria for *melancholia* [pro-
found vegetative and cognitive symptoms including psychomotor
retardation or agitation, sleep disturbance, anorexia or weight loss,
and/or excessive guilt (see DSM-IV-TR, p. 419)], or is *atypical*
[increased appetite, weight gain, hypersomnia, interpersonal rejection sensitivity, "leaden" feeling in limbs (see DSM-IV-TR, p. 420)
(1)]. These characteristics "may" be important in determining
treatment and prognosis.

CLINICAL PRESENTATION OF MOOD DISORDERS

Of the core clinical features common to affective disturbances,
the Major Mood Disorders have the greater number and severity
of symptoms and signs, whereas dysthymia and cyclothymia have
fewer. The most common symptoms and signs of mood disorders
are listed in Tables 4.1 and 4.2. A sufficient combination of these
symptoms often clinches the diagnosis. However, particularly
when the symptoms are mild, disorders of mood are frequently
missed.

Although many depressed patients complain of depression, some
do not. Moreover, other problems may obscure the diagnosis. Some
patients have alcohol or drug abuse or acting-out behavior. Others,
particularly early on, primarily demonstrate anxiety or agitation. Still
others, instead of feeling sad, complain of *fatigue, irritability,
insomnia*, dyspnea, tachycardia, and vague or chronic pains or both
[usually gastrointestinal (GI), cardiac, headaches, or backaches, all
unrelieved by analgesics] (2). People with such presentations
(known as masked depressions) often have a personal or family
history of depression and frequently respond to antidepressants.

Table 4.1 ■ *Symptoms* of Depression
Emotional features
Depressed mood, "blue"
Irritability, anxiety
Anhedonia, loss of interest
Loss of zest
Diminished emotional bonds
Interpersonal withdrawal
Preoccupation with death
Cognitive features
Self-criticism, *sense of worthlessness*, guilt
Pessimism, *hopelessness*, despair
Distractible, *poor concentration*
Uncertain and indecisive
Variable obsessions
Somatic complaints (*particularly in the elderly*)
Memory impairment
Delusions and hallucinations
Vegetative features
Fatigability, no energy
Insomnia or hypersomnia
Anorexia or hyperrexia
Weight loss or gain
Psychomotor retardation
Psychomotor agitation
Impaired libido
Frequent diumal variation
Signs of depression
Stooped and slow moving
Tearful sad facies
Dry mouth and skin
Constipation

Suspect depression in the unimproved patient who has atypical medical symptoms.

Patients with mania often do not complain of their symptoms. A few feel too good and elated to complain; others feel agitated and unpleasant but fail to notice that their behavior is outrageous. Hypomanic patients can be irritable, or "full of life," or both.

Patient rating scales can help determine the severity of a depression and can be used to measure change over time [e.g., the Beck Depression Inventory (21 questions, patient self-rates) and the Hamilton Rating Scale for Depression (17–21 questions, therapist rates)].

Table 4.2 ■ *Symptoms* of Mania (When Nonpsychotic and Not Severe Enough to Impair Social or Occupational Functioning = Hypomania)

Emotional features
    Excited elevated mood, euphoria
    Emotional *lability*
    Rapid temporary shifts to acute depression
    Irritability, low frustration tolerance
    Demanding, egocentric
Cognitive features
    Elevated self-esteem, *grandiosity*
    Speech disturbances
    Loud word rhyming (clanging)
    Pressure of speech
    Flight of ideas
    Progression to incoherence
    Poor judgment, disorganization
    Paranoia
    Delusions and/or hallucinations
Physiologic features
    Boundless energy
    Insomnia, *little need for sleep*
    Decreased appetite
Signs of mania
    Psychomotor agitation

NORMAL MOOD PROCESSES

Sadness or simple unhappiness affect us all from time to time. The cause is often obvious, the reaction understandable, and improvement follows the disappearance of the cause. However, prolonged unhappiness in response to a chronic stress may be indistinguishable from a minor affective disorder and require treatment. Support and improved life circumstances are the keys to recovery.

Grief or **BEREAVEMENT** (p. 740, V62.82) is a more profound sense of dysphoria that follows a severe loss or trauma and that may produce a full depressive syndrome, but, as time distances the precipitating event, the symptoms disappear. This process often takes weeks or months and requires a "working through," which often includes disbelief, anger, intense mourning, and eventual resolution (see Chapter 10). Some bereavement grades into and, with time (e.g., longer than 2 months), becomes a major depressive disorder.

No generally accepted equivalent nonpathologic manic process is known, although some people do react to stress with hypomania.

MINOR MOOD DISORDERS

Depression

The common *chronic* nonpsychotic disorder of lowered mood or anhedonia or both is **DYSTHYMIC DISORDER** (p. 376, 300.4) (3). These patients feel depressed, have difficulty falling asleep, characteristically feel best in the morning and despondent in the afternoon and evening, and can display any of the nonpsychotic symptoms and signs of depression. Symptoms must have been present, at least intermittently, for 2 or more years. It is more common in women (W/M ratio, 2–3:1), often develops for the first time in the late 20s or 30s, has a lifetime prevalence of 6%, and begins insidiously, frequently in a person predisposed to depression by

- major loss in childhood [e.g., of parent (maybe)]
- recent loss (e.g., health, job, spouse).
- chronic stress (e.g., medical disorder).
- psychiatric susceptibility (e.g., personality disorders of histrionic, compulsive, and dependent types; alcohol and drug abuse; major depression in partial remission; obsessive–compulsive disorder). It frequently coexists with these conditions.

It is similar to but less severe than a Major Depressive Disorder; however, 20%+ of patients who experience major depression will clear incompletely and have a chronic residue of Dysthymic Disorder ("double depression"). It tends to last for many years.

Dysthymia must be differentiated from **ADJUSTMENT DISORDER WITH DEPRESSED MOOD** (p. 669, 309.0). This disorder occurs in an adequately functioning individual shortly after a readily identifiable, causative stress, results in impaired functioning, and resolves as the stress disappears. These patients are first seen with a depressive syndrome midway between normal sadness and major depression. If feelings of anxiety commingle with those of depression, the patient may have **ADJUSTMENT DISORDER WITH MIXED ANXIETY AND DEPRESSED MOOD** (p. 679, 309.28).

Hypomania

CYCLOTHYMIC DISORDER (p. 398, 301.13) requires the presence of mild depression *and* hypomania, separately or inter-mixed, continuously or intermittently over at least a 2-year period. It usually begins in the 20s in patients (F/M ratio, 1:1) with a fam-ily history of major affective disorder and forms a chronically disabling pattern that yields troubled interpersonal relationships, job instability, occasional suicide attempts and short hospitaliza-tions, and a markedly increased risk of drug and alcohol abuse.

MAJOR MOOD DISORDERS

Patients with major mood disorders are profoundly depressed or excited. Clinical presentations and genetic studies support two dis-tinct groups, **MAJOR DEPRESSIVE DISORDER** (unipolar) (p. 369, 296.2x–.3x) and two types of bipolar disorders: **BIPOLAR I DISORDER** (p. 382, 296.xx) and **BIPOLAR II DISORDER** (p. 392, 296.89); yet some question this dichotomy (e.g., bipolar disorder *may* be a more-severe form of recurrent unipolar disorder). The lifetime risk in the general population for a major depression (4) is about 17%[+]:10 times the frequency of bipolar disorder; 15% of pa-tients kill themselves eventually.

Major Depression

These patients have many serious symptoms and signs of depression, yet their clinical presentations can vary markedly from profound retardation and withdrawal to irritable, unrelieved agitation. A pre-sumed precipitating event occurs in 25% (50% among the elderly) (5). A diurnal variation is common, with the most severe symptoms early in the day. Some fail to recognize their depression, complain-ing instead of their "insides rotting out" or their "minds going crazy," yet the profound affective disturbance is usually recognizable to the observer. A thought disorder is occasionally present. Delusions are usually affect laden and mood congruent, but need not be. Hallucinations are uncommon, auditory, and usually have a self-condemning or paranoid content. These "psychotic depressions" may represent a separate disorder or may simply be a more severe form of depression (**M.D., or B.D., WITH PSYCHOTIC FEATU-RES**). Depressed elderly may be seen primarily with retardation, memory impairment, and mild disorientation (*pseudodementia*).

The disorder can occur at any age (median age at onset is the late 20s; 10% occur after age 60), with the majority of cases spread evenly throughout the adult years and with females affected 2:1. (However, increasing numbers of teenagers and young adults seem to be afflicted.) Unlike schizophrenia, it occurs evenly in the higher social strata. Family and twin studies strongly suggest a genetic factor: increased incidence of major depression, alcoholism, and possibly antisocial personality disorder in relatives (the "depressive spectrum" disorders). The prevalence of serious affective illness in first-degree relatives is 13% contrasted with 1% to 3% in the general population. About 30% to 40% of identical twins are concordant for unipolar depression. Alcoholism and chronic stress may predispose to the development of the illness. Molecular genetic "segregation and linkage analysis" has yet to identify a gene or chromosome for major depression, in spite of the strong (suggestive) evidence that this is a genetic illness.

Fewer than 50% of patients will have only one episode (**M.D., SINGLE EPISODE**, 296.2x); 50% to 60% have two or more attacks (**M.D., RECURRENT**, 296.3x). Some patients clear between episodes; others remain mildly depressed (20%); and 10% are chronically, severely depressed. Most attacks begin gradually over a 1- to 3-week period and, untreated, last from 3 to 8 months or longer. This is often a cyclic disorder: relapse during the months or a year or two after recovery from an acute episode is common (but partly avoidable with maintenance medications). These patients are often incapacitated during an episode and are at great risk of suicide. About half of the patients with recurrent illness will recover over a period of 1 to 2 decades, whereas the rest will be chronically affected, although most at the level of dysthymia, with infrequent relapses into major depression.

Postpartum depression is a severe depression, usually beginning 1 to 2, and certainly by 4, weeks after delivery, usually of the second or third child. Affected women are at risk for repeated episodes with future deliveries.

Seasonal affective disorder (SAD) is characterized by the development of major depression with a seasonal pattern: symptoms appear each fall/winter and return to normal (or even hypomania) during the spring/summer. It afflicts predominantly younger women (F/M ratio, 2 to 4:1), displays many features of "atypical" depression (hypersomnia, weight gain, hyperphagia), and is often treated successfully with bright, artificial light (2 to 6 h/day; response in 2 to 3 days; occasionally hypomania occurs) with or without antidepressants (6). Its relation to more classical major depression is unclear.

The apparent biologic nature of many serious depressions is reflected in the recent development of several putative biologic tests for depression: the dexamethasone suppression test (DST-positive test is the failure of normal suppression of plasma cortisol 6 to 24 h after an oral dose of dexamethasone); elevated serum cortisol (30% of patients have adrenal hypertrophy); decreased urinary MHPG (3-methoxy-4-hydroxyphenylene-glycol, a catabolite of norepinephrine), and CSF 5-HIAA (a metabolite of serotonin); TRH-stimulation test [low TSH and blunted TSH and growth hormone (GH) responses to exogenous TRH suggest unipolar depression]; sleep abnormalities [*short REM latency*: time from falling asleep to start of REM sleep (a *very* good indicator); *frequent awakenings; early-morning awakenings*; decreased NREM sleep; *increased REM density*, frequency of rapid eye movements in REM sleep (all may be a trait in people prone to depression)]; and the stimulant challenge tests (some depressed patients briefly improve when given 10 mg of amphetamine). Unfortunately, these tests have little routine clinical utility [the best seem to be (a) abnormal sleep studies, (b) abnormal TSH levels and TRH responses, and (c) a *posttreatment* positive DST as a measure of poor outcome]. They all have inadequate sensitivity and specificity (too many false positives and negatives). However, each further emphasizes that biology plays a role in many depressions. (Still, environment also plays a role, because in 25% of patients with serious medical conditions and in others with marked psychosocial stress, a major depression will develop.)

Searching for the CNS site(s) of the illness with positron emission tomography (PET) and functional magnetic resonance imaging (*f*MRI) has been more promising, suggesting that major depression is associated (somehow) with decreased activity in the lateral prefrontal cortex (particularly the left side), the caudate, the putamen, and probably also the amygdala (7,8).

Bipolar Disorders

Mania, at some time severe enough to produce compromised functioning, is necessary to diagnose Bipolar I Disorder, but 90%+ of patients also have periods of depression (**B.D., DEPRESSED**, 296.5x). The manic episode typically develops over days and may become uncontrolled and psychotic (**B.D., MANIC**, 296.4x). About 20%+ of manic patients have hallucinations or delusions or both. A severe mania may be indistinguishable from an organic delirium (sudden onset, anorexia, insomnia, disorientation, paranoia, hallucinations, and delusions) or acute schizophrenia. When the bipolar patient is depressed, the depression is *usually* profound but occasionally may appear as a mild depressive syndrome. Attacks usually are separated by months or years, but the patient occasionally may cycle from one to the other over days or weeks [**WITH RAPID CYCLING** (p. 427), four or more mood episodes in a year; 10%+ of patients; F/M ratio, 4:1; younger, poorer prognosis, but the pattern may disappear] or actually have contrasting symptoms simultaneously (e.g., spirited singing intermixed with crying; **B.D., MIXED**, 296.6x)]. This is a recurrent illness; single attacks are rare. Pure manic syndromes (patients who have only mania, *unipolar mania*) occur clinically but are unusual and are probably not a separate entity.

The lifetime risk for developing bipolar disorder is approximately 1.0%+. This is a genetic disorder. First-degree relatives are at risk for bipolar disorder (5% to 10% develop it), major depression (10%+), and cyclothymia. A 70%+ concordance for bipolar illness occurs in identical twins. In contrast with major depression, M/F ratio, 1:1. The type of inheritance is uncertain—almost certainly genetically heterogeneous and polygenic. "Innumerable" linkage studies suggest at least a dozen different chromosomes and even more different locations (9).

The first manic episode is often before age 30, begins quickly, and resolves in 2 to 4 months if untreated. One or more episodes of depression usually have already occurred. Most patients go on to have a majority of depressive episodes. Suicide is the major risk during periods of depression. Legal difficulties and drug and alcohol abuse (as well as suicide) occur with manic periods.

Bipolar II Disorder occurs when a patient who has had a major depression also experiences an hypomanic episode (usually around the time of the depression), but never becomes fully manic. It occurs more frequently in women who have a family history of mood disorder; 10%+ go on to develop Bipolar I Disorder by later having a manic episode. It is relatively common—4 times as common as Bipolar I Disorder. Moreover, a treatment-resistant depression dominates the clinical picture, and such a depression is often thought to be unipolar and thus is inappropriately treated.

MOOD DISORDER DUE TO A GENERAL MEDICAL CONDITION

Various medical conditions can directly produce major depressive or manic syndromes or both (p. 401, 293.83), although in whom such a syndrome will develop is unpredictable. Some illnesses have a high likelihood of producing a mood disturbance (e.g., depression in 50%+ of patients with stroke, pancreatic carcinoma, and Cushing syndrome), whereas it is much less common, but no less direct, with other illnesses. This disorder is *not* meant for those medical conditions that produce depression or mania as a reaction to having the illness or for those patients who show a mood disturbance only when delirious. Likely medical diseases include (see Chapters 14 and 15) the following.

Depression

- Tumors: Particularly of brain and lung, carcinoma of pancreas (in 50%, psychiatric symptoms develop before the diagnosis is made).
- Infections: Influenza, mononucleosis, "flu-fatigue" syndrome [Epstein–Barr (EB) virus?], encephalitis, hepatitis.
- Endocrine disorders: Cushing disease (60% of patients; also from exogenous steroids), hypothyroidism [some experts recommend a careful thyroid evaluation in most (all?) depressed patients], apathetic hyperthyroidism, hyperparathyroidism (symptoms parallel levels of serum Ca^{2+}), diabetes, Turner syndrome.
- Blood: Anemia (particularly pernicious anemia).
- Nutrition and electrolytes: Pellagra, hyponatremia, hypokalemia, hypercalcemia, inappropriate antidiuretic hormone (ADH).
- Miscellaneous: Multiple sclerosis (MS), Parkinson disease, head trauma, stroke [poststroke depression; particularly L-frontal (?)], early Huntington disease, post–myocardial infarction (MI), premenstrual syndrome (PMS, maybe), menopause (relieved by estrogens).

Mania

- Tumors: of brain.
- Infections: Encephalitis, influenza, syphilis (20% of patients with general paresis).
- Miscellaneous: MS, Wilson disease, head trauma, psychomotor epilepsy, hyperthyroidism.

SUBSTANCE-INDUCED MOOD DISORDER

Drugs of abuse, medications, and toxins all can produce mood disorders of various types (DSM-IV, p. 405). The likelihood of mood symptoms from use of a substance and the pattern of symptoms produced varies not only with the specific drug but also with the dose, the duration of use, whether the issue is intoxication or withdrawal, and ill-specified and poorly understood individual factors in the patient. A modest list of likely agents include (see Chapter 13):

Depression

- Drugs of abuse: alcohol (often hard to tell "which is the chicken and which the egg"), sedative–hypnotics, opioids, phencyclidine (PCP).
- Medication: oral contraceptives, corticosteroids, reserpine (6% of patients), α-methyldopa, guanethidine, levodopa, indomethacin, benzodiazepines, opiates, cimetidine, propranolol, anticholinesterases, amphetamine withdrawal.
- Miscellaneous: heavy-metal poisoning.

Mania

- Drugs of abuse: Cocaine, amphetamines, hallucinogens, PCP.
- Medication: Steroids, L-dopa.
- Miscellaneous: Organophosphates, petroleum distillates.

MOOD DISORDER NOS

BIPOLAR DISORDER NOS (p. 400, 296.80) and **DEPRESSIVE DISORDER NOS** (p. 381, 311) include the remaining (unusual) affective presentations.

DIFFERENTIAL DIAGNOSIS

Depression

- Schizophrenic disorders: Particularly catatonics, but any type can look or be depressed during or after an episode. Poor premorbid adjustment, formal thought disorder with well-formed delusions and complex hallucinations, lack of cyclic history, and no family history for affective disorder all suggest schizophrenia.
- Schizoaffective disorder: A psychotic disorder that meets the criteria for schizophrenia, but with superimposed major mood symptoms for part of the time.

- Generalized anxiety disorder: Anxiety appears first and predominates. With the anxious patient, always consider depression.
- Alcoholism and drug abuse: Alcoholism and depression are both often present ("dual-diagnosis" patients).
- Obsessive–Compulsive Disorder; Histrionic and Borderline Personality Disorders: Are the full syndromes present?
- Dementia: "Pseudodepression" is common, and differentiation is tricky, particularly in the elderly. Check for memory impairment and disorientation.

Mania

- Schizophrenic disorders: Often indistinguishable in acute cases. Check personal and family history.
- Schizoaffective Disorder
- Borderline Personality Disorder

PSYCHOBIOLOGIC THEORIES

Psychoanalytic theory (Freud) postulates that a depressed patient has had a real or imagined loss of an ambivalently loved object, has reacted with unconscious rage, which has been then turned against the self, and this has resulted in a lowered self-esteem and depression. Cognitive Theory postulates a "cognitive triad" of distorted perceptions in which (a) a person's negative interpretation of his own life experiences (b) causes a devaluation of himself, which (c) causes depression.

Promising but unproven biologic theories focus on brain norepinephrine (NE) and serotonin (5-HT) abnormalities. Biologic and psychological theories need not be mutually exclusive. The catecholamine hypothesis suggests that low brain NE levels cause depression, and elevated levels cause mania; however, urinary MHPG levels (a major metabolite of NE) are low in only some depressions. The indolamine hypothesis holds that low cerebral 5-HT (or the primary metabolite, 5-HIAA) causes depression, and elevation causes mania, yet exceptions occur. The permissive hypothesis postulates that reduced NE produces depression, and increased NE causes mania only if 5-HT levels are low. The known mechanisms of action of antidepressants support these theories: tricyclics block NE and 5-HT reuptake, and monoamine oxidase inhibitors (MAOIs) block oxidation of NE. In addition, recent research suggests that frontal lobe/whole brain hypometabolism in depression, or some fundamental abnormality of the circadian rhythms of depressed patients may exist.

TREATMENT OF DEPRESSION

Evaluate medically and psychiatrically to rule out secondary depression and to attempt to identify an affective syndrome. Always ask about vegetative features, and evaluate suicidal potential (see Chapter 7). If the patient is (a) incapacitated by the disorder, (b) has a destructive home environment or limited environmental support, (c) is a suicide risk, or (d) has an associated medical illness requiring treatment, hospitalize. All depressed patients should receive psychotherapy; some must receive physical therapies in addition. The specific treatments used depend on the diagnosis, severity, patient's age, and past responses to therapy.

Psychological Therapies

Supportive psychotherapy is always indicated. Be warm, empathic, understanding, and optimistic. Help the patient to identify and express concerns and to ventilate. Identify precipitating factors and help correct. Help solve external problems (e.g., rent, job); be directive, particularly during the acute episode and if the patient is immobilized. Train the patient to recognize signs of future decompensation. See the patient frequently (1 to 3 times per week initially) and regularly, but not interminably; be available. Recognize that some depressed patients can provoke anger in you (through anger, hostility, unreasonable demands, etc); watch for it. Long-term insight-oriented psychotherapy may be of value in selected chronic minor depressions and in some conflicted patients with a major depression in remission.

Cognitive–behavior therapy is very useful with mild to moderately severe depressive patients (10). Thought by some to be "learned helplessness," depressions are treated by giving patients skill training and providing success experiences. From a cognitive perspective, the patient is trained to recognize and eliminate negative thoughts and expectations. This therapy helps prevent relapse (11,12).

Partial sleep deprivation (awaken midway through the night, and keep up until the next evening) helps lessen the symptoms of a major depression temporarily. Physical exercise (running, swimming) may produce improvement in depression, for poorly understood biologic reasons.

Physical Therapies (see Chapter 23)

All major and most chronic or unimproved minor unipolar depressions require a trial of antidepressants (70% to 80% of patients respond), even though an apparent precipitant of the depression is identified. Begin with an selective serotonin reuptake inhibitor (SSRI) or an SNRI. If that fails, try one or two more, and then consider a tricyclic antidepressant, an MAOI (particularly in "atypical" depressions), or one of numerous effective drug combinations or augmenting medications if the first two or three drugs fail. Be alert to side effects, and be aware that antidepressants "may" precipitate a manic episode in a few bipolar patients (10% with TCAs; possibly lower with SSRIs). Maintain for several months after remission from a first depressive episode, and then taper; however, most patients, after one or more relapses, may require maintenance medications for long periods. An antidepressant rarely is sufficient alone in treating a unipolar psychotic depression. Psychotic, paranoid, or very agitated patients may require an antipsychotic, alone or with an antidepressant, lithium, or electroconvulsive therapy (ECT); the newer atypical antipsychotics seem particularly effective.

Bipolar depression is often much more difficult to treat and requires a different approach: it almost always requires a mood stabilizer (lithium or lamotrigine as first choices; perhaps valproate, carbamazepine, or topiramate as alternatives), and usually, but not always, an antidepressant as well. Lithium is effective at producing a remission in bipolar disorder, mania, and it appears to be useful in treating acute bipolar depressions (and a few unipolar depressions). It is moderately effective at maintaining a remission in bipolar and some unipolar patients as well. The anticonvulsants seem to be at least as good as lithium at treating the acute conditions and perhaps at maintenance (13). Antidepressants and mood stabilizers may be started concurrently, and the mood stabilizer continued after remission. The atypical antidepressants also seem to have antidepressant qualities in this population.

ECT may be the treatment of choice for either unipolar and bipolar depression (a) if medication fails after one or more 6-week trials, (b) if the patient's condition demands an immediate remission (e.g., acutely suicidal), (c) in some psychotic depressions, or (d) in patients who cannot tolerate medication (e.g., some elderly cardiac patients). Up to 90% of patients respond.

TREATMENT OF MANIA

Evaluate carefully but quickly. Is the patient medically ill or taking drugs? Has he been manic before? Is he taking lithium? What is the blood level?

If the patient is hypomanic, use outpatient treatment, and work with the family, if possible. Consider short-term, low-dose antipsychotics (e.g., haloperidol, 2 to 5 mg/day), but rely on treatment with lithium or anticonvulsants over the longer term. If the patient is manic, hospitalize. Is the patient debilitated? Seriously sleep deprived?

1. Medicate immediately with lithium carbonate; however, as many as 30% of manics stay partially symptomatic in spite of lithium. Depending on the degree of agitation, consider an atypical antipsychotic as well. If control is not achieved, consider adding to or replacing the lithium with an anticonvulsant (valproate, carbamazepine, and lamotrigine are currently the best choices).

2. Be relaxed, reasonable, and controlled. Treat in quiet setting with minimal stimuli. Set firm limits.

REFERENCES

1. Nierenberg AA, Alpert JE, Pava J, et al. Course and treatment of atypical depression. *J Clin Psychiatry* 1998;59(suppl 18):5–9.
2. Posse M, Hällström A. Depressive disorders among somatizing patients in primary health care. *Acta Psychiatry Scand* 1998; 98:187–192.
3. Klein DN, Norden KA, Ferro T, et al. Thirty-month naturalistic follow-up study of early-onset dysthymic disorder. *J Abnorm Psychol* 1998;107:338–348.
4. Blazer DG, Kessler RC, McGonagle KA, et al. The prevalence and distribution of major depression in a national community sample: the National Comorbidity Survey. *Am J Psychiatry* 1994;151:979–986.
5. Cui X, Vaillant GE. Antecedents and consequences of negative life events in adulthood. *Am J Psychiatry* 1996;152:21–26.
6. Lewy AJ, Bauer VK, Cutler NL, et al. Morning vs evening light treatment of patients with winter depression. *Arch Gen Psychiatry* 1998;55:890–896.
7. Kennedy SH, Javanmard M, Vaccarino FJ. A review of functional neuroimaging in mood disorders: positron emission tomography and depression. *Can J Psychiatry* 1997;42:467–475.
8. Soares JC, Mann JJ. The anatomy of mood disorders: review of structural neuroimaging studies. *Biol Psychiatry* 1997;41:86–106.

9. Gershon ES, Badner JA, Goldin LR, et al. Closing in on genes for manic-depressive illness and schizophrenia. *Neuropsychopharmacology* 1998;18:233–242.
10. Jørgensen MB, Dam H, Bolwig TG. The efficacy of psychotherapy in non-bipolar depression: a review. *Acta Psychiatry Scand* 1998;98:1–13.
11. Hollon SD, DeRubeis RJ, Shelton RC, et al. Prevention of relapse following cognitive therapy vs medications in moderate to severe depression. *Arch Gen Psychiatry* 2005;62:417–422.
12. Fava GA, Rafanelli C, Grandi S, et al. Prevention of recurrent depression with cognitive behavioral therapy. *Arch Gen Psychiatry* 1998;55:816–820.
13. Keck PE, McElroy SI. Treatment of bipolar disorder. In: Schatzburg AF, Nemeroff CB, eds. *American Psychiatric Association Textbook of Psychopharmacology*, 3rd ed. Washington, DC: APPI, 2004:865–884.

Delirium and Amnestic and Other Cognitive Disorders

The psychiatric conditions in this chapter are all caused by medical (organic) pathology. The most common is delirium, but several other specific presentations occur as well. In addition, gross organic processes contribute to dementia (see Chapter 6), intoxication, and withdrawal (see Chapters 16 and 17), and many of the syndromes found in other chapters.

These syndromes are common, particularly among the elderly (20% or more of all acute medical inpatients develop some organic syndrome, usually delirium). Delirium is acute, usually brief, and reversible, whereas dementia is of slower onset, longer lasting, and more likely to be irreversible, yet none of these characterizations is completely true (e.g., 15% to 20% of dementias are at least partially reversible). These conditions are clinically defined, and their course and characteristics depend on the nature, severity, course, and location of the causative organic pathology. First, identify the syndrome, and then determine the likely organic cause.

DELIRIUM

Delirium (1,2) is a common condition that may be caused by physical illness (**D. DUE TO A GENERAL MEDICAL CONDITION**, DSM, p. 141, 293.0), drugs (**SUBSTANCE INTOXICATION OR WITHDRAWAL.**, DSM, p. 143), several causes simultaneously (**D. DUE TO MULTIPLE ETIOLOGIES**, DSM, p. 146), or by unknown organic conditions. These patients may be confused, bizarre, or even "wild," and thus can be mistakenly thought to have other psychotic illnesses. Other delirious patients may appear somnolent or perfectly normal during the day but decompensate dramatically in the evening or night. Still other patients may have increasing difficulty functioning because of a mild delirium that is revealed only by specific mental status testing. Synonyms include acute brain syndrome, toxic psychosis, acute confusional state, and metabolic encephalopathy.

Diagnosis

Delirium is a rapidly developing disorder of *disturbed attention* that fluctuates with time. Although the clinical presentation of delirium differs considerably from patient to patient, several characteristic features help to make the diagnosis:

- **Clouding of consciousness:** The patient is not normally alert and may appear bewildered and confused. Noticeably decreased alertness (grading into stupor) or hyperalertness may be present. Observe the patient.
- **Attention deficit:** The patient usually is very distractible and unable to focus attention sufficiently or for a long enough time to follow a train of thought or to understand what is occurring around him. Have the patient do serial 7s or 3s and/or a Random Letter Test.
- **Perceptual disturbances:** These are common and include misinterpretations of environmental events, illusions (e.g., the curtain blows, and the patient believes someone is climbing in the window), and hallucinations (usually visual). The patient may or may not recognize these misperceptions as unreal.
- **Sleep–wake alteration:** Insomnia is almost always present (all symptoms are usually worse at night and in the dark), and marked drowsiness may also occur.
- **Disorientation:** Most frequently to time but also to place, situation, and (finally) person. Ask for the date, time, and day of the week: "What place is this?" etc.
- **Memory impairment:** The patient typically has a recent memory deficit and usually denies it (he or she may confabulate and may want to talk about the distant past). Ask about the recent past (e.g., "Who brought you to the hospital?" "Did you have any tests yesterday?" "What did you have for breakfast?") Name four objects and two words, and ask the patient for them in 5 minutes. Does he or she remember your name?
- **Incoherence:** The patient may attempt to communicate, but the speech may be confused or even unintelligible. Verbal perseveration may occur.
- **Altered psychomotor activity:** Many delirious patients are restless and agitated, and some may display perseveration of motion, some may be excessively somnolent, and some may fluctuate from one to the other (usually restless at night and sleepy during the day).
- **Fluctuations:** Most of the characteristics listed above vary in severity *over hours* and days.

A delirium usually develops over days and *may* precede signs of the organic condition causing it. Usually it lasts less than a week (depending on the cause). Many of these patients are significantly anxious or frightened by their experiences, may become combative, and may develop some delusional ideas based on their misperceptions. A few patients become dangerously suicidal—watch for it. Environmental conditions can significantly alter the presentation of a delirium. Change of setting (e.g., moving out of familiar surroundings), overstimulation, and understimulation (e.g., darkness, sensory deprivation) can all worsen the symptoms, as can stress of any kind. Delirium seems to be an *independent* factor that significantly increases mortality among patients; thus it *must* be identified and dealt with (3).

It is necessary to have a high index of suspicion and to ask specific mental-status questions if you are going to identify delirium early. Ask questions tactfully because many patients defensively resist this probing. The early prodromal symptoms that should alert you to a developing delirium include the following:

Restlessness (particularly at night), anxiety;
Daytime somnolence;
Insomnia, vivid dreams, and nightmares;
Hypersensitivity to light and sound;
Fleeting illusions and hallucinations;
Distractibility, difficulty in thinking clearly.

The EEG (although usually not necessary to make the diagnosis) has a characteristic pattern of *diffuse slowing* that is proportional to the severity of the delirium (except for intoxication or withdrawal delirium—fast waves). It can help if a question exists about the presence of a functional psychosis, drug use, or a dissociative state. Delirium may also be accompanied by a tremor, asterixis, diaphoresis, tachycardia, elevated blood pressure (BP), tachypnea, and flushing.

Etiology and Differential Diagnosis

The presence of a delirium usually means that the patient is seriously medically ill. Delirium is a diagnosis that demands an immediate search for causes. Most causes produce diffuse cerebral impairment and lie *outside* the central nervous system (CNS)—usually due to some form of deranged metabolism (e.g., infection, fever, hypoxia, hypoglycemia, medication side effects, drug-withdrawal states, hepatic encephalopathy, postoperative changes)—but also include CNS trauma and postictal states. The specific potential etiologies are too numerous to list (consult a more complete source), although usually the cause is evident. These patients all deserve a thorough physical and laboratory examination.

Major problems in differential diagnosis include distinguishing delirium from dementia or a psychotic disorder. The presence of marked, acute confusion usually differentiates from the slow onset of dementia. Recognize, however, that (a) the presence of dementia is almost impossible to identify until an overlying delirium clears, and (b) patients (particularly elderly) in whom delirium develops when they are ill are at marked risk (more than 50% of patients) to display an early dementia within the following 2 years (4). Compared with the psychotic patient, the delirious patient is usually more ill and confused, and the hallucinations are usually more disorganized and are more likely to be visual. Typical psychotic disorders usually do not have confusion, disorientation, and illusions, and they are more likely to have a formal thought disorder. *Always* check the personal and family history for serious psychiatric illness.

Treatment

The following are guidelines in treating delirium (5):
- Of course, treat an identified medical cause of the delirium.
- Provide for the patient's safety. Maintain around-the-clock observation (particularly at night). This may require someone in the room constantly—preferably someone with whom the patient is familiar. Use restraints only if absolutely necessary (they frequently increase agitation).
- Keep the patient in a quiet, well-lighted room. Keep familiar objects around, and use the same treatment personnel, if possible. Frequently (and tactfully) reorient the patient. Introduce yourself again, and describe what you are doing and why. Anticipate the patient's anxiety, and reassure him. Be calm and sympathetic. These "preventive" measures may be helpful but will not control a serious delirium.
- Medication should be used cautiously, with aggressiveness dependent on patient age, degree of illness, and severity of delirium (and accompanying level of agitation). Use low doses in mild delirium; often p.o. but occasionally i.m. Haloperidol is still preferred (0.5 to 2 mg to begin), although atypical antipsychotics are becoming the drugs of choice [e.g., begin with olanzapine p.o. or i.m. (2.5 to 10 mg), ziprasidone p.o. or i.m. (10 to 40 mg), risperidone p.o. (0.5 to 2 mg, b.i.d.), or quetiapine p.o. (12.5 to 50 mg)] (6). For marked delirium with agitation or psychotic features or both, haloperidol remains the drug of choice; begin

with a bolus i.m. or i.v. (usually in the ICU) of 5 to 10 mg with repeats in 30 minutes until quiet. For delirium from alcohol or sedative–hypnotic withdrawal, consider a benzodiazepine (e.g., lorazepam, clonazepam). For an anticholinergic delirium/psychosis, use i.v. physostigmine very carefully (avoid a cholinergic reaction; e.g., bradycardia, hypotension) initially, and then perhaps switch to a cholinesterase inhibitor (e.g., donepezil, 5 mg).

The following organic syndromes are considerably less common than delirium, dementia, and the substance-abuse syndromes of intoxication and withdrawal. They are also more likely to be associated with focal organic pathology and with a few specific medical or neurologic diseases.

AMNESTIC SYNDROME DUE TO A GENERAL MEDICAL CONDITION (DSM, P. 175, 294.0); SUBSTANCE-INDUCED PERSISTING AMNESTIC DISORDER (DSM, P. 177)

These patients have severe memory deficits that usually appear suddenly after a CNS insult and that may become chronic. The deficits are *both* retrograde (old memories—ask about childhood, schooling, etc.) and anterograde (new memory—ask the patient to remember several facts for 5 to 10 min). The patients are often unaware that their memory is impaired. Unlike in delirium, the sensorium is usually clear, although disorientation may be present. Unlike in dementia, serious memory loss occurs without intellectual or other associated changes.

The numerous potential causes include CNS trauma, hypoxia, herpes simplex encephalitis, and some substance abuse (particularly alcohol and sedative–hypnotic abuse) (see Chapters 16 and 17). Bilateral lesions of the medial temporal or diencephalic regions or both appear to be required. Treatment consists of correcting any medical/organic causes and waiting.

CATATONIC DISORDER DUE TO A GENERAL MEDICAL CONDITION (DSM, P. 185, 393.89)

These patients display *catatonia* (immobility—stuporousness or the "waxy flexibility" of catalepsy—but sometimes extreme agitation; also mutism, slow and stereotyped movements, echolalia, echopraxia, or a combination of these) caused by a medical condition or a substance. The most common causes are neurologic and metabolic (e.g., hypercalcemia or hepatic encephalopathy). Be sure to rule out catatonic schizophrenia (history of psychosis; no medical causes), but do not assume every catatonic patient is "just schizophrenic."

PERSONALITY CHANGE DUE TO A GENERAL MEDICAL CONDITION (DSM, P. 187, 310.1)

These patients display a personality *change* or a marked exacerbation of previous personality characteristics. Often this takes the form of a loss of control over impulses and emotions or the development of apathy, irritability, aggression, paranoia, or indifference. Impairment of social judgment is common. The usual cause is frontal lobe damage (the frontal lobe syndrome) due to stroke, tumor, CNS trauma, normal-pressure hydrocephalus, general paresis, Huntington chorea, or multiple sclerosis (MS). Occasionally, right-sided strokes may be responsible. Be careful not to mistake it for mild delirium or the early changes of dementia, schizophrenia, or major affective disorder.

REFERENCES

1. Lipowski ZJ. *Delirium*. New York: Oxford University Press, 1990.
2. Inouye SK. Delirium in older persons. *N Engl J Med* 2006; 354:1157–1165.
3. Ely EW, Shintani A, Truman B, et al. Delirium as a predictor of mortality in mechanically ventilated patients in the intensive care unit. *JAMA* 2004;291:1753–1762.
4. McCusker J, Cole MG, Dendukuri N, et al. The course of delirium in older medical inpatients: a prospective study. *J Gen Intern Med* 2003;18:696–704.
5. American Psychiatric Association. Practice guideline for the treatment of patients with delirium. *Am J Psychiatry* 1999;156 (suppl):1–20.
6. Schwartz TL, Masand PS. The role of atypical antipsychotics in the treatment of delirium. *Psychosomatics* 2002;43:171–174.

Dementia

DEMENTIA (DSM, p. 147) results from a broad loss of intellectual functions due to diffuse organic disease of (a) the cerebral hemispheres (*cortical dementia*; amnesia, agnosia, apraxia, aphasia), or the (b) subcortical structures (*subcortical dementia*, e.g., Huntington and Parkinson diseases; cognitive impairment, apathy, depression, inertia, psychomotor retardation, loss of drive) of sufficient severity to impair social or occupational functioning or both. Dementia is a clinical presentation demanding a diagnosis—*not* a diagnosis itself. Causes are numerous, but clinical presentations are remarkably similar. Seventy percent of dementias are irreversible, but because 15% to 20% are controllable or reversible, treatable causes must be identified.

MAKING THE DIAGNOSIS

Dementia usually develops slowly and is easily overlooked. A rapid onset suggests a recent (and possibly treatable) insult, although frequently a mild unrecognized dementia is made worse and obvious by a medical illness [e.g., pneumonia, congestive heart failure (CHF)]. *Always* interview the family—they frequently notice changes (in personality, memory, etc.) of which the patient is unaware. Unlike delirium, clouding of consciousness is minimal (unless dementia and delirium are mixed)—make sure the patient is alert (1).

EARLY: Effects include short-term memory loss, a gradual loss of intellectual skills and acuity, subtle changes in personality, impaired social skills, a decrease in the range of interests and enthusiasms, lability and shallowness of affect, agitation, numerous somatic complaints, and vague psychiatric symptoms. These are often first noticed in work settings where high performance is required. Patients may recognize a loss of abilities initially but vigorously deny it. Early dementia may precipitate a depression or anxiety. Early dementia may appear primarily with emotional (usually depressive) rather than cognitive symptoms, *but also* emotional disorders may mimic early dementia. Do not under- or overdiagnose it.

LATE: Parts of the full picture emerge:

- **Memory loss:** Usually immediate and recent memory loss (hippocampus) but gradually involves remote recall (medial temporal and diencephalic regions involved). Does the patient forget appointments, the news, people he or she has just met, or places he or she has just been? Patient may confabulate, so check the information. Ask the patient to (a) repeat digits (normal, remember 6 forward, 4 backward), and (b) recall two words and three objects after 5 minutes. Does the patient know your name? the nurse? this place? the names of his or her visitors? last night's meal? Does the patient know his or her birth date? hometown? the name of his or her high school?

- **Changes in mood and personality:** Often exaggeration of previous personality (e.g., more compulsive or more excitable). *Depression*, anxiety, irritability, or a combination of these early on—later, withdrawal and apathy. Has the patient become sloppy, belligerent, thoughtless of others, *paranoid*, socially inappropriate, fearful? Does he lack initiative or interest? Use vulgar language or jokes?

- **Loss of orientation:** Particularly time (of day, day of week, date, season) but also place ("What place is this?") and, when severe, person. Has the patient been getting lost—in new places, in the former neighborhood, or at home? Does the patient know why he or she is here (situation)? The patient may not sleep well, wander around at night, and get lost.

- **Intellectual impairment:** Patient is "less sharp" than he or she used to be. Does the patient have trouble doing things he or she could previously do easily? General information (last five presidents, six large U.S. cities), calculations (multiplication tables, serial 7s or 3s, make change), similarities (how are a ball and an orange alike? a mouse and an elephant? a fly and a tree?).

- **Compromised judgment:** Does not anticipate consequences. Does the patient act impulsively? "What should you do if you find a stamped addressed envelope?" "If you noticed a fire in a theater?"

- **Psychotic symptoms:** Hallucinations (usually simple), illusions, delusions, unshakable preoccupations, ideas of reference.

- **Language impairment:** Often vague and imprecise; occasionally almost mute. Is there perseveration, blocking, or aphasia? (With early aphasia, suspect focal pathology.)

Ask about history of chronic medical or psychiatric disease, family psychiatric illness, drug or alcohol abuse, head injury, and exposure to toxins.

Physical Examination

Examine for the numerous medical causes of dementia (e.g., endocrine, heart, kidney, lung, liver, infection). Always perform a careful neurologic examination, and identify any focal CNS causes of dementia. Always test for sense of smell (first cranial nerve)—may identify a large unrecognized frontal lobe lesion. Always test hearing. Advanced diffuse disease displays ataxia, facial grimaces, agnosias, apraxias, motor impersistence, and/or perseveration and pathologic reflexes (grasp, snout, suck, glabella tap, tonic foot, etc.). Recognize that all types of physical illnesses occur more frequently in the demented patient (reasons for this are unclear). Survival time is reduced.

Laboratory Examination

Selected tests based on suspected etiology. Consider screening with ESR, CBC, STS, SMA-12, T_3 and T_4, vitamin B_{12} and folate assays, UA, chest radiograph, and CT or MRI scan. Other tests based on likely causes include drug levels, EEG (20% of all elderly have an abnormal EEG), LP (rarely), arteriography, HIV, and heavy metal screen, etc. The EEG is useful for identifying pathology in the usually silent CNS areas (frontal and temporal lobes)—investigate further if the dementia is mild, but the EEG is grossly abnormal.

Psychological Testing

These can (a) help identify a focal lesion, (b) provide a baseline, (c) help with the diagnosis, and (d) identify strengths to be used in planning treatment. Useful tests include the WAIS, Bender-Gestalt Test, the Luria test, and the Halstead and Reitan Batteries (very time consuming; do not use routinely). A brief but useful screening test is the Mini-Mental State Exam (2); numerous others exist. Patients with even mild dementia often will show impaired *constructional ability*; thus have them draw simple figures (e.g., a diamond, a cross, and a cube or the face of a clock set at a certain time—can be done on initial interview). Repeated drawings can be used to track the illness over time (3).

CAUSES: MAJOR TYPES OF DEMENTIAS

Dementia of the Alzheimer Type (AD) (DSM, p. 154, 294.xx)

Approximately 50%+ of all dementias (5% to 10% of people older than 65; 50% of those older than 85), but usually it is a diagnosis by exclusion. AD is the "classic cortical dementia." It is frequently overdiagnosed. Typically begins insidiously in the 50s (early onset, familial, presenile form—2% of cases) or later in the 60s to 80s (much more common late-onset form) and progresses to death in 6 to 10 years (4). Look initially for impaired recent memory, language problems, mild mood and personality changes, impaired problem solving. These all worsen over the next several years, becomes severe in 5+ years. Ceaseless pacing and a shuffling gait are common; social responses become simplistic but often remain intact until very late. Look for cortical atrophy and enlarged ventricles by MRI. The EEG is often normal for age early on but is a good screening test because it is often abnormal with reversible causes of dementia [except for general paresis and normal-pressure hydrocephalus (NPH)]. Histologically, senile plaques (degenerated nerve terminals surrounding a neurotoxic β-amyloid core), neurofibrillary tangles, and neuronal granulovacuolar degeneration are found. Recent evidence implicates primary degeneration of cholinergic neurons of the basal forebrain, particularly the nucleus basalis (although serotonergic and other neurons are increasingly being implicated—very heterogeneous).

An increased incidence is found in women (1.5:1; first-degree relatives threefold, particularly with presenile dementia), and Down syndrome. Moreover, a few *early-onset* familial cases (all autosomal dominant) have been related to the amyloid precursor protein gene (*APP* gene; increased production or deposition or both of amyloid β-protein over years or decades) on the portion of chromosome 21 near the region associated with Down syndrome. Other cases have been associated with chromosome 14 (presenilin 1 gene), and a third group, with the presenilin 2 gene on chromosome 1. Conversely, "normal" (98% of cases) *late-onset* AD has been associated with the apolipoprotein E type 4 (apoE4) allele on chromosome 19 (5) (heterozygote, 3x risk; homozygote, 10x risk; monozygotic twins, 50% concordance rate) and recently with the *A2M* gene on chromosome 12. Clearly, other genes are yet to be found for late-onset AD.

Perhaps 20% of dementias thought to be AD are really **Lewy body dementia** or Lewy body variant of AD (pathology of AD plus eosinophilic cytoplasmic "Lewy body" inclusions; cortical and subcortical symptoms, day-to-day cognitive fluctuations, visual hallucinations). A common, subsyndromal form of AD is *mild cognitive impairment* (a high percentage slowly develop into AD) (6).

Vascular Dementia (DSM, p. 158, 290.4x)

These are 10% to 20% of dementias (M:F = 2:1). Differentiate from AD by a history of rapid-onset and stepwise deterioration (can be difficult) in a patient in his 50s or early 60s and by the presence of focal neurologic impairment. EEG may show focal abnormalities. It is caused by multiple thromboembolic episodes (numerous small cerebral infarcts pathologically) in a patient with atherosclerotic disease of the major vessels or valvular disease of the heart. Hypertension is usually present. Pseudobulbar phenomena are common: emotional lability, dysarthria, and dysphagia. Controlling blood pressure may help slow progression. It is commonly found with AD pathology, and is comorbid with MDD in 50% to 60% of patients.

DEMENTIA DUE TO OTHER GENERAL MEDICAL CONDITIONS (DSM, P. 162, 294.1X)

Normal-pressure hydrocephalus: A "classic triad" of *gait ataxia*, *incontinence*, and *progressive dementia*—either idiopathic or after cerebral trauma, hemorrhage, or infection. Normal CSF pressure but dilated ventricles are seen on MRI. Treat with a lumboperitoneal or ventriculoatrial shunt; 55% show improvement.

Creutzfeldt–Jakob disease: Very rapid cognitive deterioration caused by infection by a *prion*. Spongiform changes in affected neurons. Marked extrapyramidal signs, jerks, rigidity, and ataxia. Death usually within 1 year.

Huntington chorea: This is a subcortical dementia; atrophy of the caudate nucleus. Psychiatric symptoms, ranging from neurotic to psychotic (including dementia), may precede the chorea. Dementia always occurs terminally. This disease is autosomal dominant (short arm of chromosome 4), so check family history.

Parkinson disease: Lesion in the basal ganglia (subcortical). Depression (40%) or dementia or both occur in 30% of patients. Severe apathy is common. Levodopa relieves temporarily only.

Brain tumors: Primarily metastatic tumors (from lung and breast) and meningiomas. Focal signs are usually present, except in frontal lobe. Get cerebrospinal fluid (CSF) pressure and protein, EEG, and MRI. EEG may be localizing.

Brain trauma: Cognitive impairment and memory loss usually improve over weeks after mild to moderate traumatic brain injury (TBI). The more severe the injury and longer the loss of consciousness (LOC of weeks $^+$), the more severe and chronic the dementia. Symptoms from a *subdural hematoma* that is treated quickly and aggressively usually disappear. Do not do an LP. Get CT or MRI.

Infection: Any significant infection [e.g., pneumonia, urinary tract infection (UTI)] can produce delirium and worsen a dementia in the elderly. Dementia can be caused by brain abscess, CNS syphilis (general paresis: serologic tests of blood and CSF usually positive), tuberculosis, and cryptococcal meningitis.

HIV-associated dementia: This is the most common dementia caused by an infection. Cognitive impairment may be the first symptom of HIV infection and, because HIV damages both cortical and subcortical tissue, depression from subcortical damage is common as well.

Metabolic disorders: Most common are thyroid disorders: *hypothyroidism* (dementia even with near-normal hormone levels; may be reversible; look for diffuse slowing on EEG) and also *hyperthyroidism* ("apathetic thyrotoxicosis," particularly in the elderly). Electrolyte imbalances are also common causes in the elderly (e.g., hypo- and hypernatremia and hypercalcemia). Suspect Wilson disease if signs of liver failure, tremor, rigidity, and convulsions are present in a person younger than 40. Also consider Cushing syndrome, hypoglycemia, and hyper- and hypoparathyroidism.

Disorders of heart, lung, liver, and kidney: Particularly congestive heart failure (CHF), arrhythmias, subacute bacterial endocarditis (SBE), chronic hypoxia and hypercapnia (e.g., emphysema), hepatic encephalopathy, uremia, and dialysis dementia.

Other: Malnutrition (particularly vitamin B_{12} and folate deficiencies—check for pernicious anemia and combined system disease), remote effects of carcinoma, systemic lupus erythematosus (SLE), epilepsy, progressive supranuclear palsy, spinocerebellar degenerations, parkinsonism–dementia complex of Guam, subacute sclerosing panendocarditis (SSPE), herpes simplex encephalitis, and multiple sclerosis (MS).

Substance-induced Persisting Dementia (DSM, p. 168)

This is a diagnosis by exclusion. It most commonly follows many years of heavy drinking or substance use/exposure and may be partly reversible with good nutrition and abstinence. The dementia may persist long after the absence of the substance. Possible causes include chronic sedative–hypnotic abuse, exposure to toxins like lead, mercury, solvents, carbon monoxide, and organophosphates, and medications like some anticonvulsants and antihypertensives.

DIFFERENTIAL DIAGNOSIS

Normal aging may mimic mild dementia, particularly if the patient is stressed by *environmental changes, social isolation, fatigue,* or *visual and hearing disorders* (sensory deprivation). Many elderly will develop mild *anxiety, depressive,* or *hypochondriac* disorders that mimic dementia, but with persistent questioning and encouragement, normal memory, orientation, etc., can be seen. Intellectual deterioration with schizophrenia is differentiated from dementia by a history of psychosis and social withdrawal and by the presence of a characteristic thought disorder. An Amytal interview may help distinguish dementia from *catatonic schizophrenia*. In *delirium,* an altered and fluctuating level of consciousness is noted. **Delirium and dementia frequently coexist; delirium usually must clear before the diagnosis of dementia can be made**.

A *major depression* is the most common cause of *pseudodementia*. Unlike the demented patient, these patients have a rapid recent onset (family can usually date it), *complain* of a severe memory loss (usually mild when tested), have marked affective changes, emphasize their inabilities and failings, and frequently answer simple questions with "I don't know" (the demented patient usually attempts an answer). A temporary clearing during an interview and the lack of a deteriorating course helps identify these patients. Consider a DST and MRI. These patients usually improve with antidepressants or electroconvulsive therapy (ECT). Do not mistake an aphasia due to a focal lesion for a dementia (although perhaps 10% of severely demented patients have a related aphasia).

TREATMENT

Supportive Treatment

- Provide good physical care [e.g., good nutrition, eye glasses, hearing aids, protection (e.g., stairs, stoves, medication)], and so on. Physical restraint is necessary at times.
- Keep in familiar settings, if possible. Surround with familiar objects; keep old friends engaged. Encourage the family's participation and understanding.
- Keep the patient involved—through personal contact, frequent orientation (remind them of the day, of the time). Discuss the news. Use calendars, radio, television. Structure daily activities—make them predictable.
- Help maintain patient's self-esteem. Treat him like an adult. Plan toward his strengths. Be accepting, tolerant.
- Avoid dark, isolated settings; avoid overstimulation.

Symptomatic Treatment

Psychiatric conditions may require *small* doses of appropriate medication.
- Severe anxiety, psychosis, aggression, agitation: for example, haloperidol, 0.5 mg p.o. t.i.d.; risperidone, 0.5 to 2.0 mg p.o. daily; quetiapine, 25 to 100 mg p.o. daily (7)
- Nonpsychotic anxiety, agitation, insomnia: usually avoid benzodiazepines; consider low-dose trazodone for sleep and very low-dose haloperidol or an atypical antipsychotic for agitation. If a benzodiazepine is necessary, use a short-acting one such as lorazepam or oxazepam.
- Depression: Selective serotonin reuptake inhibitors (SSRIs) and other new antidepressants are the antidepressants of choice (8). Avoid tricyclic antidepressants (TCAs) because of their anticholinergic effects.

Specific Treatment

- Identify and correct any treatable condition.
- Both the cognitive and behavioral deficits of dementia, AD, and several other forms are believed to be due to a decrease in CNS acetylcholine (ACh) secondary to the destruction of cholinergic neurons. The goal of the most-effective medications currently

available that reverse the symptoms of dementia is to increase the amount of synaptic ACh. This is done by inhibiting the enzyme (acetylcholinesterase) that hydrolyzes ACh. Four cholinesterase inhibitors are available; all are moderately effective in mild to moderate dementia and seem to work for many months or a year or two. In spite of contrary early research findings, none is specific for particular dementias. Three are almost free of side effects: some nausea, vomiting, diarrhea, flushing, sweating. **Tacrine** (Cognex) is not recommended because of hepatotoxicity and alanine aminotransferase (ALT) elevations. **Donepezil** (Aricept) is widely used, taken once daily, 5 to 10 mg daily. **Rivastigmine** (Exelon) is taken b.i.d., 6 to 12 mg daily. **Galantamine** (Razadyne) is taken at 24 mg daily, but several recent studies have raised the question that it possibly has a slight tendency to promote cardiovascular mortality.

A new medication, **memantine** (Namenda), seems to be safe and effective and to work through a different mechanism; it blocks abnormal glutamate activity found in dementia, permitting glutamate to exercise its normal beneficial effect on learning and memory. This is the only medication approved for moderate to severe AD and has been used to date beneficially with donepezil. The target dose is 20 mg daily, but increase slowly. A number of other substances are being tried for dementia (e.g., vitamin E, selegiline, estrogens, ginkgo), but none has found a place in the routine treatment of dementia.

REFERENCES

1. Corey-Bloom J, Thal LJ, Galasko D, et al. Diagnosis and evaluation of dementia. *Neurology* 1995;45:211–218.
2. Folstein MF, Folstein SE, McHugh PR. Mini-Mental State: a practical method for grading the mental state of patients for the clinician. *J Psychiatry Res* 1975;12:189–198.
3. Rouleau I, Salmon DP, Butters N. Longitudinal analysis of clock drawing in Alzheimer's disease patients. *Brain Cogn* 1996;31:17–34.
4. Stern RG, Mohs RC, Davidson M, et al. A longitudinal study of Alzheimer's disease. *Am J Psychiatry* 1994;151:390–396.
5. Evans DA, Beckett LA, Field TS, et al. Apolipoprotein Ee4 and incidence of Alzheimer disease in a community population of older persons. *JAMA* 1997;277:822–824.
6. Palmer K, Fratiglioni L, Winblad B. What is mild cognitive impairment? Variations in definitions and evolutions of nondemented persons with cognitive impairment. *Acta Neurol Scand Suppl* 2003;179:14–20.

7. Takahashi H, Yoshida K, Sugita T, et al. Quetiapine treatment of psychotic symptoms and aggressive behavior in patients with dementia with Lewy bodies: a case series. *Prog Neuropharmacol Biol Psychiatry* 2003;27:549–553.
8. Lyketsos CG, DelCampo L, Steinberg M, et al. Treating depression in Alzheimer disease: efficacy and safety of sertraline therapy, and the benefits of depression reduction: the DIADS. *Arch Gen Psychiatry* 2003;60:737–746.

Suicidal and Assaultive Behaviors

THE SUICIDAL PATIENT

Epidemiology

- Reported suicides in the United States number 31,000 per year (12 per 100,000; 300,000 attempts annually).
- Suicide is underreported and often is listed as accidental.
- The attempted suicide/successful suicide ratio is 10 to 20:1.
- Suicide increases with age; it is the third leading cause of death in male adolescents and college students.
- The ratio of completers is 3:1 (M/F); that of attempters is 3:1 (F/M).
- The most common attempt is by drug ingestion; most likely to be fatal is by shooting.
- Most patients are *not* psychotic or incompetent; most *are* depressed.

All clinicians will encounter suicidal patients. Many will not recognize them. Some of those patients will kill themselves.

Identifying the Potentially Suicidal Patient

One fifth of suicides are unanticipated. Accurate prediction is difficult, if not impossible, with present knowledge. Entertain the possibility when (1)

1. The patient has made a suicide attempt [seen in the emergency department (ED), medical ward, etc.];
2. The patient makes overt or indirect suicide talk or threats: "You won't be bothered by me much longer" (most often made to family members);
3. The patient is in a depressed or anxious mood due to an observable depression;
4. The patient has experienced a significant recent loss (e.g., spouse, job, self-esteem);
5. The patient demonstrates an unexpected change in behavior: making a will, intense talks with friends, giving away possessions;

6. The patient shows an unexpected change in attitude: suddenly cheerful, angry, or withdrawn.

Assessing Suicidal Risk

■ Assessment Procedure

First, build rapport during a supportive nonjudgmental interview. If they are not volunteered, investigate suicidal thoughts by asking questions of increasing specificity (e.g., "Have you been feeling sad?" "Have you thought of doing away with yourself?" "How?"). Asking about suicide does not precipitate it. After a serious attempt, wait until the patient is alert enough to cooperate. Always ask about suicidality during a psychiatric assessment.

The following must be learned about *all* suicidal patients:

1. The patient's intention: Why does he or she want to die?
2. Is a suicide plan made? The more specific the plan, the more likely the act.
3. Method: The more lethal the technique, the more serious the plan.
4. Presence of psychiatric or organic factors (e.g., psychotic depression, thought disorder, sedative self-medication, organicity).
5. Determine the role of impulsivity versus premeditation.
6. Is the precipitating crisis resolving?
7. Take an "inventory of loss."
8. Does the patient have plans for the future?
9. Does the patient have caring family or other supports?
10. Does the patient think she or he is going to commit suicide?

■ Population Risk Factors

- Males
- Elderly
- Isolated individuals
- Whites
- American Indians
- Policemen

■ Individual Risk Factors

- Sense of **hopelessness** [*particularly* in a patient with major depression (2)], helplessness, loneliness, exhaustion, "unbearable" psychological pain.

- Psychiatric illness (3) (in 90% of suicide patients), mainly:
  1. **Major mood disorder** (either first or second degree; 50% of all suicides), particularly with vegetative signs or constriction of thought; 15% lifetime suicide risk.
  2. **Alcoholism** (suicide rate 50 times normal; 25% of all suicides) mostly those with chronic alcoholism, mostly men, often after interpersonal loss, 3% to 4% lifetime risk. Much higher if they also are depressed and with poor social supports (i.e., many patients). Drug addiction (10% die by suicide).
  3. **Schizophrenia**, particularly when lonely, depressed, with chronic illness, or with persecutory delusions or self-destructive command hallucinations; 10% or more lifetime risk.
  4. Other: Psychoses due to organic conditions; personality disorders (borderline, antisocial), *panic disorder* with comorbid depression.
- Failing health, particularly if previously independent (5% of all suicides); chronic medical impairment; HIV/AIDS.
- Intoxication; active use (abuse) of *alcohol* and other drugs.
- Impaired impulse control for any reason; hostility.
- **History of suicide attempts**, particularly serious attempts.
- Nature of past or present suicide attempts (e.g., shooting or jumping more lethal than most ingestions or wrist cutting. Warning given? Help available at the time?
- Family history of suicide; personal exposure to suicide; suicide itself may run in families genetically.
- Widowed, divorced, separated, *single, unemployed,* retired.
- Medical patients receiving renal dialysis.
- Family stresses or instability; few external supports.
- A change in status—*up* or down.
- Recent loss or rejection.
- Parental loss during childhood.

■ **Other Risk Factors**

- Holidays, spring, anniversaries.
- Possible biochemical measures of suicide potential (4): *decreased CSF 5-HIAA* (4) and HVA and increased MHPG; decreased urine NE/E ratio; increased adrenal weight; positive DST.

Initiating Appropriate Treatment

The first question often is "Should you hospitalize?" If the patient has pressing suicidal thoughts or decreased impulse control or both coupled with several risk factors, hospitalize, if only overnight. Be conservative. Do not write off patients as "just manipulative"—all statements of suicide intent initially should be taken seriously (particularly from adolescents). Manipulative suicide patients (parasuicide) have "accidentally" killed themselves after being denied admission—60% of successful suicides have had previous suicide attempts. The most emotionally upset patient is not necessarily the most suicidal. The suicidal state is episodic; a patient may be "safe" just hours after a serious suicide attempt. Be very cautious of the patient who has trouble considering any alternative to suicide.

The decision *to* hospitalize should be communicated to the patient decisively but optimistically. Hospitalization should be involuntary if necessary. Ensure the patient's physical safety in the hospital through appropriate "suicide precautions" (e.g., close supervision, no isolation, no dangerous objects).

A patient of lesser risk may be followed up as an outpatient if a reliable family member is able to help with monitoring—assess that support. If the patient is *not* to be hospitalized, specific plans for follow-up must be made with the patient. Be absolutely clear about this with him or her.

Treatment Principles

1. Identify and treat psychiatric or medical conditions. Treat depression vigorously. Treat psychotic depressions with an antidepressant *and* antipsychotic. If the patient is determinedly suicidal, use electroconvulsive therapy (ECT) rather than wait for a medication response. Antipsychotics and benzodiazepines may be briefly useful with the agitated patient.
2. Develop a therapeutic alliance with the patient. Be concerned and accepting. Attempt to understand why the patient wants to die. Allow the patient to express anger, "unacceptable" thoughts, and feelings of rejection and hopelessness. These patients often feel misunderstood and trapped but unable to ask for help. Reduce the psychological pain any way you can.
3. Suicidal patients are usually *ambivalent about death* and may not know why they are trying to kill themselves. Point out that ambivalence to them—show them evidence of their desire to live. Be hopeful. Be definite. Make specific plans with and for the patient. Appeal to his or her mature rather than regressive side.
4. The patients are often bewildered and have a narrowed focus of thought—deal with reality issues.
5. Do not minimize the seriousness of a suicide attempt to the patient.

6. Never agree to hold a suicide plan in confidence.
7. Help the patient to grieve over losses.
8. Do not explain away the patient's symptoms (e.g., "I'd feel the same way myself").
9. Suicide potential can change rapidly. Reassess the patient's state of mind frequently.
10. Use community resources. Involve the family and significant others in treatment; use family therapy when appropriate. Actively try to reduce social isolation and withdrawal. Help make changes in the patient's environment where it is pathologic.
11. Many suicides in depressives occur during the first 3 to 6 months after hospital discharge. *Do not lose contact* with the patient. Monitor closely during holidays.
12. Be active, but insist that the patient ultimately take responsibility for his or her own life.
13. Tricyclics, monoamine oxidase inhibitors, and many sedative–hypnotics have serious overdose potential. Some depressed outpatients store medication, so track drugs prescribed. If an antidepressant is required, use a newer safer one.

Theoretic explanations of suicide include the loss of a sense of identity with the social group (Durkheim), hostility turned against the self (Freud), a "cry for help," and a reflection of biologic psychiatric conditions.

THE VIOLENT PATIENT

Human aggression has complex and uncertain biologic, psychosocial, and cultural roots. Implicated in violent behavior are lesions of the prefrontal cortex (frontal lobe syndrome) and stimulation of the amygdala and limbic system (5). Also present may be decreased cerebrospinal fluid (CSF) serotonin (similar to "violent" suicide) and possibly elevated androgens and CSF norepinephrine or decreased γ-aminobutyric acid (GABA) (6,7).

Prediction of violence is difficult. Anyone can become violent, yet some *groups* are at risk: young males aged 15 to 25; urban, black, and/or violent cultural subgroups; and alcoholics. Key *individual* predictors of violent behavior include the following:

1. A history of violence;
2. Active use of alcohol;
3. Physical abuse as a child;
4. Some form of brain injury.

Mental Disorders with Associated Violent Behavior

Although most mentally ill are not dangerous, some patients present an increased risk. (Note: Serious medical illness can first appear with violent behavior.)

1. Organic brain syndromes, particularly with confusion or decreased impulse control (e.g., the demented, drugs in the elderly, hypoglycemia, CNS infections, anoxia, metabolic acidosis).
2. Alcohol and drug abuse, particularly with intoxication, delirium, or delusional states of ETOH, amphetamines, cocaine, or phencyclidine (PCP); also with intoxication from inhalants or "downers" or with prolonged use of high-dose anabolic steroids.
3. Schizophrenia, paranoid and undifferentiated types, particularly with command hallucinations or in patients who drink.
4. Mania; acute psychotic states of any origin, particularly if comorbid with substance abuse.
5. Certain mentally retarded; XYY karyotype (possibly), and others.
6. Personality disorders, most likely antisocial and borderline types.
7. Severe attention deficit disorder with hyperactivity, in adults; post-traumatic stress disorder (PTSD) patients (occasionally).

Several Recognizable Patterns of Violence

1. **Chronic, aggressive, self-aggrandizing lifestyle**: Seen with **ANTISOCIAL PERSONALITY DISORDER** and thus associated with drug and alcohol abuse, onset in youth, delinquency and adult crime, truancy, and school failure. Patients fight frequently and are "constantly in trouble." Serious affective disorders are common in this population.
2. **Episodic violence**: Explosive rages with little provocation, daily to several times a year; brief occasional amnesia for the event and remorse about it. A mixed group of clinical presentations; CNS abnormalities in most. If violence is *directed*, consider

   • **INTERMITTENT EXPLOSIVE DISORDER** (DSM, p. 663, 312.34): usually in males with history of violent outbursts and numerous axis I problems, including mood disorders (8,9), family history of violence, neurologic soft signs, abnormal EEGs. Normal between episodes.

- **PERSONALITY CHANGE DUE TO A GENERAL MEDICAL CONDITION, Disinhibited Type** (DSM, p. 187, 310.1): neurologic origin [encephalitis, epilepsy, multiple sclerosis (MS), tumor, poststroke, etc.], disturbed personality between episodes.
- Rages in borderline or histrionic personality disorders, particularly when intoxicated.

If violence is *poorly directed*, consider temporal lobe epilepsy (get NP leads), alcohol idiosyncratic intoxication, or other neurologic syndromes.

Evaluating Threats of Violence

Take all ideas or threats of violence seriously. Assess risk factors. What is the patient's current mental state? Can he or she control impulses and rage? Does the patient feel under great tension and fear losing control? Is there an intended victim? Is the victim covertly provoking the attack? Are specific plans made? Are sadistic fantasies present? Are weapons available? Is the patient armed (always check)? Is a family support system present?

Management of the Acutely Violent Patient

1. First decide whether the patient is out of control. If so, treat immediately with restraint and medication, not talk. See immediately; do not keep him or her waiting.
2. Approach an unfamiliar patient cautiously and from a position of strength (help available, open door). Be alert to warning signs (e.g., restless, demanding). If talking appears useful, try, but set clear limits during interview. Use physical controls if the patient cannot maintain control, but emphasize their temporary helping nature. If the patient arrives in restraints, *do not remove* until rapport is established and some evaluation is done; however, many patients do better without restraints. Restraints may increase agitation and cause hyperthermia. If force is needed to subdue, use overwhelming force—one person to each limb. Do not take chances.
3. Medication for most acutely agitated patients: *lorazepam*, 1 to 2 mg i.m. (well absorbed) or p.o. q2–4 h, maximum of three doses, and/or *haloperidol*, 5 mg i.m. hourly for three to four doses; droperidol, 2.5 mg i.m./i.v. q3–4 h, two to three doses (not approved by the FDA for that purpose, however) (10); olanzapine, 5 mg p.o./i.m. q3–4 h; or ziprasidone, 20 mg

p.o./i.m. q3–4 h. Has patient taken CNS depressants, is he or she delirious, or is a medical condition responsible for behavior? If so, hold medications and observe. Electroconvulsive therapy (ECT) can control psychotic violence.

4. If patient is threatening and agitated but not wild, treat with respect—be civil, direct, confident, calm, reassuring. Do not challenge, provoke, or openly disagree with the patient. Eliminate red tape. *Always* explain what you are doing, and why. Violent patients are often frightened—find out why and of what.

5. Determine etiology of violence. Is a mental illness present? A brain injury? Are drugs involved (get urine screen)? Are identifiable environmental precipitants present? Expect to intervene directly with the psychotic patient.

6. Most patients can be "talked down" with support and understanding (and medication); however, hospitalize involuntarily if necessary. Is this really a criminal matter, and should the police be involved instead?

Ongoing Care

1. The chronically violent patient should receive medication trials. Treat psychosis with antipsychotics, and seizures with anticonvulsants. For continued aggression, consider the following (11,12).

   - Haloperidol (decanoate), risperidone, or clozapine.
   - SSRIs [e.g., fluoxetine, 10 to 20 mg (13)] for a wide variety of conditions; buspirone (head injury, mental retardation).
   - Propranolol (20 mg t.i.d., divided doses; slowly increase to 600 mg if needed), nadolol (up to 120 mg/day), or pindolol; may take 4 to 6 weeks for effect.
   - Carbamazepine (600 to 1,200 mg/day, divided doses), valproic acid, and lithium (blood level, 0.6 to 1.2 mEq/L) *may* be useful in violent patients with bipolar disorder, schizophrenia, mental retardation, intermittent explosive disorder; consider stimulants in hyperactive adults.
   - Benzodiazepines can be useful during times of stress, but paradoxic rages occur in some patients.

2. Teach the patient to recognize early signs of increasing anger and to develop ways to discharge tension. The severely brain damaged may need a structured environment and behavioral techniques.

3. Help the patient develop a support system and learn to control environmental stresses. Maintain a channel of communication with the potentially violent patient—be available by phone. You also have some legal responsibility.

REFERENCES

1. Bryan CJ, Rudd MD. Advances in the assessment of suicide risk. *J Clin Psychol* 2006;62:185–200.
2. Mendonca JD, Holden RR. Are all suicidal ideas closely linked to hopelessness? *Acta Psychiatry Scand* 1996;93:246–251.
3. Beautrais AL, Joyce PR, Mulder RT, et al. Prevalence and comorbidity of mental disorders in persons making serious suicide attempts. *Am J Psychiatry* 1996;153:1009–1014.
4. Franke L, Uebelhack R, Muller-Oerlinghausen B. Low CSF 5-HIAA level in high-lethality suicide attempters: fact or artifact? *Biol Psychiatry* 2002;52:375–376.
5. Krakowski M. Neurologic and neuropsychologic correlates of violence. *Psychiatr Ann* 1997;674–678.
6. Niehoff D. *The Biology of Violence*. New York: The Free Press, 2002.
7. Volavka J. *Neurobiology of Violence*. Washington, DC: American Psychiatric Press, 2002.
8. Coccaro EF, Kavoussi RJ, Berman ME, et al. Intermittent explosive disorder; revised: development, reliability, and validity of research criteria. *Comp Psychiatry* 1998;39:368–376.
9. McElroy SL, Soutullo CA, Beckman DA, et al. DSM-IV intermittent explosive disorder: a report of 27 cases. *J Clin Psychiatry* 1998;59:203–210.
10. Shale JH, Shale CM, Mastin WD. A review of the safety and efficacy of droperidol for the rapid sedation of severely agitated and violent patients. *J Clin Psychiatry* 2003;64:500–505.
11. Citrome L, Volavka J. Psychopharmacology of violence, part II. *Psychiatr Ann* 1997;27:696–703.
12. Ratey JJ, Gordon A. The psychopharmacology of aggression. *Psychopharmacol Bull* 1993;29:65–73.
13. New AS, Buchsbaum MS, Hazlett EA, et al. Fluoxetine increases relative metabolic rate in prefrontal cortex in impulsive aggression. *Psychopharmacology* (Berl) 2004;176:451–458.

Anxiety Disorders

Anxiety is ubiquitous; anxiety disorders are not. *Anxiety* is an unpleasant and unjustified sense of apprehension often accompanied by physiologic symptoms, whereas *anxiety disorder* connotes significant distress and dysfunction due to the anxiety. An anxiety disorder may be characterized by only anxiety, or it may display another symptom such as a phobia or an obsession, and show anxiety when the primary symptom is resisted. *Fear* also is universal and can produce the symptom picture of acute anxiety states, yet, in contrast to anxiety, the cause is obvious and understandable. A feature common to all of the anxiety disorders is the unpleasant and unnatural quality of the symptoms (anxiety, phobia, obsession)—they are *ego-alien* or *ego-dystonic*. These tend to be chronic, relapsing conditions: be alert for suicide.

Anxiety is mediated through a complex system that involves (at least) the limbic system (amygdala, hippocampus), thalamus, and frontal cortex anatomically and norepinephrine (locus ceruleus), serotonin (dorsal raphe nucleus), and γ-aminobutyric acid (GABA; $GABA_A$ receptor coupled with the benzodiazepine receptor) neurochemically. We do not yet know how these parts work.

CHRONIC, MILD ANXIETY

Tension, irritability, apprehension, and mild distractibility are common (particularly in medical and psychiatric patients), often related to environmental factors, and treated with supportive and reality-oriented therapy. Medications are of little value over the long term, and iatrogenic addiction is a serious problem. Environmentally induced, short-lived, mild anxiety (**ADJUSTMENT DISORDER WITH ANXIETY** p. 679, 309.24) usually resolves with the disappearance of the stress.

CHRONIC, MODERATELY SEVERE ANXIETY

A diagnosis of **GENERALIZED ANXIETY DISORDER** (p. 472, 300.02) is made with more severe, chronic anxiety (longer than 6 months; usually years, but waxing and waning) and including symptoms such as autonomic responses (palpitations, diarrhea, cold clammy extremities, sweating, urinary frequency), insomnia, poor concentration, fatigue, sighing, trembling, hypervigilance, marked apprehension, or a combination of these. It tends to run in families, has a moderate genetic component, prevalence of 3% and lifetime prevalence of 5%, and is associated with simple and social phobias and with major depression (50%[+] of patients at some time; elevated risk for suicide) (1). Usually no convincing etiologic stress is found, but look anyway.

Consider both medication and psychotherapy. The antidepressant, venlafaxine, seems to be particularly effective and safe for treating generalized anxiety disorder (GAD) (2). Also consider selective serotonin reuptake inhibitors (SSRIs) as a first-line treatment. Use benzodiazepines sparingly (diazepam, 5 mg, p.o., t.i.d.–q.i.d., or 10 mg hs) and for short periods (weeks to several months); allow medication use to follow the fluctuating course of the illness. Consider buspirone for a first medication or for long-term use (20 to 30 mg/day; divided doses); a patient may not find it effective after the "instant relief" of a benzodiazepine. Tricyclic antidepressants and monoamine oxidase inhibitors (MAOIs) are useful in selected patients (particularly those who have depressive symptoms), whereas some patients with autonomic symptoms improve with β-blockers (e.g., propranolol, 80 to 160 mg/day).

Encourage self-reliance, maintenance of productive activity, and reality-based cognitions. Train the patient in relaxation techniques (e.g., biofeedback, meditation, self-hypnosis). More than 50% of patients become asymptomatic with time (months, years), but the rest retain a significant degree of impairment. It is common in old age. Help the patient understand the chronic nature of the illness and the likelihood of having to live with some symptoms (3).

ACUTE ANXIETY: PANIC ATTACKS

A **PANIC DISORDER WITHOUT AGORAPHOBIA** (p. 433, 300.01) has dramatic, acute symptoms lasting minutes to hours, is self-limited, and occurs in patients with or without chronic anxiety. Symptoms often are perceived by the patient as medical and are characteristic of strong autonomic discharge—hyperventilation, heart pounding, chest pains, trembling, choking, abdominal pain, sweating, dizziness—as well as disorganization, confusion, dread, and often a sense of impending doom, terror, or death. Attacks may come "out of the blue," usually in young adults, or may be initiated by crowds, stressful situations, or anticipation ("anticipatory anxiety"). They may be repeated several times daily, weekly, or monthly, and wax and wane, often disappearing for months at a time (but may become chronic; 20% of patients). A typical panic attack can be produced in 50% to 75% of patients with panic disorder (but not in normal patients) by the intravenous infusion of sodium lactate or by breathing CO_2. (Panic patients seem to be hypersensitive to a sense of breathlessness, whether chemically or environmentally produced.)

Like other anxiety conditions, it runs in families (15%+ of first-degree relatives; 30%+ of monozygotic twins), is probably genetic, but no linkage to a particular gene has been found. It is comorbid with *major depression* (50%), suicide, social and specific phobias, and alcoholism (however, family members are at risk only for panic disorder and social phobia). It occurs in women more frequently than in men (2:1), particularly in those who have had a disturbed childhood and early difficulty separating from their parents (separation anxiety disorder). In its milder forms, panic disorder tends to grade into the GAD clinically, although it appears to be a distinct disorder. Etiology is unclear, but an overactive locus coeruleus with excessive norepinephrine (NE) in panic attacks is often involved. In addition, the majority of patients with panic also have agoraphobia (**PANIC DISORDER WITH AGORAPHOBIA**, p. 433, 300.21; see later): combined, these conditions afflict about 3% of the population. Patients often receive the "million dollar workup" for angina, thyrotoxicosis, or abdominal complaints. Hyper- and hypothyroidism and stimulant drug abuse may initiate a first panic attack. Effective treatment exists.

1. Medication is essential for panic disorder. Several effective drugs are available, although response to any one is unpredictable. Some patients respond to initial doses of medication with dysphoria or marked jitteriness, so *always start slowly*. Likewise, discontinue slowly. Consider:
   a. SSRIs, but also other serotonergic drugs such as clomipramine (4).
   b. Tricyclic antidepressants (e.g., imipramine or desipramine, 150 to 300 mg/day); expect 2 to 3 weeks for response.

c. Benzodiazepines [e.g., clonazepam (1 to 5 mg/day, b.i.d.); sedative but useful; alprazolam (0.5 to 2 mg/day, t.i.d.–q.i.d.) (patients respond rapidly, but depression, potential addiction, and need for frequent doses can be problems)].

d. MAOIs (particularly phenelzine, 30 to 75$^+$ mg/day); effective with a broad spectrum of patients but may take 4 to 6 weeks for a response.

e. Other medications occasionally effective include venlafaxine (200 to 450$^+$ mg), β-blockers (propranolol), and possibly carbamazepine (400 to 1,200 mg/d) or valproate (500 to 3,000 mg/d).

A valuable approach is to combine a benzodiazepine (e.g., clonazepam) with either an SSRI or a TCA initially, and then discontinue the benzodiazepine over a 3- to 4-week period. Typical practice is to maintain medications for 6 months after improvement, and then slowly discontinue. Unfortunately, the relapse rate is high: "half-dose" maintenance may work better.

2. Cognitive–behavioral therapy *should* be coupled with medication (see discussion under "agoraphobia") (5). Supportive psychotherapy is of use in the short term but does not correct the condition or prevent relapses.

ANXIETY WITH SPECIFIC FEARS: PHOBIC DISORDERS

Phobias are fears that are persistent and intense, are out of proportion to the stimulus, make little sense even to the sufferer, lead to avoidance of the feared object or situation, and when sufficiently distressful or disabling are termed a *phobic disorder*. Common, mild, frequently transient fears (of the dark, heights, snakes) receive no diagnosis. Phobias may wax and wane over months or years and may disappear spontaneously, but serious cases may continue for decades and gradually take the form of a depressive disorder. The fears may generalize during their developing stages (e.g., fear of a store generalizes to the street in front of the store and then to the entire shopping area).

More than 12% of the population may have a phobic disorder in some circumstances, yet in fewer than 1% is it significantly disabling. Many begin suddenly in women (F/M, 2:1) from stable families and of ages 15 to 30 years. Anxiety with ruminations may dominate the day-to-day picture, or anxiety may occur only when the phobic object is encountered directly. Relief occurs with escape, thus reinforcing the avoidance pattern—a vicious cycle.

Phobics are at risk to abuse alcohol and drugs as self-medication. Three subtypes have been identified, all of which have a moderate genetic component:

1. AGORAPHOBIA WITHOUT HISTORY OF PANIC DISORDER (p. 441, 300.22): Multiple phobias with chronic anxiety: specifically fears of open and/or closed spaces, crowded places, being trapped (in crowds or waiting in line), being away from home, being in unfamiliar places, being alone, and, more generally, of a loss of a sense of security. Many other fears and hypochondriacal concerns may be present, as well as multiple other symptoms including fainting, obsessional thoughts, depersonalization (feel unreal, detached), and derealization (feel surroundings are unreal). Depression is common. This is the most disabling phobic disorder.

This may actually be a subset of panic disorder, because *most* patients with agoraphobia also have panic attacks:

PANIC DISORDER WITH AGORAPHOBIA. Typically, in these combined patients, the agoraphobia develops as an extension of a panic disorder [i.e., unpredictable *panic attacks* cause them to avoid public places for fear of having an attack (*anticipatory anxiety*), which then reinforces the behavior (*phobic avoidance*)]. This is even more disabling than agoraphobia alone. It most commonly develops during the 20s, with a F/M ratio of 2:1. Genetics are similar to panic disorder (10%+ of first-degree relatives are similarly affected). Fix the panic, and often (with help) the agoraphobia will disappear.

2. SOCIAL PHOBIA (p. 450, 300.23): Fear of scrutiny from others during public speaking, while using public lavatories, during blushing, eating in public, etc. Typically begins during adolescence and is found in 2% to 4% of the population (F/M, 2:1). Some patients are troubled by *specific* and limited social activities while others suffer from *generalized* social exposure. Marked general anxiety is common in severe cases: patient controls by avoidance, which can be socially crippling. It is frequently associated with substance abuse and depression, but do not mistake it for the social withdrawal of primary depression, schizophrenia, or paranoid states; if symptoms have been present lifelong, consider Avoidant Personality Disorder.

3. SPECIFIC PHOBIAS (p. 443, 300.29): Monophobias of animals, storms, heights, blood, needles, etc. These usually begin in adolescence, are found in 10%+ of the population (more frequent among women; 2:1), and have few associated symptoms or syndromes.

Treatment: twofold

1. Cognitive–behavior therapy is essential in all three types of phobias (6). The key to treatment is *exposure* to the feared object or situation coupled with a reversing of the fearful expectations ("cognitions") about the upcoming encounter. *Cognitive restructuring* helps patients to reassess the troublesome events that precipitate panic. *Systematic desensitization* (by reciprocal inhibition) uses a graded hierarchy of frightening stimuli, allowing the patient to "work up" to facing the phobic object. In *flooding*, the patient faces the feared object or situation directly, whereas with *implosion*, the exposure is to the idea of the object or a vivid account of the "terrible" consequences expected. Social-skills training may also be required for those who are socially inept. Such treatment may require (and be enhanced by) support or antianxiety medication or both. Early evidence suggests that exposure is most effective at decreasing agoraphobia but not panic attacks, whereas cognitive therapy works primarily on the panic attacks.

2. Medication: Minor tranquilizers are used temporarily to help the patient confront the phobia. In social phobias, SSRIs are effective with generalized social phobias (7), as is gabapentin (900 to 3,000 mg/day), whereas β-blockers [1] (e.g., propranolol, atenolol) can be used to help control incapacitating autonomic symptoms (e.g., before a speech or a piano concert) if the symptoms are specific.

In the agoraphobic, with or without panic attacks, use medication for panic disorder (SSRIs, TCAs, SNRIs, benzodiazepines). Once the panic attacks are controlled with medications, an agoraphobic usually needs supportive exposure to the feared situations (without experiencing panic) before the phobia resolves. "Half-dose" maintenance medications may be necessary as well. Medication has not yet been proven useful in specific phobias.

POSTTRAUMATIC STRESS DISORDER (P. 463, 309.81)

If a patient has a severe loss or stress (e.g., rape, serious car accident, harm to a child or spouse, natural disaster, combat, prison camp), the clinical syndrome of **POSTTRAUMATIC STRESS DISORDER** (8) may develop. A mixture of the following symptoms are present initially; usually folded within the three categories of

(a) reexperiencing the event, (b) avoiding event-related cues and psychological numbing, and (c) emotional arousal (9):

Marked anxiety

Personality change with irritability and poor concentration

An exaggerated startle response

Insomnia and nightmares

Intrusive thoughts of the event

Reliving the feelings experienced at the time

Avoidance of anything associated with the trauma

Emotional blunting, which can impair interpersonal relationships and day-to-day functioning

Later, depression, emotional numbing, and preoccupation with the trauma may predominate. The more severe the stress, the more likely PTSD is (a) to develop and (b) to be long-lasting. It may resolve after months (*acute*, lasts 1 to 3 months) or, untreated, last for decades (*chronic*, 3 months). Occasional patients are first seen primarily with physical symptoms or chronic pain. Comorbid psychiatric conditions include depression, OCD, anxiety and panic disorders, dissociative states, and substance abuse.

Patients in whom PTSD develops are more likely to have a personality disorder, a history of depression and/or earlier trauma and/or substance abuse, a childhood history of physical abuse, or a family history of psychopathology, but presumably PTSD can occur in anyone who has experienced sufficient stress (found in 1% to 9% of the general population; slightly higher in women; 20% with severe stress). Psychophysiologic arousal at the time of the stress seems to be important in developing PTSD, whereas conditioned arousal keeps it going.

PTSD patients are often noncompliant: as many as 70% to 80%+ drop out of treatment, partly because they cannot tolerate reliving the event in therapy. Medication is useful in some cases: primarily SSRIs of any kind as first choice, and then TCAs (e.g., imipramine, 150 to 300 mg/day). Augmentation can be done by using a variety of medications: carbamazepine perhaps is useful in controlling flashbacks, nightmares, and intrusive recollections (400 to 600 mg/day; 5 to 10 g/ml); propranolol (80 to 160 mg/day) to reduce sympathetic hyperarousal; clonidine (0.2 to 0.4 mg/day) for treating symptoms of hyperarousal and reexperiencing (10); lithium; valproate for intrusion and hyperarousal; lamotrigine; buspirone; or cyproheptadine (nightmares?). Psychotherapy should accompany medication: primarily exposure therapy, but also education, support, and cognitive–behavioral therapy. The rape victim needs special and sensitive care—often in the emergency department (ED)—after the assault, for psychiatric as well as legal reasons. Many of her interpersonal relationships may have been altered by that episode. Work with the family; the married victim often needs to establish a new equilibrium with her partner.]

ACUTE STRESS DISORDER (P. 469, 308.3)

Acute Stress Disorder (ASD) is an expected reaction of anyone experiencing an adequately severe trauma, yet individuals require different amounts and types of stress to develop it. PTSD symptoms predominate: nightmares, reexperiencing the event, avoiding stimuli that remind one of the trauma, and symptoms of increased arousal, such as irritability, hypervigilance, poor concentration, and marked startle response. In addition, patients may respond for several days with derealization, depersonalization, and as though they are in a daze.

Typically, ASD will disappear after 1 to 2 weeks (if that long), but if it lasts for longer than 1 month, the diagnosis must be changed to PTSD. The most useful therapy is to get the patient to come to terms with his acute stressor as soon as possible by having him "talk it through" and realize that life can return (and is returning) to normal. Sometimes it is necessary to use benzodiazepines briefly to facilitate this process. Failure to put the trauma into perspective and get on with life all too often results in the development of PTSD.

ANXIETY DISORDER DUE TO A GENERAL MEDICAL CONDITION (P. 476, 293.84)

Medical conditions (most commonly cardiac disorders) can produce anxiety states, although often they generate no sense of apprehension or foreboding. If suggestive physical symptoms accompany anxiety, remember the following:

1. Abnormal ECGs and heart sounds help identify cardiac symptoms (chest pain, palpitations) due to *angina* pectoris, prolapse of the mitral valve, and cardiac *arrhythmias* [e.g., paroxysmal atrial tachycardia (PAT)]. *Mitral valve prolapse syndrome* (MVPS; midsystolic click, late systolic murmur, and echocardiographic findings) occurs with increased frequency (15% to 40%+) in patients with panic disorder; however, anxiety and

panic disorders may *not* be increased in patients with MVPS. Thus the relation between the two is not clear.

2. The apprehension and dyspnea associated with bronchial *asthma* or COLD ("pink puffers") usually has accompanying wheezing or characteristic spirometric and radiographic features.

3. Acute Intermittent *Porphyria*: anxiety with abdominal focus; look for fever, leukocytosis, pain in extremities, prior drug exposure, elevated urine porphobilinogen; Watson–Schwartz Test is positive.

4. Characteristic findings usually occur with *duodenal ulcer* (bleeding, relief of pain with food, persistent crater by radiograph, suggestive gastric analysis) and *ulcerative colitis* (bloody diarrhea, fever, weight loss, sigmoidoscopic findings), but without them, differentiation is sometimes difficult. *Internal hemorrhage* may be accompanied by pain and restlessness; the picture develops quickly.

5. The vertiginous, anxious patient with Ménière *disease* also has deafness, tinnitus, and nystagmus during the attack.

If no localizing features accompany the acute attack, or if the anxiety is chronic, consider:

6. *Hypoglycemia*, at times indistinguishable from chronic or acute psychogenic anxiety; obtain blood glucose at the time of the episode; 5-hour glucose tolerance test (GTT).

7. *Hyperthyroidism*: anxiety symptoms occur with rapid-onset type; skin warm and moist rather than cold and clammy; look for exophthalmos; get T_3 and T_4; check for goiter; consider TRH stimulation test.

8. *Pheochromocytoma*: anxiety attacks with hypertension; visual blurring, headache, perspiration, palpitations; get 24-hour urinary VMA or free catecholamines.

Other medical conditions can produce an anxiety syndrome: intracranial tumors, menstrual irregularities, hypothyroidism, hyper- and hypoparathyroidism, postconcussion syndrome, psychomotor epilepsy, and Cushing disease. Appropriate tests help differentiate these.

SUBSTANCE-INDUCED ANXIETY DISORDER (P. 479)

Many drugs of abuse can produce an anxiety syndrome on intoxication, whereas anxiety symptoms commonly predominate on withdrawal from alcohol, hypnotic–sedatives, and cocaine. Likewise, a number of medications can produce anxiety with use [e.g., antihypertensives and other cardiac drugs, thyroid, sympathomimetics and bronchodilators, anticholinergics, antiparkinsonian medications, lithium, and antipsychotics (see Chapter 13)]. Once the cause is identified and corrected, the anxiety usually promptly disappears.

ANXIETY WITH OBSESSIONS AND COMPULSIONS

Obsessive–Compulsive Disorder (p. 456, 300.3)

Obsessions are repetitive ideas, images, and impulses that intrude on a patient who feels powerless to stop them. They are unwanted, distressful, occasionally frightening or violent (e.g., the impulse to leap before a car; the thought that he may attack his spouse; that he may molest a child), and often impair functioning. The patient can ruminate endlessly ("Did I lock the door?"); most develop rituals or *compulsions* (counting, touching, cleaning) to ward off unwanted happenings or to satisfy an obsession (e.g., an obsession with dirt leading to hand-washing rituals). Compulsions are thus obsessions made manifest and occur in 75%+ of obsessive patients (11–13). The performance of the ritual temporarily relieves the anxiety from the obsession. Thinking is often magical ("My son won't have an accident if I stamp each foot 30 times."), and the patient is aware of this.

OCD afflicts 2% of the population, has varying degrees of severity, and is chronic, with some spontaneous cures. OCD patients have depressive feelings (80%), major depression (30%), and Tourette syndrome (5%); 8% of first-degree relatives have OCD. First symptoms occur by the 20s in 75%, may begin suddenly or slowly, and often have an episodic course. The clinical picture may be dominated by the rituals, which require direct treatment.

The cause of OCD is unknown, but CNS serotonin neurons are implicated in some cases. Moreover, CNS damage (e.g., head trauma), the orbitofrontal cortex, caudate, neostriatum, globus pallidus, and thalamus play roles. An increase in anxiety disorders occurs in family members (15%), but only slightly increased OCD.

■ Differential

Obsessive–compulsive problems are common in serious psychiatric illnesses. About 20% of serious depressions have obsessive symptoms—major symptoms and family history help separate them—treatment may be identical. Schizophrenics have bizarre obsessions and are usually comfortable with them. (Be cautious: OCD can reach psychotic proportions, so do not overdiagnose schizophrenia.) Some organic conditions may be seen early with obsessions and compulsions.

A number of disorders seem to share some characteristics with OCD and are sometimes referred to as part of the Obsessive–Compulsive Spectrum Disorders. This loose confederation includes conditions such as compulsive gambling, sexual addiction, eating disorders, hypochondriasis, body dysmorphic disorder, Tourette syndrome, trichotillomania, onychophagia, and other impulse-control disorders. Much more research will be required to define the relations among these conditions.

■ Treatment

Medication partially reduces symptoms in 40% to 60%+ and should be tried: start with an SSRI in high dose for 8+ weeks; clomipramine (Anafranil) is effective (150 to 250 mg/day) but, because of side effects, is not used until at least two unsuccessful trials of SSRIs. Later if there is a (common) partial response, augment with clonazepam (0.5 to 2.5 mg b.i.d.–t.i.d.), atypical antipsychotics, pindolol (2.5 mg t.i.d.), i.v. clomipramine, or an SSRI + clomipramine. Behavior therapy should be considered an essential complement to medications. For ritualizers, use a combination of *exposure* to the feared situation and response prevention (blocking the compulsive behaviors). For patients with just obsessions, use *imaginal exposure* (mentally experiencing what "could happen") and *thought stopping* (the therapist, and then later the patient, interrupts obsessional thought with the shouted word "Stop!").

From the combination of medications and psychotherapy, expect moderate to significant improvement in some. Medications promote rapid change, but exposure sustains that change and may make medications unnecessary in the long term. For the chronic, treatment-resistant, and disabled patient, consider very localized psychosurgery: either cingulotomy or bilateral anterior capsulotomy.

REFERENCES

1. Judd LL, Kessler RC, Paulus MP, et al. Comorbidity as a fundamental feature of generalized anxiety disorders. *Acta Psychiatry Scand* 1998;98(suppl 393):6–11.

2. Rudolph RL, Entsuah R, Chitra R. A meta-analysis of the effects of venlafaxine on anxiety associated with depression. *J Clin Psychopharmacol* 1998;18:136–144.
3. Gorman JM. Treating generalized anxiety disorder. *J Clin Psychiatry* 2003;64(suppl 2):24–29.
4. Bocola V, Trecco MD, Fabbrini G, et al. Antipanic effect of fluoxetine measured by CO_2 challenge test. *Biol Psychiatry* 1998;43: 612–615.
5. Taylor CB. Panic disorder. *Br Med J* 2006;332:951–955.
6. Shear MK, Beidel DC. Psychotherapy in the overall management strategy for social anxiety disorder. *J Clin Psychiatry* 1998;59 (suppl 17):39–44.
7. Davidson JRT. Pharmacotherapy of social anxiety disorder. *J Clin Psychiatry* 2006;67(suppl 12):20–26.
8. Yehuda R. *Psychological trauma*. Washington, DC: American Psychiatric Press, 1998.
9. Tomb D. The phenomenology of post-traumatic stress disorder. *Psychiatric Clin North Am* 1994;17:237–250.
10. Friedman MJ. Current and future drug treatment for posttraumatic stress disorder patients. *Psychiatr Ann* 1998;28:461–468.
11. Fineberg N, Marazziti D, Stein DJ. *Obsessive compulsive disorder*. London: Martin Dunitz, 2001.
12. Jenike MA, Baer L, Minichiello WE. *Obsessive-compulsive disorders*. St. Louis: Mosby, 1998.
13. Pato MT, Zohar J. *Current treatments of obsessive compulsive disorder*. Washington, DC: American Psychiatric Publishing, 2001.

Dissociative Disorders

Dissociation is the splitting off of specific mental activities from the rest of normal consciousness, such as the splitting of thoughts or feelings from behavior (e.g., to daydream through a boring lecture and yet end with a complete set of notes without being aware of having taken them) (1). Minor dissociation is a common human phenomenon (2). *Dissociative disorders* demonstrate severe dissociation that produces significant and diverse symptoms and impairs functioning. Such disorders are fairly common (10% lifetime risk), often occur within the context of childhood physical or sexual abuse or both or associated with acute trauma, and are frequently comorbid with major depression, somatization disorder, affective spectrum disorder (ASD), posttraumatic stress disorder (PTSD), substance abuse, borderline personality disorder, conduct disorder, and antisocial personality disorder (3).

A biologic basis for dissociation is suggested by data such as a variety of functional magnetic resonance imaging (fMRI) and positron emission tomography (PET) studies of dissociative patients who display increased activity compared with normal persons in the right frontal cortex and parietal association areas, whereas others show decreased activity bilaterally in the orbitofrontal region and perhaps the hippocampi. Neurotransmitters involved in dissociation are just being identified, with a focus on increased glutamate (4), as well as others. Much work remains to be done.

AMNESIA

Organic processes (usually involving the temporal lobes) account for most cases of significant memory loss in adults. These processes include intoxication or withdrawal from drugs or alcohol (e.g., alcoholic blackouts for acute amnesia; Korsakoff syndrome for **SUBSTANCE-INDUCED PERSISTING AMNESTIC DISORDER**), various dementias, acute or chronic metabolic conditions (e.g., hypoglycemia, hepatic encephalopathy), brain trauma (i.e., postconcussive amnesia), brain tumors (particularly in the temporal lobes), cerebrovascular accidents, epilepsy (particularly temporal lobe epilepsy), and various degenerative or infectious CNS diseases. *Transient global amnesia* (TGA) is a sudden, self-limited, massive loss of memory in middle-aged or elderly patients due to a temporary (presumably vascular) cause. Always look for an organic cause for amnesia first.

DISSOCIATIVE AMNESIA (DSM, p. 520, 300.12) is a retrograde, usually reversible loss of memory from psychological causes. Immediately, a sudden loss of emotion-laden information occurs for the time surrounding a severe physical or psychosocial stress. It occurs more frequently in women in their teens or 20s or in men during the stress of war. The patient often appears confused and puzzled during the attack, but recovery is typically rapid (hours to 1 to 2 months), spontaneous, and complete. However, other people have amnesia, partial or complete, for past periods in their lives (often associated with past trauma) that may last for months or years, be associated with current psychiatric symptoms, and be discovered only during a careful history (5). Therapy or hypnosis or both may help revive memories (delayed recall) or may create false ones [i.e., the *false memory syndrome* (6)].

If, usually after an acute stress, the patient has a severe memory loss, leaves home, and acts like a different person, he has **DISSOCIATIVE FUGUE** (DSM, p. 523, 300.13). Although patients present themselves well to strangers, on questioning they are usually unaware of their previous (real) identity and may seem somewhat perplexed about their current personal identity. However, occasional patients function for long periods in complex roles, undetected. The return of old memories and the old identity usually occurs abruptly within hours or days but may not happen for months (or longer); then they have no memory for life during the fugue. Fugue seems more common in alcohol abusers (7).

The differential diagnosis of both conditions includes
1. Various organic conditions (see earlier).
2. Psychiatric conditions. Amnesia may often accompany severe depressive or anxiety states. Somnambulism may superficially resemble some fugues but has marked clouding of consciousness. PTSD, somatoform disorders, and other dissociative states often include amnesia as well.
3. Malingering and secondary gain in patients with antisocial personality disorder.

Evaluate these patients with a careful history and physical examination, liver enzymes, blood alcohol level, and drug screen.

Further evaluation may include a computed tomography (CT) scan and a sleep-deprived EEG with nasopharyngeal (NP) leads. Are old skills preserved during the attack (uncommon in organic conditions)? Is obvious secondary gain present? Is a personal or family history for mental illness or epilepsy known? The Amytal interview is occasionally diagnostic—organic patients usually become more confused, whereas patients with psychological amnesia may have a return of memory.

DISSOCIATIVE IDENTITY DISORDER (DID) (DSM, P. 526, 300.14)

This was formerly known as multiple personality disorder (MPD). Patients with this dramatic disorder (e.g., *The Three Faces of Eve*) have at least two (and frequently several) personalities within themselves. One of the personalities is usually dominant, yet any one of them may dominate from time to time, and the patient may "switch" among "alters" over seconds to a few minutes, usually when under stress. The patient's behavior is consistent with whatever personality is in "control" at that moment. Each personality may or may not be aware of the presence of the others. When checking for episodes of dissociation, always ask about past "blackouts" or periods of "lost time," because patients often have no memory for when they have been dissociated.

This poorly understood (and hotly debated) psychiatric condition begins in childhood (likely in response to abuse), is more common among female patients (3 to 9:1), tends to be chronic, and is replete with multiple symptoms such as anxiety, depression with suicidal impulses and acts, trances and amnesia, a multitude of somatic complaints, substance abuse and other "misbehavior," and psychotic-like symptoms. Once considered rare, it may be relatively common, particularly in milder forms, and is frequently mistaken for the more flamboyant personality disorders (particularly borderline), somatization disorder, major depression, anxiety and panic disorders, and schizophrenia. DSM-IV-TR criteria are often fulfilled for DID and several of these conditions as well.

Proper treatment (8,9) *may or may not* center around a careful integration of the different personalities and personality fragments through 1–3 times/week psychotherapy and hypnotherapy over years. This may be the best treatment, or it may worsen the condition by helping to generate inaccurate memories (6)—treatment remains uncertain. Once personalities have been integrated or fused (considered a "cure" by the therapist), stress can fragment the personality again (Eve of *The Three Faces of Eve* is a good example). Sometimes supportive or cognitive behavioral therapy is preferable. Avoid hospitalization if possible, or make the stay brief.

DEPERSONALIZATION DISORDER (DSM, P. 530, 300.6)

These patients experience periods during which they have a strong and unpleasant sense of their own unreality (depersonalization), often coupled with a sense that the environment is also unreal (derealization). The patient may feel mechanical and separated from his or her own thoughts, emotions, and identity. Although many people transiently experience this phenomenon in a mild form at some time (perhaps 40% to 50% of population) or experience it as a symptom of another psychiatric condition (e.g., anxiety disorder and particularly panic disorder and depression), the experience for those receiving this clinical diagnosis is much more intense and recurrent. An episode occurs suddenly (often during relaxation after stress); usually in persons in their teens or 20s; may last for minutes, hours, or days; and then gradually disappears. It may return many times over the years and is frequently accompanied by anxiety or depression. "Perhaps" (10) $♀:♂ = 2:1$.

Psychotherapy, except supportive, has been of little value. Recently, however, anxiolytics and antidepressants (e.g., SSRIs) have seen some success. Rule out the symptom of depersonalization that may accompany psychiatric disorders and organic conditions (e.g., delirium, temporal lobe epilepsy, drug and alcohol use, brain tumor), and then try medication. Success is usually moderate, and the full condition is chronic.

REFERENCES

1. Coons PM. The dissociative disorders: rarely considered and underdiagnosed. *Psychiatry Clin North Am* 1998;21:637–648.
2. Ross CA, Joshi S, Currie R. Dissociative experiences in the general population. *Am J Psychiatry* 1990;147:1547–1552.
3. Allen JG, Smith WH. Diagnosing dissociative disorders. *Bull Menninger Clin* 1993;57:328–343.
4. Chambers RA, Bremner JD, Moghaddam B, et al. Glutamate and post-traumatic stress disorder: toward a psychobiology of dissociation. *Semin Clin Neuropsychiatry* 1999;4:274–281.

5. Merckelbach H, Dekhers T, Wessel I, et al. Dissociative symptoms and amnesia in Dutch concentration camp survivors. *Comp Psychiatry* 2003;44:65–69.
6. Brainerd CJ, Reyna VF. *The science of false memory*. Oxford: Oxford University Press, 2005.
7. Akhtar S, Brenner I. Differential diagnosis of fugue-like states. *J Clin Psychiatry* 1979;40:381–384.[1]
8. Chu JA. The rational treatment of multiple personality disorder. *Psychotherapy* 1994;31:94–100.
9. Spira JL, Yalom ID. *Treating dissociative identity disorder*. New York: Jossey-Bass, 1996.
10. Simeon D, Knutelska M, Nelson D, et al. Feeling unreal: a depersonalization disorder update of 117 cases. *J Clin Psychiatry* 2003;64:990–997.

Chapter 10

Grief and the Dying Patient

Everyone endures personal losses; many suffer chronic illnesses. Everyone dies. Physicians attend at all of these events and need to recognize normal and abnormal human responses to loss (grief reaction and unresolved grief), illness, and death.

GRIEF REACTION

Normal Grief

■ Symptoms

BEREAVEMENT (DSM, p. 740, V62.82) (grief, mourning) is a normal response to a significant loss (of spouse, parent, child—but also of health, limb, career, savings, status, etc.) (1). *Expect* to see it with major losses—be alert for future problems if the patient does not grieve (although 30% of widows mourn briefly and very little) (2,3). If a loss is obviously approaching, mourning may begin before the loss actually occurs (*anticipatory grief*). Symptoms associated with divorce may also be coded as **PARTNER RELATIONAL PROBLEM** (DSM, p. 737, V61.10).

Recognize grief by restlessness, distractibility, disorganization, preoccupation, "numbness," feelings of sadness, apathy, crying, anxious pining, a need to talk about the dead, and intense mental pain during the days, weeks, and months after a loss. Somatic distress is common and includes generalized weakness, a tightness in the throat, choking, shortness of breath, palpitations, headaches, and gastrointestinal (GI) complaints. Do not be surprised if the patient displays marked but short-lived irritability, hostility, or anger toward you, others, or the dead (you did not "do enough," they do not "care enough," he died, etc.). This often alternates with listlessness, social withdrawal, depression, and feelings of guilt (about that which was left undone or could have been done differently). Patients become preoccupied with their loss. They constantly think about the dead and review past experiences, visit the grave, and may even briefly deny the death.

About 25% to 35% of patients have symptoms that suggest a major depression: anorexia, feelings of worthlessness, impaired memory, suicidal thoughts, and hopelessness. Nearly 10% have delusional thoughts or hallucinations or both. Be careful not to "overread" temporary bizarre behavior in the bereaved. Some patients develop psychophysiologic disorders, hypochondriasis, major anxiety symptoms, or phobias. A few begin to drink too much; some deteriorate physically; and major psychiatric illnesses (e.g., acute schizophrenia) may be precipitated in those predisposed (e.g., with a family history). Moreover, bereavement has been associated with increased adrenocorticotropic hormone (ACTH) and cortisol, decreased immune function and natural killer cell activity, and an increased rate of heart disease and malignancy (4). Recent magnetic resonance imaging (MRI) studies (5) implicate the cerebellum, posterior cingulate gyrus, and medial-superior frontal gyrus in grief. Death from suicide and illness is increased during the first year after the loss.

Unresolved Grief

Loss not dealt with through a normal mourning process *may* produce chronic symptoms (6,7):

- **Prolonged grief:** Grief develops into a chronic depression or a subsyndromal depression that lasts for more than 1 year in as many as 30%. Lowered self-esteem and guilt tend to be prominent (8).
- **Delayed grief:** The patient who does not grieve at the time of a loss is at risk for later depression, social withdrawal, anxiety disorders, panic attacks, overt or covert self-destructive behavior, alcoholism, and psychophysiologic syndromes. Chronic anger and hostility, marked emotional inhibition, or distorted interpersonal relationships also may be displayed. Unresolved grief *may* be an unsuspected cause of psychiatric disability in many people—always inquire about a history of significant losses.
- **Distorted grief:** Exaggerated (bizarre, hysterical, euphoric, or psychosis-like) reactions that occur in a few patients have the effect of postponing the normal grieving process. Alternately, the patient may have physical complaints (e.g., pain or "chronic illness behavior") and may be mistaken for having a primary medical problem.

Persons at risk for developing an abnormal grief reaction include those who

1. Received little support or understanding from others after their loss (e.g., abortion, suicide, death of an illicit lover);
2. Are social isolates, either "psychological loners" or those without family or friends nearby—multiple strong supports help truncate the mourning process;
3. Are inhibited, compulsive, or uncomfortable with any form of emotion;
4. Have experienced *multiple* recent losses or a sudden, severe, unexpected loss;
5. Have unresolved past losses;
6. Had ambivalent feelings about the deceased when alive and have reacted to the death with guilt.

Treatment

Encouraging satisfactory mourning is an important activity for the physician.

- Encourage mourning. Say it is *okay*. Say it is *important* and necessary. Explain that the anguish undoubtedly experienced during this process is essential and curative. However, do *not* force the patient—let him or her set the pace.
- Help the patient identify and experience his emotions—sadness, hopelessness, despair, anxiety, fear, anger. Assure the patient that these are normal, expected, and understandable. Do not be embarrassed by these emotions yourself.
- Help the patient review the loss. Be an active listener. Ask for a description of the deceased—ask for particulars, details, shared intimacies, etc. Become a support.
- See the patient frequently. Be interested. Be available, particularly over time. Recognize and tolerate relapses. Be alert to the presence of anniversaries.
- Do *not* use medication to attenuate normal grief—help the patient work through the grief instead. Sleeping medication may be useful. If anxiety or restlessness is excessive, consider a temporary use of minor tranquilizers (e.g., diazepam, 5 mg PO, t.i.d.) *as therapy is begun.* Treat a major depression or psychosis with medication (9).
- Work with the family. Help develop a sympathetic support system. Mourners are social outcasts—help decrease "the social

isolation of the bereaved." Self-help groups can be very valuable (e.g., groups of parents who have lost a child).
- Keep the mourner "involved in life"—slowly at first, but insist on increasing independence.

THE DYING PATIENT

Few patients stress physicians as much as do those who are dying. This need not be. Even if little can be done to change a fatal outcome, *care*ful handling by the physician and crucial others can help turn a patient's dying (whether expected or untimely) into a time of genuine relief, satisfaction, and (even) growth. When time is so limited, new realities and priorities emerge that must be dealt with if life is to be concluded satisfactorily (10).

Normal Responses in the Dying

The news that one is dying produces a special kind of grief reaction. A typical series of "stages" or psychological reactions to the threat of imminent death are seen frequently (11):
- **First Stage, Shock and Denial:** Denial is the initial reaction of many patients to being told that they are dying and is particularly severe in those "caught by surprise." They may refuse to believe the diagnosis, actively begin doctor shopping, or be dazed and appear oblivious to the significance of the diagnosis. This may be fleeting, but some patients may never pass beyond this stage.
- **Second Stage, Anger:** A frustrated, hopeless, angry, bitter, "Why me?" response often accompanies the realization of impending death. The anger is directed at the physicians (or family, God, fate, etc.) for the "unfairness" of this turn of events.
- **Third Stage, Bargaining:** The patient attempts to bargain with physicians or God for more time—promising good behavior, good intentions, etc., in exchange for "a chance to see my boy graduate from college."
- **Fourth Stage, Depression:** The patient despairs and begins to grieve. Be alert to suicide, particularly in the irritable, demanding, agitated depression.
- **Fifth Stage, Acceptance:** The patient is quiet and resigned. He or she has few outside interests but seeks the presence of loved ones or a few close friends.

These stages are not necessarily stepwise and invariable. Just as often, the person will shift back and forth among stages (e.g., from denial to anger and then back to denial), exhibit varying degrees of denial throughout, but gradually become more detached. The younger the adult, the more likely the stages are to be turbulent, and the problems, severe.

Specific psychiatric problems occur often and should be identified and treated:

1. Depression is common but not "normal"; thus if a depression is not relieved by support and time, a major depression may develop. Consider treatment with antidepressants.
2. Organic brain syndromes (usually waxing and waning) develop frequently and can be frightening to patients. Help them see the disorders as separate from themselves—as just another thing to be experienced.
3. Acute anxiety is common but usually temporary, particularly if treated with medication.
4. Communication failures between the patient and loved ones are very common and troublesome —often taking the form of a "tyranny of silence" or a lack of understanding on either one's part about the distress of the other. These must be dealt with directly.

Treatment

■ Telling the Patient

- Choose a quiet and private spot, be relaxed, sit down with the patient, and briefly reveal the diagnosis. Use the patient's response as an indicator of how much to tell.
- Patients need to know and need a chance to ask questions, but, most of all, they need someone (usually the physician, but also spouse, pastor, etc.) *available*—someone to help them grieve.
- Be truthful (but allow them to deny if they insist on it) and realistically hopeful ("We will begin treatment. Sometimes remissions occur."). *Do not* encourage false hopes, but do not dwell on the fatal outcome.
- Strong negative reactions do occur. Sedation can be helpful temporarily.

■ Treating the Patient

- Be supportive, empathic, warm, a good listener, hopeful (e.g., about goals to be achieved before death), and available. Get to know the patient as a person—attention to exclusively medical matters is "dehumanizing." Be tolerant of ups and downs. Recognize that the patient may become hostile toward you—be patient.

- *Always* take your lead from the patient. Some days, some topics are too stressful. Other days, patients "have" to talk. Force the issue only if their denial, anxiety, or anger is seriously obstructing good care. Occasionally confrontation may be required.
- Make them comfortable. Treat pain aggressively—narcotics are okay. Attend fastidiously to basic physical needs. Make their room pleasant and cheerful.
- Certain fears are common and must to be looked for and dealt with [e.g., fear of pain, of physical dependency, of being isolated, of losing control (emotional and physical), of being helpless, of the unknown, or of leaving loved ones to flounder (financially or emotionally)].
- It is essential to help the patient "work through" the process of dying. Help him set new priorities and goals (e.g., get his affairs in order). Help the patient resolve old problems and feel good about current relationships. Help him be responsible. Encourage the patient to consider not only how he will die but also how he will live out the rest of life.
- Do *not* insist that patients march through the "stages of dying" in a set order and on schedule.
- Allow the patient "terminal dependency"—it is okay finally to regress.

■ Treating the Family

- Family members show many of the signs of grief. Like the patient, they also may be angry, hostile, or denying. They may need treatment—help *them* mourn.
- It is important to keep the family (i.e., loved ones) involved. Help the patient die "with their blessing."
- It can be enormously beneficial (to the patient, to the family) if the patient can be supportive to the family members in their grieving.

■ Treating the Staff

- Recognize that the physician, nurses, aides, etc., are all affected by death. Anxiety, intellectualization, avoidance, and grieving frequently occur among staff—do not let this stress impair care. Staff conferences to ventilate and explore these issues may help.

THE CHRONICALLY ILL PATIENT

Chronic illness is another form of stress that entails grieving. Like the dying patient, these patients may deny their illness, become angry and resentful, regress, or become depressed. Common to all these reactions is anxiety associated with a loss of health and attractiveness, a loss of self-esteem, and the threat of dependency or even death. Certain personality types are at risk (e.g., the narcissistic or the very independent). Treatment principles useful with the grieving or dying patient apply here as well.

REFERENCES

1. Bonanno GA, Kaltman S. The varieties of grief experience. *Clin Psychol Rev* 2001;21:705.
2. Marmar CR, Horowitz MJ, Weiss DS, et al. A controlled trial of brief psychotherapy and mutual-help group treatment of conjugal bereavement. *Am J Psychiatry* 1988;145:203–209.
3. Zisook S, Shuchter SR, Sledge PA, et al. The spectrum of depressive phenomena after spousal bereavement. *J Clin Psychiatry* 1994;55(suppl 4):29–36.
4. Spurrell MT, Creed FH. Lymphocyte response in depressed patients and subjects anticipating bereavement. *Br J Psychiatry* 1993;162:60–64.
5. Gundel H, O'Connor MF, Littrell L, et al. Functional neuroanatomy of grief: an fMRI study. *Am J Psychiatry* 2003;160:1946.
6. Rynearson EK. Pathologic grief: the queen's croquet ground. *Psychiatr Ann* 1990;20:295–303.
7. Prigerson HG, Bierhals AJ, Kasl SV, et al. Complicated grief as a disorder distinct from bereavement-related depression and anxiety. *Am J Psychiatry* 1996;153:1484–1486.
8. Barry MJ. Therapeutic experience with patients referred for prolonged grief reaction: some second thoughts. *Mayo Clin Proc* 1981;56:744–747.
9. Zisook S, Shuchter SR. Treatment of the depression of bereavement. *Am Behav Sci* 2001;44:782.
10. Brown JH, Henteleff P, Barakat S, et al. Is it normal for terminally ill patients to desire death? *Am J Psychiatry* 1986;143:208–211.
11. Kubler-Ross E. *On death and dying.* London: Tavistock, 1970.

Conditions That Mimic Physical Disease

It is essential to differentiate organic illness from psychogenic illness in patients complaining of physical symptoms. Patients with physical complaints in whom no medical illness can be found or who do not improve with treatment (or both) are common (1). These frustrating patients often exhaust one doctor after another and usually are finally labeled "hysterics" or "crocks." This occasionally angry response by the physician does a disservice to these patients because, although some may be consciously "faking it" (e.g., malingering), most patients have as yet undiagnosed organic conditions or have symptoms that are unconsciously and involuntarily produced.

Several discrete involuntary psychiatric syndromes (somatoform disorders; see later) mimic organic disease. These disorders have typical clinical presentations, family histories, recommended treatments, and likely prognoses.

Failure to identify an organic etiology for a physical symptom does not necessitate a diagnosis of a somatoform disorder or malingering; these are not diagnoses by exclusion but rather should be based on specific characteristics. Consider the following diagnoses in any patient with a poorly specified or uncertain medical condition.

UNDETECTED PHYSICAL ILLNESS

The possibility of an underlying unrecognized illness must continue to be considered throughout the course of diagnosis and treatment, however long. Follow-up studies find 15% to 30% of conversion reaction diagnoses to represent misdiagnosed organic disease. Physical illness may produce symptoms that mimic a somatoform disorder or may predispose susceptible patients to concurrent psychiatric conditions (it's not "*either, or*"). Some patients with subtle central nervous system (CNS) disease are at risk for conversion symptoms, so always carefully evaluate neurologically. The physical conditions

commonly found (on follow-up) among these "false-positive hysterics" include
- CNS disease, particularly epilepsy, multiple sclerosis (MS), and postconcussion syndrome, but also CNS infections (e.g., encephalitis), dementia, brain tumor, and cerebrovascular disease.
- Degenerative disorders of musculoskeletal and connective tissues, including systemic lupus erythematosus (SLE), polyarteritis nodosa, early rheumatoid arthritis, and myasthenia gravis.
- Others: Syphilis, tuberculosis (TB), hyper- and hypothyroidism, hyperparathyroidism, porphyria, hypoglycemia, duodenal and gallbladder disease, pancreatic disease, etc.

Be suspicious of any somatoform disorder that *develops late in life*—very unlikely. Psychological testing is of little help in differentiation; do not be misled by a "neurotic" picture on the Minnesota Multiphasic Personality Inventory (MMPI) into prematurely abandoning the search for a physical cause.

SOMATOFORM DISORDERS

Conversion Disorder (DSM, p. 492, 300.11)

A patient whose predominant problem is an obvious loss of function, incompatible with known physiology and anatomy, of some part of the nervous system that no identified organic pathology can completely explain (conversion symptom) may have a conversion disorder (2). Conversion symptoms include, among others:
- Motor: Paralysis, astasia–abasia, seizures, urinary retention, aphonia, globus hystericus (a very distressing "lump in the throat" that makes swallowing difficult);
- Sensory: Paresthesia, anesthesia, anosmia, blindness, tunnel vision, deafness;
- Other: Unconsciousness, vomiting.

In addition, the particular symptom appears to serve one of two specific psychological purposes.
1. As *primary gain*, the symptom "buries" an unconscious mental conflict. An unacceptable painful thought is repressed, and the emotional energy is converted to a physical symptom. Usually the specific symptom "chosen" represents the conflict symbolically (e.g., in the negligent mother of a burned child, anesthesia develops over the corresponding part of her body).

2. As *secondary gain*, the symptom gets the patient something he or she wants (e.g., paralysis permits dependency on wife or justifies workman's compensation) or allows him or her to avoid something unwanted (e.g., seizures prevent a court appearance).

As obvious as these relationships may be to the observer, the patient is unaware of them (unconscious), and the patient does not grasp their significance, even if explained (lacks insight).

Diagnosis

In the apparent absence of organic pathology, it is necessary to identify features in addition to a presumed conversion symptom before making the diagnosis. Realize also that as many as 25% of patients with conversion disorders have associated organic pathology (e.g., epilepsy in a patient with pseudoseizures is common), so also investigate symptoms only partially explained by the physical abnormalities. Features associated with conversion disorders include the following:

- The symptom occurs abruptly and frequently follows an acute stress.
- Often a history exists of the same or a different conversion symptom.
- The disorder usually is seen first during adolescence or in the 20s and in a person predisposed by a dependent, histrionic, antisocial, or passive–aggressive personality disorder.
- The patients often have associated moderate anxiety and depression.
- The patients are frequently immature, shallow, and demanding, although they tend to cooperate with examinations. They tend to have lower intelligence, limited insight, and lower socioeconomic status. This occurs primarily in women.
- Indifference to the symptom may be found (*la belle indifférence*).

The individual neurologic symptoms usually have some characteristics that distinguish them from those of an organic etiology. In general, they tend to be variable, atypical, and inconsistent with anatomy.

▓ Conversion Seizures

Seizures (3) are often atypical and bizarre (the patient may laugh or cry throughout the seizure) but usually purposeful. Only infrequently is there incontinence, cyanosis, physical self-harm, tongue biting, or complete loss of consciousness during the seizure.

Awareness of surroundings and good muscle tone are preserved during the typically brief postictal stage (arm dropped onto face may land lightly or miss the face altogether; patient may resist eye opening). The seizure onset may be slow but also often dramatic, and seizures usually occur when the patient is around others. Set the patient quickly upright—seizures often stop.

■ Conversion Unconsciousness

The loss of consciousness is usually light and incomplete, with the patient showing some awareness of environmental events, particularly when he or she feels unobserved. VS and reflexes are normal, and the patient usually responds to painful stimuli. The eyes are held tightly shut, and some movements may be purposive (e.g., move to keep from falling from examination table).

■ Conversion Paralysis

The paralysis is often variable, even during one examination. Paralysis of one limb, part of a limb, or hemiparesis is most common, but the specific involvement is often inconsistent with anatomy, and the related changes (e.g., tone) are atypical. DTR changes are variable, and pathologic reflexes (e.g., Babinski) are not present. The paralyzed limbs often show little resistance to passive movement but resist the pull of gravity. If resistance to a forced movement occurs, it tends to give way abruptly (vs. gradually, as in organic conditions). Movement may occur when the patient is startled by a painful stimulus. Palpate the antagonists— they often contract to simulate agonist weakness. Usually associated conversion sensory changes are found.

■ Astasia–Abasia

This exaggerated and bizarre conversion ataxia varies from moment to moment. The patient falls toward walls and people, rarely falls to the floor, and rarely hurts himself, despite a dramatic presentation.

■ Conversion Sensory Changes

These are often dramatic, sometimes vague, and usually inconsistent with anatomy (e.g., "stocking and glove" anesthesia, loss of *all* senses on one side or below a certain level on a limb, loss of which stops *exactly* at midline). Careful testing differentiates most cases.

■ Conversion Blindness

Visual disturbances are usually blurring, double vision, or tunnel loss, but may be total blindness. Response to a bright light (check with EEG) and avoidance of objects in the room are often inconsistent with the degree of presumed visual loss.

When the diagnosis is in doubt, a single dose of i.v. sodium amobarbital (Amytal) often temporarily removes the conversion symptom, thus clarifying the diagnosis. Slowly give a 10% solution i.v. (1 ml/min, maximum of 500 mg). When the patient's words begin to slur, stop administration, and observe for disappearance of symptom.

Differential Diagnosis

- Carefully rule out physical illness.
- Some patients with conversion symptoms require a primary diagnosis of major depression or schizophrenia.
- Two somatoform disorders (see later) have features in common with conversion disorders: somatization disorder and psychogenic pain disorder.
- Differentiation from malingering is difficult (see later).

Treatment

Some patients have a short course and are "spontaneous cures"; a few may be chronic (e.g., in some paralyzed patients, contractures actually develop), but most improve over weeks or months. A physical process is later identified in a significant minority (25%). Temporary improvement may be produced by hypnosis (4).

It is uncertain what treatment is best. Long-term psychoanalysis appears to effect real change in a few but is not for most patients. Use minor tranquilizers if anxiety predominates. Behavior modification has had mixed success.

Crucial to any therapy is the formation of a supportive therapeutic alliance, but these patients are generally resistant to treatment. Direct confrontation about the "hysterical" nature of the symptom rarely works—the patient usually withdraws. Always provide support and the confident expectation of improvement/cure. Help the patient ventilate. Help the patient explore areas of stress in life, but relate that to symptoms only after an alliance has been formed. Gradually identify the symbolic nature of the symptoms, if present.

Work with the family. Help restructure the patient's environment to remove the secondary gain, if possible. Educate other involved medical personnel about the disorder—help them avoid countertherapeutic hostility.

SOMATIZATION DISORDER (DSM, P. 486, 300.81)

This syndrome, historically called Briquet syndrome, describes patients who have *numerous* vague and often dramatically presented physical symptoms that must involve several organ systems and have no adequate medical explanation despite extensive workups:

- Vague and ill-defined *pains*; at least one each at four different sites;
- At least one *neurologic* symptom (e.g., conversion or dissociative type or loss of consciousness);
- Menstrual/*sexual* problems, inhibited orgasm;
- At least two GI symptoms, often vague (e.g., bloating, nausea)

The clinical picture must be evident by age 30; the symptoms wax and wane, have a very chronic course, and usually are presented forcefully by the patients, who insist on examination and treatment. They rarely feel they are well enough to be active or to work. These patients demand and often receive multiple evaluations, medications, treatments, and even operations, and are at risk for iatrogenically induced medical complications and drug side effects or addiction or both.

Analytically oriented researchers argue that symptoms are produced when forbidden impulses are repressed, and the emotional energy associated with those drives is converted (conversion) into a physical symptom. Although definitive information remains incomplete, features currently associated with Somatization Disorder include the following:

- Occurs primarily in women (1% of all women);
- Anxiety, irritability, impulsiveness, and depression are common; frequent suicide attempts;
- Lower intelligence and lower socioeconomic groups;
- Frequent interpersonal and marital problems; chaotic lifestyles;
- Often previous or concurrent history of antisocial behavior and a poor school history;
- Patients may have histrionic, dependent, or antisocial personality disorder;
- First-degree female relatives have a 20% incidence of somatization disorder. First-degree male relatives have increased prevalence of alcoholism and antisocial personality disorder.

Somatization disorder is difficult to distinguish from factitious disorder or malingering: occasionally a combination is present. It is essential to rule out inconstant and confusing medical syndromes (e.g., SLE, acute intermittent porphyria, sarcoidosis, lymphoma, TLE, MS, thyroid disease, hyperparathyroidism), although most can be differentiated from the full Briquet syndrome (reliable diagnostic screening tests are available). Look for early onset, chronic course, multiple organ system involvement, and negative workups. Follow-up studies find few cases of undiagnosed organic illness (unlike conversion disorder). Common comorbid psychiatric conditions (75% of somatization patients) include MDD, panic disorder, substance abuse, and histrionic, borderline, and antisocial personality disorders.

A similar but subsyndromal picture (e.g., nonspecific weakness, fatigue, vague but incapacitating medical symptoms) that lasts longer than 6 months may qualify for **UNDIFFERENTIATED SOMATOFORM DISORDER (DSM, p. 490, 300.82)**, and if lasting fewer than 6 months, **SOMATOFORM DISORDER NOS (DSM, p. 511, 300.82)**. Perhaps 5% to 10% of the general population qualify for one of these disorders at some time.

Treatment

Treatment success is limited. Focus usually should be placed on management rather than on cure. Develop a therapeutic alliance by being sympathetic and interested in the patient and his or her health, but do not make that your exclusive focus. Gradually encourage an examination of the patient's general life problems and coping styles. Help the patient develop mature social, occupational, and intimate interpersonal skills. CBT is showing increasing success, however (5). Treat depression and anxiety with medication (SSRIs preferred), but recognize the risk for addiction when treating pain and medical conditions.

PAIN DISORDER (DSM, P. 498, 307.8X)

These patients experience pain for which no cause can be found. Acute pain is most typically comorbid with anxiety disorders, and chronic pain with depressive disorders. It appears suddenly, usually after a stress, and may disappear in days or last for years. It is frequently accompanied by organic illness that, however, does not adequately explain the severity of the pain. The lifetime prevalence is 10%[+] in the general population; once established, it may become the central factor in the patient's life. This condition is very similar to conversion disorder, and the patients may differ only by experiencing pain rather than a neurologic deficit as the predominant symptom. Treatments are similar, although (a) it is essential to keep the patient engaged in regular life activities despite the pain; and (b) newer antidepressants may be useful.

HYPOCHONDRIASIS (DSM, P. 504, 300.7)

Although many people may mentally expand a minor symptom into a major physical illness (particularly during times of stress), they rarely become preoccupied with it and can easily be dissuaded when examination and laboratory tests are normal. The hypochondriac, conversely, is "bodily preoccupied" and is (a) convinced he has a serious and unrecognized physical illness, rejects evidence to the contrary, insists on further tests and treatments, doctor shops, appears pleased only if assured of sickness, and eagerly seeks additional medical attention; and (b) is consoled temporarily when reassured but resurrects old or new symptoms in days or weeks (a variant of OCD?) (6). This common (1% to 5% in general population; 5%+ among medical patients, $\male:\female = 1:1$) chronic condition begins in adolescence or middle age, is common among the elderly, and is resistant to therapy. The patient rarely sees a psychiatrist but rather drifts from internist to surgeon to neurologist, etc.

The patient is hyperalert to symptoms and presents them in great detail ("compulsively" rather than "dramatically" as in somatization disorder) during the history. These patients usually have some specific idea of "what the trouble is" and merely may want the physician to concur. Physicians frequently become angry and rejecting toward the patient, which leads to further "shopping around." In severe cases, the patient becomes an invalid, and in many patients, the illness disrupts social and occupational functioning.

Many of these patients display anxiety or depression. Hypochondriacal features occur frequently in serious psychiatric conditions like schizophrenia, major depression, dysthymic disorder, and organic brain syndromes. Rule out other somatoform disorders, chronic factitious disorder, and malingering.

Treatment to "cure" is unlikely, and lengthy or complete remissions are very uncommon. Symptoms may disappear if an associated depression or psychosis is successfully treated. Do not expect a cure, but rather work with the patient to help *control* the symptoms. Reassure the patient that the problem is persistent but not debilitating or fatal. See the patient frequently for short periods. Assure the patient that you will be available if needed, but schedule regular appointments (to be kept whether or not he or she is feeling ill). Formal CBT may help. Avoid extensive medical testing or interventions. Consider giving a mild medication (e.g., antihistamine, vitamin) that can be a focus of attention during appointments and will be evidence that he or she is taken seriously. This form of palliation can restore the patient to functional health more readily than any definitive medical treatment. Early evidence suggests that SSRIs are useful.

BODY DYSMORPHIC DISORDER (DSM, P. 507, 300.7)

This disorder of young adults can be minor or incapacitating: patients can become preoccupied with an imagined physical defect (face most common), which they feel negatively affects their appearance, and seek surgical correction or become socially withdrawn or even housebound. The "affected" part of the body may change with time. "Most" BDD patients have comorbid MDD or OCD. Although in its minor forms, it is surprisingly common, little is known of its etiology, family patterns, biology, or treatment. It has some characteristics of OCD and may be an element of the obsessive–compulsive spectrum disorders. The preoccupation not infrequently becomes delusional and reaches psychotic proportions. SSRIs and clomipramine may help (7) with both psychotic and nonpsychotic forms. Plastic surgery is often requested, rarely successful, and may generate a lawsuit.

SIMULATION OF PHYSICAL SYMPTOMS

Two categories of patients *voluntarily* mimic physical symptoms.
1. **MALINGERING (DSM, p. 739, V65.2)** (8) These people knowingly fake symptoms for some obvious gain. They may be trying to get drugs, avoid the law, get a bed for the night, etc. Despite their physical complaints, they tend to be evasive and uncooperative during evaluation and therapy, and they avoid medical procedures. When exposed, they may angrily give up their symptoms and sign out against medical advice (AMA). Antisocial personality disorder and drug abuse are common associated conditions.

2. **FACTITIOUS DISORDER With PREDOMINANTLY PHYS-ICAL SIGNS AND SYMPTOMS (DSM, p. 513, 300.19)**
These patients also knowingly fake symptoms but do so for psychological reasons: They usually prefer the sick role and may move from hospital to hospital to receive care. They are usually loners with an early childhood background of trauma and deprivation. They have difficulty establishing close interpersonal relationships and generally have severe personality disorders (e.g., borderline). Unlike many malingerers, they demand and follow through with medical procedures and are at risk for drug addiction and for the complications of multiple operations.

Both groups of patients can be difficult to distinguish from those with the somatoform disorders and from those with organic illness, yet careful and *repeated* examinations will usually uncover their deceptions. The most common presentations include

- Abdominal pain: May have an abdomen "like a railroad yard."
- Heart: Complains of pain. May induce arrhythmias with digitalis or produce tachycardia with amphetamines or thyroid.
- Bleeding: Patient may take anticoagulants or add blood from a scratch to laboratory samples.
- Neurologic: Weakness, seizures, unconsciousness—difficult to differentiate from conversion symptoms.
- Fever: Produced by manipulating the thermometer (e.g., hot coffee in the mouth).
- Skin: Look for lesions in a linear pattern in areas the patient can reach.

Although both groups produce symptoms consciously, they should be dealt with differently. The malingerer should be handled formally (and often legally). The patient with a factitious disorder should be treated sympathetically, and every effort made to convince him or her to enter psychotherapy (difficult). Unlike the malingerer, these patients are unable to control their self-destructive behavior, and that should be tactfully pointed out to them.

REFERENCES

1. Phillips KA. *Somatoform and factitious disorders.* Washington, DC: American Psychiatric Publishing, 2001.
2. Halligan PW, Bass C, Wade DT. New approaches to conversion hysteria. *Br Med J* 2000;320:1488–1489.

3. Iriarte J, Parra J, Urrestarazu E, et al. Controversies in thee diagnosis and management of psychogenic pseudoseizures. *Epilepsy Behav* 2003;4:354–359.
4. Moene FC, Spinhoven P, Hoogduin KA, et al. A randomized controlled clinical trial on the additional effect of hypnosis in a comprehensive treatment programme for in-patients with conversion disorder of the motor type. *Psychother Psychosom* 2002;71:66–76.
5. Kroenke K, Swindle R. Cognitive-behavioral therapy for somatization and symptoms syndromes: a critical review of controlled clinical trials. *Psychother Psychosom* 2000;69:205–215.
6. Barksy AJ. The patient with hypochondriasis. *N Engl J Med* 2001;345:1395–1399.
7. Phillips KA, Albertini RS, Rasmussen SA. A randomized placebo-controlled trial of fluoxetine in body dysmorphic disorder. *Arch Gen Psychiatry* 2002;59:381–388.
8. LoPiccolo CJ, Goodkin K, Baldewicz TT. Current issues in the diagnosis and management of malingering. *Ann Med* 1999; 31:166–174.

Psychosomatic Disorders

Two overlapping classifications exist here. A PSYCHOSO-MATIC DISORDER (not in DSM-IV) is a physical disease *partially* caused or exacerbated by psychological factors, whereas the new DSM-IV category, **PSYCHOLOGICAL FACTORS AFFECTING MEDICAL CONDITION** (p. 731, 316), broadly identifies those psychological and social factors that influence the development and maintenance of medical disease (1,2). Both classifications apply only to those conditions in which psychological or behavioral influence (or both) is of *major* significance (but be aware that *any* physical disease may be modified by psychological stress). Neither the term "psychosomatic" nor the DSM-IV category refers to (a) a physical symptom or clinical presentation caused by psychological factors for which no organic basis exists (e.g., conversion disorder, pain disorder, somatization disorder); or (b) a patient with knowingly spurious physical complaints (e.g., factitious disorder, malingering), but the DSM-IV condition does allow physical complaints due to habit disorders (e.g., dyspnea due to excessive smoking, problems from obesity).

MECHANISMS OF DISEASE PRODUCTION

Many specific diseases are influenced greatly by the "psyche" (see later), but although much studied, the mechanisms by which the brain produces such organic pathology are unclear.

Psychological Mechanisms

"*Stress*," either internal or external, is required but is much more likely to cause disease if

1. The stress is severe (e.g., death of a loved one, divorce or separation, major illness or injury, financial crisis, incarceration). Holmes and Rahe developed a ranked scale of stressful life events (rated by life change units; LCUs) and found a close

correlation between an event's stress (in LCUs) and the patient's likelihood of a physical illness developing.

2. The stress is chronic.
3. The patient perceives the stress as stressful.
4. The patient has an increased level of general instability (e.g., difficult job, troubled marriage, urban dweller, socially disrupted environment).

It was once thought (F. Dunbar) that *specific* superficial personality traits produced specific organic diseases (e.g., that a "coronary personality" or an "ulcer personality" exists). It was also held (F. Alexander) that specific deep and unconscious, unresolved neurotic conflicts caused specific physical disorders. Currently, the specificity that is generally accepted associates the "type A" personality (i.e., sense of time urgency, impatience, aggressiveness, upward striving, competitiveness, tendency to anger when frustrated, and particularly a "*cynical hostility*") with coronary artery disease. More generally accepted are *nonspecific* hypotheses that link a wide variety of stresses to the development of disease in an individual placed at risk by one or more of the following:

1. A genetic susceptibility.
2. A degree of chronic debilitation, a current illness, or "an organ vulnerability."
3. A tendency to react to stress with anger, resentment, frustration, anxiety, or depression.
4. A "psychological susceptibility" (e.g., patient is pessimistic and "expects the worst" vs. being optimistic and actively working to overcome stress) (3).
5. An "alexithymic" personality (4) (e.g., a person who is in poor contact with his emotions and has an impoverished fantasy life).

Physiological Mechanisms

These mechanisms are poorly understood, and only the broad outline can be sketched. Stress is perceived cognitively (by the cerebral cortex) but, once recognized, is meditated primarily by the limbic system, which, under chronic stress, stimulates the hypothalamus and the vegetative centers in the brainstem over the long term. This stimulation produces a direct effect on the various organs by

1. Activation of the autonomic nervous system (sympathetic and adrenal medulla; parasympathetic).

2. Involvement of the neuroendocrine system i.e., *releasing hormones* from the hypothalamus travel through the pituitary portal system to the anterior pituitary, where they cause the release of the tropic hormones [e.g., adrenocorticotropic hormone (ACTH), thyroid-stimulating hormone (TSH), growth hormone (GH), follicle-stimulating hormone (FSH)], which either act directly or release other hormones from the endocrine glands [e.g., cortisol, thyroxin, epinephrine, norepinephrine (NE), sex hormones]. These produce a variety of changes in structures throughout the body. Hans Selye (1976) emphasized the central role of cortisol as a primary mediator of the body's stress response (general adaptation syndrome; GAS). If cortisol is released over too long a period, various organs are damaged, producing psychosomatic diseases.

The details have yet to be worked out: more questions than answers remain. The recently identified hormones, endorphins, may play a major role in stress-response regulation. Central to all of these physiologic systems is the concept of homeostasis: psychosomatic diseases occur when the body's "natural balance" is upset, particularly if it is chronically upset.

Although psychosomatic medicine has been concerned primarily with those diseases thought to be "psychosomatic," recently the concept has been broadened to include (or overlap with) the field of behavioral medicine. The essence of behavioral medicine is the application of behavior-modification techniques derived from learning theory to various medical problems (e.g., chronic pain, hypertension and other psychosomatic diseases, habit disorders). Techniques used include behavioral self-management methods, biofeedback, hypnosis, and various relaxation procedures.

SPECIFIC PSYCHOSOMATIC DISORDERS

Although (a) stress can increase the susceptibility to any disease, and (b) most diseases are currently viewed as multifactorially determined, those that most clearly have a major psychosomatic contribution include the following disorders.

Cardiovascular

Coronary artery disease: This is more common in "type A" personalities. These patients have increased serum cholesterol, low-density lipoproteins, and triglycerides; also increased urinary 17-ketosteroids, 17-hydroxycorticosteroids, and NE. Sudden death by myocardial infarction (MI) is increased in patients experiencing a severe recent loss (first 6 months). Likewise, depression is correlated with increased risk for heart disease (5).

Hypertension: Chronic psychosocial stress *probably* plays a role in its development in genetically predisposed patients. Mechanism is uncertain but may not be related to the brief hypertension that occurs during periods of acute stress. May occur more frequently in type A people and in compulsive people who "store resentment" and who handle angry feelings poorly. Treat first with antihypertensives. Relaxation therapy (e.g., progressive relaxation, meditation, hypnosis) is an effective adjunct to drugs; biofeedback also may help.

Arrhythmias: Palpitation, sinus tachycardia, and worsening of preexisting arrhythmias may all be produced by stress, probably through a sympathetic–parasympathetic imbalance.

Hypotension (fainting): Produced by fear, probably due to peripheral vasodilation and a decreased ventricular filling.

Congestive heart failure: Frequently develops after periods of stress. Anxiety tends to exacerbate the condition.

Raynaud disease: Can often be treated effectively with progressive relaxation or biofeedback.

Migraine: Attacks are often precipitated by stress. Treatment should include medication *and* biofeedback. Consider relaxation and psychotherapy also.

Respiratory

Bronchial asthma: Occurs in people with a genetic predisposition. It is made worse by acute and chronic stress. These patients are at risk for developing neurotic emotional reactions secondary to the respiratory disorder. Good evidence exists that a wide variety of problem-solving and stress-reducing techniques (e.g., psychotherapy, family therapy, systematic desensitization, hypnosis) are effective at preventing attacks in many asthmatics and should be used in conjunction with medication.

Hay fever: Patients have an increased sensitivity to their allergens when stressed, but characteristic symptoms also may develop when no allergens can be identified.

Tuberculosis: Chronic stress often precedes development of the disease.

Hyperventilation syndrome: A common ER presentation (see Chapter 8). Differentiate from panic disorder.

Gastrointestinal

Peptic ulcer: Stress contributes to ulcer development, probably through its influence on the hypothalamic–pituitary–adrenal axis. The chronically frustrated and angry patient with increased gastric HCl (hypersecretor) is at risk. Help the patient develop more stress-free life patterns. Relaxation therapy may be of value.

Ulcerative colitis: Stressful emotional factors often precede disease development and can induce a relapse, but the mechanism is unclear. Nonconfrontive, supportive psychotherapy is indicated to help the patient adapt better to stress and to the illness and to help him deal with the frequently associated anxiety and depression, but psychiatric care alone will not prevent relapses. Other intestinal conditions that are markedly influenced by psychosocial stress include *regional enteritis* (Crohn disease) and *irritable bowel syndrome.* "Functional gastrointestinal disorders" may be associated with a history of physical and sexual abuse in women.

Obesity: Genetic and psychological factors interact. Improper conditioning around food habits, an overvaluation of food, and a negative body image (e.g., "fatso") are central. "Binge eaters" are particularly susceptible to stress. Supportive psychotherapy may be of some value, but behavior modification is most useful. Long-term success is limited; initial weight loss is frequent, but relapses are very common. A change in lifestyle appears essential.

ANOREXIA NERVOSA (p. 583, 307.1): This disorder of profound weight loss without loss of appetite usually develops in adolescence (F:M, 10 to 20:1), continues through the early 20s, and may end in death by starvation (5% over a 5-year period; 20% over a 20-year period). It is increasingly common in upper-middle-class female patients. These patients have a disturbed body image (feel fat in spite of dramatic visual evidence to the contrary) and are preoccupied with losing weight. They diet, exercise, and dangerously abuse diuretics and laxatives, even while family members and professionals attempt to stop them. Many anorexic patients (50% at some time during their course) also binge eat. Major depression, alcoholism, and anxiety disorders are likely to occur at some point (6).

A related condition, **BULIMIA NERVOSA** (p. 589, 307.51), is a chronic disorder characterized primarily by episodic eating binges in adolescent or early adult females (F:M, 5 to 10:1) *of normal weight,* who follow the gorging by self-induced vomiting (purging) or by inducing diarrhea with laxatives. These individuals are weight conscious and markedly depressed by their uncontrolled eating: self-deprecation, major depression, and suicidal ruminations are common, as is substance abuse (25%). Endocrinologic, family history, and treatment findings are similar to those of anorexia, and some patients slip back and forth between the two conditions over time.

Anorexic patients often have hormone imbalances (e.g., amenorrhea), numerous signs of starvation (e.g., edema, bradycardia, and hypothermia), and associated features like ritual behavior (e.g., hand washing). The etiology is uncertain. In a few patients, anorexia is comorbid with avoidant, and bulimia, comorbid with borderline personality disorders. The families frequently have disturbed interpersonal patterns and an increased incidence of eating and affective disorders. Be certain to rule out a primary affective or schizophrenic disorder. Treatment should be comprehensive: hospitalization for severe cases, individual *and* family therapy, behavior modification, and (maybe) antidepressants. In its early stages, this condition is frequently overlooked, yet treatment can be lifesaving. Develop a high index of suspicion in thin, young female patients. The primary treatment goal for anorexic patients is to gain weight: all else is secondary. Anorexic patients, if they survive, tend to be chronically thin women. Bulimics, conversely, benefit most from the combination of outpatient cognitive–behavioral therapy *and* antidepressants (7) [e.g., fluoxetine, 20 to 60 mg/d (8)], but relapses are frequent, whereas a few require antipsychotics. Short-term relapse rate (1 to 2 years) is close to 75% to 80%, but long-term (10+ years) outcome of bulimic patients finds 50%+ symptom free and most of the rest with reduced symptoms.

Musculoskeletal

Rheumatoid arthritis: Symptoms frequently worsen after emotional stress. Stress may be acting as an immunosuppressant. Depression is common in these patients. Psychotherapy is of little value in altering the course of the disease.

Tension headaches: These are caused by chronic muscular tension. Treat with mild analgesics and electromyogram (EMG) feedback from the frontalis muscles or with relaxation techniques (often coupled with vigorous activity).

Spasmodic torticollis: Exacerbated by stress. EMG biofeedback may be useful.

Fibromyalgia: This is a common (3 to 6,000,000 patients in the United States) condition with widespread musculoskeletal aches, stiffness, and points of tenderness ("trigger points") that tend to respond to amitriptyline and multimodal psychotherapy, which includes cognitive–behavioral methods (9).

Low back pain: Treat multimodally.

Endocrine

Conditions that are exacerbated by stress include *hyperthyroidism* and *diabetes mellitus*. Acute and chronic stress may precipitate a thyroid crisis in genetically predisposed patients. Ketosis may be produced and maintained by stress in diabetic patients. Patients with either condition should receive psychotherapy if they have adopted self-destructive life habits and if they experience frequent relapses.

Genitourinary

Most gynecologic disorders reflect primarily an endocrine imbalance, but many of these conditions also can be influenced significantly by psychosocial stress. Psychosomatic influences are most evident for: menstrual disorders (premenstrual tension, amenorrhea, oligomenorrhea), dyspareunia, frigidity pseudocyesis, premature ejaculation, and impotence. Spontaneous abortion can be produced by major stress.

Chronic Pain

Chronic pain patients are common. The sources of their pain may or may not be identifiable. They often have been thoroughly evaluated medically, have experienced several unsuccessful surgical or medical procedures, and may or may not be currently iatrogenically addicted to analgesics [be wary of requests for meperidine (Demerol), oxycodone (Percodan), codeine, propoxyphene (Darvon), pentazocine (Talwin), diazepam (Valium), etc.]. Nothing has helped, and the patients show evidence of depression, hopelessness, chronic anxiety, insomnia, chronic anger, interpersonal withdrawal, somatic preoccupation, or a combination of these. Their lives may be totally dominated by the pain.

Be certain that you are not dealing with conditions that mimic or complicate chronic pain (see Chapter 11):

1. Unrecognized, treatable organic pathology.
2. Primary depression, anxiety disorder, or psychosis.
3. Unrecognized, early delirium or dementia.
4. Drug addiction.

5. Conversion disorder.
6. Somatization disorder.
7. Pain disorder.
8. Hypochondriasis.
9. Histrionic personality disorder.
10. Malingering.
11. Compensation factors.

Always treat the chronic pain patient globally. Do not become overly concerned about whether the pain is "real" or "psychological"—it invariably will have elements of both, and treatments will be similar. Use whatever medical and surgical means are of value but *do not* stop there. Always explore and apply the multiplicity of psychological treatments that are available.

- First, detoxify the patient, if necessary.
- Take the patient and the pain seriously. Be interested, sympathetic, and hopeful. Be a continuing presence; see the patient regularly, and do not abandon him.
- Help the patient identify and accept reasonable expectations. Encourage him to continue functioning; avoid hospitalization.
- Recognize that prolonged administration of analgesics has limited usefulness and great risks, yet can be done therapeutically. Attempt to use no drugs or nonaddicting drugs (e.g., antidepressants, major tranquilizers, antihistamines). Codeine is the preferable narcotic.
- Have the patient keep a pain diary. Work with the patient over time to help him determine what variables improve or worsen the pain.
- Consider the variety of psychological techniques available (e.g., hypnosis, biofeedback, relaxation therapy). Encourage the patient to discover that he is "in control of his own pain." Use these methods within the context of a good therapeutic alliance. Consider family and group therapy. Help others in the patient's environment become more appropriately responsive to the pain.
- Consider some physical procedures (e.g., nerve block dorsal column stimulators, acupuncture, rhizotomy). Avoid surgery if possible.
- Recognize that not all patients will improve markedly.

Other

Skin: A wide variety of psychosocial stressors can exacerbate certain skin conditions, including psoriasis, chronic urticaria, pruritus, and neurodermatitis (eczema). Research suggests that (a) warts (a contagious disease) respond to hypnosis, and (b) **TRICHOTILLOMANIA** (p. 674, 312.39); hair pulling, 1%+ of population (maybe); F/M, 10^+:1; try venlafaxine [37.5 to 450 mg/day (10)], fluoxetine, or clomipramine [related to OCD?].

Malignant disease: Psychological stressors appear to influence the development (but perhaps not the course) of a malignancy. Isolation and depression are mild risk factors for cancer; their repair decreases that risk (11). This may be related to the effect of stress on the immune system. Much work remains to be done, yet some suggestion exists that psychological treatments (e.g., hypnosis) may play a future role in cancer treatment.

Hematologic: Stress may aid clotting among hemophiliac patients. Changes in levels of various blood elements may occur in normal patients under acute stress.

Accident proneness: Some people are at risk for accidental trauma due to psychological characteristics (e.g., impulsive, anxious, hostile).

Chronic fatigue syndrome (CFS): In spite of extensive research, CFS remains a puzzle (12). It is a chronic illness (longer than 6 months; 1% of the population) of unknown etiology (medical? psychological?) characterized by chronic fatigue (particularly after exercise), generalized pain and myalgia, fever and lymphadenopathy, insomnia and hypersomnia, and poor concentration and anterograde memory deficits. Depression is common (13), but antidepressants seldom produce marked improvement. Treatment is supportive, although cognitive–behavioral approaches seem to help (14). With luck, the future will bring clarity.

Seizures: Emotional stress can trigger seizures (both neurogenic and conversion). Psychotherapy and stress management is effective in helping to control seizure disorders, particularly in patients with partial seizures.

REFERENCES

1. Sapolsky RM. *Why zebras don't get ulcers*. New York: WH Freeman, 1998.
2. Levenson JL. *Textbook of psychosomatic medicine*. Washington, DC: American Psychiatric Publishing, 2005.
3. Denollet J, Sys SU, Brutsaert DL. Personality and mortality after myocardial infarction. *Psychosomat Med* 1995;57:582–591.
4. Sifneos PE. Alexithymia: past and present. *Am J Psychiatry* 1996;153:137–142.

5. Glassman AH, Shapiro PA. Depression and the course of coronary artery disease. *Am J Psychiatry* 1998;155:4–11.
6. Sullivan PF, Bulik CM, Fear JL, et al. Outcome of anorexia nervosa: a case-control study. *Am J Psychiatry* 1998;155:939–946.
7. Walsh BT, Wilson GT, Loeb KL, et al. Medication and psychotherapy in the treatment of bulimia nervosa. *Am J Psychiatry* 1997;154:523–531.
8. Mayer LES, Walsh BT. The use of selective serotonin reuptake inhibitors in eating disorders. *J Clin Psychiatry* 1998;59(suppl 15):28–34.
9. Mason LW, Goolkasian P, McCain GA. Evaluation of a multimodal treatment program for fibromyalgia. *J Behav Med* 1998; 21:163–178.
10. O'Sullivan RL, Keuthen NJ, Rodriguez D, et al. Venlafaxine treatment of trichotillomania: an open series of ten cases. *SNS Spectrum* 1998;3:56–63.
11. Spiegel D, Sephton SE, Terr AI, et al. Effects of psychosocial treatment in prolonging cancer survival may be mediated by neuroimmune pathways. *Ann N Y Acad Sci* 1998;840:674–683.
12. Johnson H. *Osler's web*. New York: Penguin Books, 1996.
13. Saltzstein BJ, Wyshak G, Hubbuch JT, et al. A naturalistic study of the chronic fatigue syndrome among women in primary care. *Gen Hosp Psychiatry* 1998;20:307–316.
14. Hotopf M, Wessely S. Chronic fatigue syndrome: mapping the interior. *Psychol Med* 1999;29:255–258.

Chapter 13

Psychiatric Symptoms of Nonpsychiatric Medication

In many medical patients, psychiatric symptoms (1,2) develop because of common side effects of medical drugs, as an idiosyncratic response, from administration of excessive amounts, or as the result of an untoward combination of drugs. Unrecognized, the responsible medications might be continued. Likely offenders (among many) are explored here.

ANTICONVULSANTS

Anticonvulsants as a group typically produce neuropsychiatric symptoms of various kinds when the dose exceeds the usual therapeutic range. Some, however, produce problems in a few patients even at normal doses. Dementia, macrocytic anemia, and lower limb neuropathy may be due to anticonvulsant-induced folic acid deficiency.

- Carbamazepine: Sedation, irritability, and depression at the start of treatment; on to psychosis.
- Phenacemide: Emotional lability, agitation, and confusion in a few.
- Phenobarbital: Normal blood levels (5 to 40 µg/ml) occasionally may produce irritability and mood disturbance, cognitive impairment, confusion, or a combination of these, whereas excessive dosage will produce sedation grading into ataxia and coma. Symptoms of withdrawal may occur if phenobarbital is stopped abruptly.
- Phenytoin: Irritability, nystagmus, tremor, and ataxia often begin at 20 µg/ml and worsen as the dose climbs. Psychosis may occur.
- Primidone: More than 50% of patients experience sedation, irritability, weakness, vertigo, or a combination of these on beginning the medication.

ANTI-INFLAMMATORY AGENTS

- Salicylates: High doses can produce elation and euphoria grading into depression, confusion, and delirium.
- Nonsteroidal anti-inflammatory drugs (NSAIDs): About 50% of patients experience sedation, headache, and dizziness. In high doses, a few will produce anxiety, disorientation, and confusion.

HORMONES

- Exogenous thyroid: Excess can result in symptoms varying from restlessness and anxiety to a psychosis mimicking mania or acute schizophrenia. Inadequately treated patients may display symptoms of hypothyroidism [e.g., fatigue, depression, psychosis (*myxedema madness*)].
- Adrenal corticosteroids (e.g., cortisone, dexamethasone, prednisone): In addition to physical complications, excessive or prolonged use can produce widely varying affective syndromes (e.g., euphoria and hypomania, fatigue, and *depression*) or degrees of a toxic psychosis or both. Steroid withdrawal can produce complaints of weakness and fatigue—suspect *pseudotumor cerebri* if coupled with headache, vomiting, and confusion.
- Estrogens: Restlessness, a sense of well-being, or euphoria may be present.
- Progesterones: May produce fatigue, irritability, tearfulness, and depression when given either alone or in combination as oral contraceptives (2% to 30% of patients).
- Androgens: Restlessness, agitation, aggressiveness, euphoria may occur.

ANTICHOLINERGICS

Anticholinergics are contained in numerous medications and can produce mild peripheral (dry mouth, hypotension) and central (lability, distractibility, restlessness) side effects. For a start, consider
- Antihistamines: diphenhydramine (Benadryl), promethazine (Phenergan), chlorpheniramine (Teldrin), phenylpropanolamine (Ornade), dimenhydrinate (Dramamine).

- Antispasmodics: propantheline (Pro-Banthine).
- Ophthalmic drops: *atropine*, homatropine, cyclopentolate.
- Antiparkinsonian drugs: benztropine (Cogentin), trihexyphenidyl (Artane), 1-cyclohexyl-1-phenyl-3-(1-piperidyl)propan-1-ol hydrochloride (Tremin), procyclidine (Kemadrin), biperiden (Akineton).
- Others: Compoz, Excedrin PM, Sleep-Eze, Sominex, and others containing *scopolamine*.

At higher doses, an *anticholinergic psychosis* (see Chapter 23) can be caused by a variety of these drugs. Treat psychosis with physostigmine, 1 to 2 mg i.m. or slowly i.v.; repeat in 20 minutes if needed.

ANTIHYPERTENSIVES AND CARDIAC DRUGS

- Rauwolfia alkaloids (reserpine): Can cause nightmares, confusion, and profound depression in susceptible patients taking normal doses. Impotence may occur.
- Diuretics (thiazides, furosemide, ethacrynic acid): Fatigue may be found.
- Methyldopa (Aldomet): Persistent lassitude, verbal memory impairment, depression with obtundation and confusion (on normal dosage). Impotence may occur.
- Guanethidine (Ismelin): Mild depression, erectile dysfunction may be found.
- Calcium-channel blockers (flunarizine, cinnarizine; nifedipine, verapamil): Dizziness, lethargy, and euphoria are common with some medications; *depression* with others.
- Clonidine: Sedation, depression; antagonized by tricyclic antidepressants; hypomania on withdrawal occurs sometimes.
- Propranolol (Inderal) and other β-blockers: Fatigue, insomnia, nightmares, verbal memory impairment, impotence, and *depression*; hyperactivity, paranoia, rarely confusion, and a toxic psychosis may occur.
- Digitalis and the cardiac glycosides: Fatigue, apathy, *depression*, toxic delirium, psychosis, or a combination of these may be found, particularly in the elderly.
- Antiarrhythmics (quinidine, procainamide, lidocaine): Mild confusion, mild-to-major delirium, psychotic symptoms, occasionally depression occur.

SYMPATHOMIMETICS

Both catecholamine and noncatecholamine stimulants may produce restlessness, anxiety, fear and panic, weakness, dizziness, irritability, and insomnia in recommended dosages.

BROMIDE

Intoxication is rare; availability of bromide in medications has decreased to almost nothing. Chronic intoxication (weeks, months; "bromism") occurs very infrequently: symptoms range from mild disorientation to full toxic psychosis and dementia. Look for "classic" acneiform rash of face and hair roots (30% of patients).

LEVODOPA

The depression and apathy of Parkinson disease may be relieved, but anxiety and agitation are produced frequently. In about 15% of patients, more serious psychiatric problems develop, including an acute organic brain syndrome with confusion or frank delirium, hypomania, acute psychosis, or major depression. These are often hard to differentiate from the progression of the disease.

HYPOGLYCEMICS (INSULIN, TOLBUTAMIDE)

Symptoms of hypoglycemia occur, including restlessness, anxiety, and disorientation.

ANTIBIOTICS AND RELATED DRUGS

- Tetracyclines: Can produce emotional lability, depression, and confusion—from vitamin deficiencies secondary to alteration of colonic bacteria.
- Nalidixic acid and nitrofurantoin: Lethargy, but rarely confusion is found.

- Isoniazid (INH): Euphoria, transient memory loss, agitation, psychotic reaction, paranoia, catatonic-like syndrome may occur.
- Antimalarials: psychosis may be present.
- Cycloserine: Lethargy and confusion, agitation, severe depression, psychosis, paranoid reactions may occur.

ANTINEOPLASTICS

Depression, acute organic brain syndromes, and psychosis can be produced by a variety of these agents, either by a direct CNS effect or because of involvement of other systems (e.g., anemia).

REFERENCES

1. Brown TM, Stoudemire A. *Psychiatric side effects of prescription and over-the-counter medications*. Washington, DC: American Psychiatric Press, 1998.
2. Patten SB, Love EJ. Drug-induced depression. *Psychother Psychosom* 1997;66:63–73.

Psychiatric Presentations of Medical Disease

Physical and psychiatric illnesses are closely interwoven (1,2). Both medical and psychiatric physicians should know the specifics of these interrelations.

- Of patients needing mental health care, 60% are being treated by medical physicians.
- From 50% to 80% of the patients treated in medical clinics have a diagnosable psychiatric illness, and 10% to 20% of medical patients primarily have an emotional disorder.
- Of patients in psychiatric clinic populations, 50% have undiagnosed medical conditions.
- Of self-referred psychiatric patients, 10% have symptoms solely due to a medical illness.

Always evaluate psychiatric patients medically. Be particularly alert to patients first seen with depression, confusion, memory loss, anxiety, personality changes, psychosis of rapid onset, visual hallucinations, and illusions. Always be suspicious of symptoms of sudden onset in a patient, particularly one older than 35 years, who previously had been problem free. Recognize that patients (or their physicians) often can identify a "precipitating event" for even the most organic of psychiatric conditions—do not be fooled.

Always consider psychiatric possibilities for physical symptoms in medical patients. Take a good history, including past emotional problems. Why is the patient coming for help now?

PSYCHIATRIC SYMPTOMS

Only a few typical psychiatric presentations exist, and many different medical illnesses can cause them. Some of the most common associations are listed later, although almost any physical condition can contribute to symptom production (Table 14.1).

Table 14.1 ■ Common Associations for Psychiatric Symptoms	
Presentation	**Disease**
Anxiety	Hyperthyroidism
	Hypoglycemia
	Pneumonia
	Acute intermittent porphyria
	Pheochromocytoma
	Mitral valve prolapse
	Angina pectoris
	Cardiac arrhythmias
	Hyper- and hypoparathyroidism
	Hypothyroidism
	Cushing disease
	Menstrual irregularities
Depression	Hypothyroidism
	Debilitating disease
	Pneumonia, other infections
	Cushing disease
	Addison disease
	Pancreatic carcinoma
	Intracranial tumors
	Pernicious anemia
	Hyper- and hypoparathyroidism
Confusion, memory loss	Numerous medical conditions (see Chapters 5 and 6)
Mixed psychotic–hysterical symptoms	MS
	Wilson disease
	SLE
	Intracranial tumors
	Hyperthyroidism
	Psychomotor epilepsy
	General paresis
	Huntington chorea
	Metachromatic leukodystrophy
	Porphyria

MEDICAL DISEASES

No medical illness produces pathognomonic psychiatric symptoms, yet each has a typical *range* of presentations. Some of the most characteristic are listed, but more comprehensive sources are available. In many of these diseases, psychiatric pathology develops before any medical signs or symptoms are noticed.

Cardiovascular Disease

Serious heart problems *very* commonly produce psychiatric symptoms, particularly in the elderly (3). The most common heart-related symptom is probably *depression*, regardless of whether the medical situation is congestive heart failure (CHF), survival after a myocardial infarction (MI), or postcardiotomy recovery. Heart patients in whom depression develops are at markedly increased risk for further heart problems (4), making treatment of the depression mandatory; selective serotonin reuptake inhibitors (SSRIs) are currently the medications of choice. In addition to depression, serious heart disease increases the incidence of apathy, disinhibition, and cognitive impairment. Finally, a well-recognized syndrome, **postcardiotomy delirium**, occurs in *one third* of patients after open-heart surgery and is characterized by symptoms that range from mild disorientation through hallucinations and paranoid delusions (5).

Endocrine

- Hyperthyroidism: Anxiety [70%+ meet criteria for generalized anxiety disorder (GAD) at some point], *depression* is common (25% to 50% of patients), with fatigue but restless, emotional lability, irritability, weight loss, and sweating. The elderly are more likely to have apathy, cognitive impairment, and depression. Check for free and bound T_4 levels as well as $\downarrow$TSH; $\male \gg \female$ psychiatric symptoms usually resolve with successful treatment of the hyperthyroidism.
- Hypothyroidism: *depression* (to some degree in most hypothyroid patients), anxiety, irritability, fatigue, apathy, occasionally psychosis ("myxedema madness" in severe cases), dry and puffy skin, EEG slowing, cold intolerance, and persistent cognitive defects are found [even after return to normal hormone levels in some chronic patients (6)]. Look for markedly slowed speech and movement in women (2% of $\female$ population at some time; $\female/\male$ 20:1) with other classic symptoms. Thyroid hormone replacement usually reverses psychiatric symptoms; always look for an abnormal thyroid-stimulating hormone (TSH) concentration and free T_4.
- Hyperparathyroidism: Psychiatric symptoms begin above 12 mg/mL and worsen with $\uparrow$ Ca^{2+} from $\downarrow$ spontaneity and apathy, to anxiety, depression, irritability, and mild to moderate cognitive changes, and on to agitation, confusion, paranoia, hallucinations, delusions, and lethargy worsening to coma (18 mg/ml or so) (7).

- Hypoparathyroidism: Psychiatric symptoms with decreasing Ca^{2+} levels (usually 7 to 8 ml/dl and less) begin with irritability, anxiety, and emotional lability, on through depression, and on to hallucinations, delusions, and delirium. Additional symptoms tend to be medical: muscle cramping (e.g., carpal spasms), paresthesias, seizures, tetany.

- Hyperadrenalism (Cushing syndrome): Psychiatric symptoms may precede other symptoms, particularly in chronic onset. Most common are the full spectrum of *depression* symptoms (50%+, usually the agitated type) and *cognitive impairment* (80%, most commonly memory loss and concentration). Also look for hypomania or mania [usually from exogenous steroids (e.g., prednisone)], anxiety (may grade into depression as the disease progresses), and numerous "psychotic-like" presentations (8).

- Hypoadrenalism (Addison disease): If "acute" the patient is obviously medically ill; however, if "chronic," the patient may have (60%+ of afflicted patients) fatigue, apathy, depression (40%+), irritability, weakness, occasional confusion, and in primary patients, hyperpigmentation.

- Pheochromocytoma: Anxiety, restlessness, apprehension and panic, flushing, headaches; all are found during attacks.

- Hypoglycemia: Usually appears with glucose levels less than 50 mg/dl. Symptoms vary with blood sugar; episodic anxiety, tremor, sweating, fatigue, personality changes, various grades of delirium and bizarre behavior.

- Diabetes mellitus: Depression, apathy, confusion, intellectual dullness.

- Premenstrual syndrome (PMS): In as many as 25% of women, significant physical/psychological discomfort develops during the week before menses, ending shortly after flow begins. Common symptoms include irritability, tension, tearfulness, moderate depression, a sense of bloating, swelling of the extremities, and headaches, but may include more severe symptoms such as profound depression, aggressiveness, and even psychosis. Patients with the more severe symptoms may meet criteria for **PREMENSTRUAL DYSPHORIC DISORDER** (currently classed as **Depressive Disorder NOS**) (9). The etiology is unknown but may be related to hormonal imbalance: possibly prolactin, estrogen, or prostaglandins. Women with a preexisting mood disorder may be at risk for problems. No treatment is certain, but the SSRIs (fluoxetine, paroxetine, and sertraline are currently FDA approved) are by far the most effective.

Infections

Depression, anxiety, organic brain syndrome (OBS), and acute psychosis all can occur because of a variety of infectious processes, depending on the patient's sensitivity, age, and physical condition, the site of the infection, and the agent. Particularly common are symptoms with pneumonia (particularly delirium with bacterial and depression with viral; most common in elderly), infectious mononucleosis (anxiety and psychosis may be the first symptoms; depression is commonly late), viral hepatitis (the posthepatitic syndrome: weakness, irritability, lethargy, depression), syphilis (general paresis), human immunodeficiency virus (HIV), and tuberculosis (TB). The reverse may also be true; psychiatric disorders such as depression may increase the risk for developing infections [e.g., herpes simplex virus (8)].

Other

- Acute intermittent porphyria (10): Psychiatric symptoms are seen first in 15% of cases, whereas 20% to 40% have such symptoms at some time: episodic bouts (days, weeks) of anxiety, irritability, *delirium*, emotional outbursts, depression, acute psychosis; *abdominal pain*, peripheral *motor neuropathies*, *seizures*. Autosomal dominant mutation on chromosome 11; $\female > \male$.
- Hepatolenticular degeneration (Wilson disease): May be seen with a labile mood, explosive outbursts, and psychotic behavior in a young man before the development of cirrhosis, portal hypertension, rigidity, Kayser–Fleischer rings, and dementia.
- Pellagra: A deficiency of niacin (vitamin B_3) may produce the complete syndrome of *dementia*, *diarrhea*, and *dermatitis*; also depression, personality changes, and a confusional psychosis. The proper laboratory diagnosis is the level of N-methylniacinamide, a metabolite of niacin.
- Systematic lupus erythematosus (SLE): Patients (mostly women) may have *depression* (50%), irritability, emotional lability, delirium, dementia, and impaired concentration and attention; sometimes these symptoms appear before physical signs.
- Pernicious anemia: Depression and fatigue but also an organic psychosis. Look at blood for characteristic megaloblastic anemia due to B_{12} deficiency.
- Pancreatic carcinoma: Severe depression in 40% or more of patients; depression, restlessness, and anxiety often precede awareness of the cancer (11). (Anxiety is common as well.) Depression appears more common with CA of lung and brain

as well as with the use of a number of cancer chemotherapeutic drugs.

- Prolapse of the mitral valve: Has been associated with generalized anxiety disorder, panic disorder, and agoraphobia with panic attacks, but the significance of the association is questioned.
- Chronic obstructive pulmonary disease (COPD): Anxiety, depression, and mild to moderate organicity are common.
- Irritable bowel syndrome (12): Gastrointestinal (GI) pain, distention, and gas; *also* psychiatric symptoms of autonomic arousal such as anxiety, panic, weakness, fatigue, headaches, tremor, insomnia, etc. (Is this fundamentally a psychiatric illness?)

REFERENCES

1. Lishman WA. *Organic psychiatry*, 3rd ed. Oxford: Blackwell Publishers, 1998.
2. Levenson JL. *Textbook of psychosomatic medicine*. Washington, DC: American Psychiatric Publishing, 2005.
3. Musselman DL, Evans DL, Nemeroff CB. The relationship of depression to cardiovascular disease: epidemiology, biology, and treatment. *Arch Gen Psychiatry* 1998;7:580–592.
4. Carney RM, Blumenthal JA, Catellier D, et al. Depression as a risk factor for mortality after acute myocardial infarction. *Am J Cardiol* 2003;92:1277–1281.
5. Smith LW, Dimsdale JE. Postcardiotomy delirium: conclusions after 25 years? *Am J Psychiatry* 1989;146:452–458.
6. Leentjens AFG, Kappers EJ. Persistent cognitive defects after corrected hypothyroidism. *Psychopathology* 1995;28:235–237.
7. Watson LC, Marx CE. New onset with neuropsychiatric symptoms in the elderly: possible primary hyperparathyroidism. *Psychosomatics* 2002;43:413–417.
8. Sonino N, Fava GA. Psychiatric disorders associated with Cushing's syndrome: epidemiology, pathophysiology and treatment. *CNS Drugs* 2001;15:361–373.
9. Grady-Weliky TA. Premenstrual dysphoric disorder. *N Engl J Med* 2003;248:433–438.
10. Gonzalez-Arriaza HL, Bostwick JM. Acute porphyrias: a case report and review. *Am J Psychiatry* 2003;160:450–459.
11. Carney CP, Jones L, Woolson RF, et al. Relationship between depression and pancreatic cancer in the general population. *Psychosom Med* 2003;65:884–888.
12. Gaynes BN, Drossman DA. The role of the mental health professional in the assessment and management of irritable bowel syndrome. *CNS Spectrums* 1999;4:19–30.

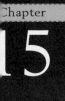

Psychiatric Presentations of Neurologic Disease

Many psychiatric symptoms caused by various neurologic diseases [e.g., central nervous system (CNS) tumor, trauma, seizure, infection] can be correlated directly to the CNS site involved.

FRONTAL LOBES

In prefrontal damage, the *frontal lobe syndrome* occurs with unilateral or bilateral damage (personality changes, irritability, euphoria, apathy, depression, impulsivity, social inappropriateness). Do not mistake this for depression or mania. Intelligence is usually unimpaired in unilateral damage, although memory can be affected. Symptoms are milder if only one side is involved. If the premotor area is involved (on the left), apraxia of the left hand and Broca (expressive) aphasia also may be present. Do not confuse with psychosis.

TEMPORAL LOBES

The hippocampal complex of the temporal lobe mediates recent (anterograde) memory and learning (left side is primarily verbal; right side, primarily visual); the amygdala mediates emotion-laden memories; the temporal poles and inferotemporal regions coordinate retrograde memory. Stimulation or lesions may produce auditory or visual hallucinations or emotions such as fear, anxiety, and perhaps OCD. Bilateral lesions may result in the amnesia of Korsakoff and the Kluver-Bucy syndrome (placidity and hypersexuality).

PARIETAL LOBES

Dominant lobe lesions may produce language difficulties (e.g., inability to express or understand spoken words, perform simple tasks, read or write or both), tactile agnosia, apraxia, and intellectual deterioration. Nondominant lobe lesions may produce anosognosia.

OCCIPITAL LOBES

Some lesions produce crude visual illusions (distortions) and hallucinations.

LIMBIC SYSTEM

Effects are diverse but usually involve primitive and emotional behavior (e.g., emotional lability, fear, rage, impulsivity, irritability, depression, memory loss). Also, amnestic syndrome is seen when mammillary bodies are involved (Korsakoff syndrome).

NEUROLOGIC DISEASES

Neurologic disorders can produce a variety of psychiatric symptoms. Consult a comprehensive source for detailed descriptions of specific conditions. Some major diseases include the following:

- **Parkinson disease:** *Depression* [50%, do not confuse with motor symptoms (1)], dementia [40%, psychosis in 30%+ (2)], and anxiety (30%).
- **Huntington chorea:** May present first with psychiatric symptoms (e.g., emotional lability, impulsiveness, depression (up to 40%), hallucinations, delusions). Do not mistake for *schizophrenia*. Look for family history (autosomal dominant, chromosome 4), chorea, and dementia (subcortical type).
- **Multiple sclerosis** (MS): Psychiatric symptoms are common, particularly early *depression* (50%) (3), emotional lability, euphoria, and late-onset subcortical depression. Differentiate from the very common *fatigue* (80%+) and acute or chronic pain (4).
- **Intracranial tumors:** 50% of patients develop psychiatric symptoms, and occasionally they may be the presenting symptoms. Pattern is site related, although usually a degree of generalized organicity is seen. Early personality changes are often subtle (e.g., "He's not the same person anymore"). Temporal and

ventral frontal tumors produce most mood and psychotic abnormalities, with occipital tumors likely responsible for visual disturbances.

- **Head trauma** (5): If a postconcussion syndrome follows the confusion and perhaps brief loss of consciousness (LOC) of a mild head trauma, it may be accompanied by some combination of decreased memory and attention, fatigue, apathy, headache, dizziness, insomnia, irritability, emotional lability or anxiety or both, depression, and personality changes. The course may be brief or long-lasting.

- **CNS infection:** Meningitis and encephalitis can produce the most psychiatric symptoms; be alert to an initial rapid onset of delirium, fever, headache, stiff neck, focal signs. Herpes simplex encephalitis often has mood and cognitive changes and high fatality. Lyme disease meningitis displays a wide variety of psychiatric symptoms (6), with depression most common (30%+). General paresis (chronic CNS syphilis) usually is seen as a gradually developing dementia.

- **Stroke:** *Poststroke depression* is common (50%+ of patients) and associated with specific (moderately well-localized) anatomic locations of damage (7); major depression and dysthymia with L-frontal, L-basal ganglia, and L-posterior sites. Do not mistake for Broca (expressive) aphasia (dominant frontotemporal area) or aprosodia (nondominant frontotemporal area). Inappropriate cheerfulness, anxiety, and anhedonia may result from R-orbitofrontal damage. Major depression lasts for 9 to 12 months, and dysthymia, for 2 years, but both often respond to antidepressants or electroconvulsive therapy (ECT). Treat aggressively.

- **HIV/AIDS** (8): The brain becomes involved within days of HIV infection with a concentration on subcortical structures. Early, subsyndromal HIV infection may display mild cognitive problems in a few patients, but, with worsening, mild to moderate cognitive impairment occurs in 15%+, and HIV-associated dementia, in 7%+. As HIV infection worsens, psychiatric symptoms become more prominent and severe: depression (most common; suicide is a major risk), delirium, various anxiety presentations, insomnia, substance abuse, psychosis. Some combination of apathy and depression, anxiety and agitation, and denial occur in many AIDS patients and requires therapy. Minor memory, language, and concentration abnormalities develop in many as HIV grades into AIDS; in 50% or more, serious neurologic complications develop late that may become delirium or dementia or both. Always rule out other medical causes for the neuropsychiatric presentations such as neoplasms, medication side effects, hepatic or renal problems, metabolic abnormalities, etc.

- **Epilepsy:** Depression (50%+ lifetime among epilepsy patients), psychosis, schizophrenia-like psychotic syndrome, anxiety, and panic all can develop as interictal problems among patients with epilepsy. Temporal lobe seizures (TLE) and partial seizures (both simple and complex) can produce bizarre behavior and experiences during the event. Patients with these forms of seizures are also at highest risk for postictal abnormal behavior as well as the interictal psychiatric syndromes listed earlier (9).

- **TOURETTE DISORDER** (DSM p. 111, 307.23): This neuropsychiatric syndrome of uncertain etiology usually develops in latency or early adolescence (before age 18; ♂:♀ = 3:1) with the onset of vocal and multiple motor tics such as head or extremity tics, eye blinks, and the spasmodic production of coughs, grunts, or "barks" that occasionally can progress to phrases and verbal obscenities (coprolalia; 10% of patients) (10). Symptoms must last 1 year for diagnosis. TD may be severe and lifelong, is familial (along with other tic phenomena), appears to have a major genetic component, and is associated within families (genetically?) with OCD and chronic tic disorder and also possibly with hyperactivity (ADHD) and learning disorders. All symptoms are worsened by stress and may be improved by psychotherapy. The primary treatment is pharmacologic (11) [e.g., begin with an atypical antipsychotic and progress to a traditional antipsychotic if needed: haloperidol (past mainstay; 60% to 70% of patients improve; 1 to 5 mg/day) but consider pimozide (2 to 12 mg/day), risperidone (2 to 4 mg/day, may produce depression) (12), ziprasidone (20 to 30 mg/day), olanzapine (5 to 15 mg/day). To avoid an antipsychotic, try clonidine (0.1 to 0.5 mg/day; 30% to 40%+ respond), desipramine (to a maximum of 100 mg/day), and clonazepam (maximum of 2 to 3 mg/day). Stimulant medication for ADHD can precipitate or worsen Tourette symptoms (usually reversibly) in some patients but can also help, so use cautiously, if at all].

REFERENCES

1. Brooks DJ, Dodor M. Depression in Parkinson's disease. *Curr Opin Neurol* 2001;14:465–470.
2. Aarsland D, Ballard C, Larsen JP, et al. A comparative study of psychiatric symptoms in dementia with Lewy bodies and

Parkinson's disease with and without dementia. *Int J Geriatr Psychiatry* 2001;16:528–536.

3. Sadovnick AD, Remick RA, Allen J, et al. Depression and multiple sclerosis. *Neurology* 1996;46:628–632.

4. Ehde DM, Gibbons LE, Chwastiak PG, et al. Chronic pain in a large community sample of persons with multiple sclerosis. *Mult Scler* 2003;9:605–611.

5. Silver JM, McAllister TW, Yudofsky SC. *Textbook of traumatic brain injury.* Washington, DC: American Psychiatric Publishing, 2005.

6. Fallon BA, Nields JA. Lyme disease: a neuropsychiatric illness. *Am J Psychiatry* 1994;151:1571–1583.

7. Singh A, Herrmann N, Black SE. The importance of lesion location in poststroke depression: a critical review. *Can J Psychiatry* 1998;43:921–927.

8. Treisman GJ, Angelino AF, Hutton HE. Psychiatric issues in the management of patients with HIV infection. *JAMA* 2001; 286:2857–2864.

9. Trimble MR, Mendez MF, Cummings JL. Neuropsychiatric symptoms from the temporolimbic lobes. In: Salloway S, Malloy P, Cummings JL, eds. *The neuropsychiatry of limbic and subcortical disorders.* Washington, DC: American Psychiatric Press, 1997: 123–132.

10. Leckman JF. Tourette's syndrome. *Lancet* 2002;360:1577–1586.

11. Jimenez-Jimenez FJ, Garcia-Ruiz PJ. Pharmacological options for the treatment of Tourette's disorder. *Drugs* 2001;61:2207–2220.

12. Scahill L, Leckman JF, Schultz RT, et al. A placebo-controlled trial of risperidone in Tourette syndrome. *Neurology* 2003; 60:1130–1135.

Alcohol is *the* major substance of abuse. About 55% of Americans drink; 7% are heavy drinkers (men, 3:1); 20%+ have alcohol-abuse problems at some time (peak at age 21); the lifetime risk for alcoholism is 10% to 14%; and 40% of homicides and automobile deaths are alcohol related (1). Certain populations are at risk (e.g., elderly urban blacks, urban Indians, bartenders, musicians). Finally, mixed abuse of alcohol and other drugs is extremely common.

CLASSIFICATION

Normal (recreational) drinking grades into pathologic use. **ALCOHOL ABUSE** (DSM p. 214, 305.00) exists if clearly recurrent (not continuous) impaired social and occupational functioning due to alcohol use is present over a 1-year period. Individual patterns can vary from steady sporadic consumption to periodic binges. All demonstrate the inability to abstain from drinking or to stop drinking once started, despite an obvious downward spiral. Such drinking may result in depression and anxiety. Beginning often as evening and weekend drinking, the pattern usually becomes established by the late 20s in men (later in women) with gradual deterioration in some during their 30s and 40s. Spontaneous remissions can occur: they are the norm, but they are temporary. *Blackouts* (anterograde amnesia for events that occurred during acute intoxication but while the patient was conscious, functional, and appearing normal to those around him or her) often develop as abusive drinking becomes more serious.

If the patient also demonstrates tolerance (increased amounts needed to achieve effect), withdrawal, compulsive and continuous use, or a combination of these, he has **ALCOHOL DEPENDENCE (ALCOHOLISM)** (DSM p. 213, 303.90). Cultural groups are differently affected [e.g., low among Jews and Asians: 50%+ of Asians have genetic polymorphisms that metabolize alcohol (ethanol) rapidly and its metabolite, acetaldehyde, slowly, producing unpleasant acetaldehyde side effects such as "flushing"]. All social strata are affected—fewer than 5% are "skid row" types. No "typical alcoholic personality" exists. Alcoholism is comorbid with chronic anxiety disorders, mood disorders (particularly in women), schizophrenia, dementia, and antisocial personality disorder; the presence of these conditions is often both (and/or) an effort to "self-medicate" with alcohol and the aftereffect of primary alcoholism. Nevertheless, always rule out (or treat) these psychiatric disorders.

The etiology of alcoholism is unknown. Evidence for genetic biologic characteristics grows but is not without controversy (risk of developing alcoholism: one alcoholic parent, 4 times normal risk; both parents alcoholic, 60% risk). Adoption studies indicate a genetic factor in some families: increased frequency of alcohol abuse and sociopathy among male relatives and possibly increased somatization among female relatives of alcoholics. Recent research identifies two groups of alcoholics (2):

Type 1: adult onset; steady, gradually escalating consumption; guilty, worried, rigid, perfectionistic, dependent, introverted; modest family history; both men and women; some recover completely; 75% of alcoholics.

Type 2: alcohol seeking from adolescence and early adulthood; impulsive; distractible; risk taking; antisocial characteristics with recklessness and aggression; *strong* family history; primarily men; very treatment resistant; 25% of all alcoholics.

Moreover, certain predictive biologic features of future alcoholism may be inherited by some first-degree relatives (particularly men) of alcoholics [e.g., a *resistance to intoxication* (the person who can "really hold his liquor" from an early age is at a *very* high risk to develop alcoholism), a subnormal cortisol increase after drinking, and a subnormal epinephrine release after stress]. Alcohol stimulates the release of dopamine from the nucleus accumbens, producing euphoria. Over time, the dopaminergic neurons atrophy and natural level of dopamine decreases, producing malaise unless the level is stimulated by alcohol (i.e., very reinforcing). With abstinence, the alcoholic's dopamine level may take months or years to recover.

RECOGNIZING THE ALCOHOLIC

Clinical Markers

The *majority* of alcoholics function fairly well most of the time and go unrecognized by physicians until their social and occupational lives and their physical health have been significantly harmed. Early recognition is important. These patients frequently conceal alcohol use; keep a high index of suspicion if the predominant complaints include chronic anxiety and tension, insomnia, chronic depression, headaches, blackouts, nausea and vomiting, vague gastrointestinal problems, tachycardia, palpitations, and frequent falls or minor injuries. Ask about absenteeism, job loss, financial difficulties, and family trouble. Ask "Do you drink?" Be encouraging and nonjudgmental. Get drinking specifics (number of beers per day, oz/glass, drink alone?, etc). Interview relatives and friends, if possible.

Screening Tests

Use a brief screening questionnaire (but remember, patients often "fake good"). Two that are quick and reliable are the *SAAST* (Self-Administered Alcoholic Screening Test; can be computer scored; takes 10 minutes; accurate when completed by a relative) and the *CAGE* (consists of four "mnemonic" questions; two or more positive answers are suggestive of alcoholism) (3):
1. "Have you ever felt you should Cut down on your drinking?"
2. "Have people Annoyed you by criticizing your drinking?"
3. "Have you ever felt bad or Guilty about your drinking?"
4. "Have you ever had a drink first thing in the morning to steady your nerves or get rid of a hangover (Eye opener)?"

A subscale of the MMPI, the MacAndrew Scale (Mac), consists of 49 MMPI items and provides a degree of reliability when coupled with the MMPI validity scales.

Biologic Markers

Chronic drinking frequently elevates serum γ-glutamyltransferase (GGT) and RBC MCV (together they identify 90% of alcoholics). These measures, coupled with evidence of more acute alcoholic insult (protein, Alk Phos, LDH, SGOT, SGPT, etc.), constitute a fairly reliable laboratory screen for alcoholism. A new blood test, carbohydrate-deficient transferrin (CDT), has demonstrated a sensitivity of 82% and specificity of 97%. It could be very useful but primarily when used with other tests because its sensitivity is very high, and it is likely to pick up "normal heavy drinkers" (like college students).

CLINICAL PRESENTATIONS OF ALCOHOL SYNDROMES

When suspecting alcohol problems, always determine whether (a) the patient is *currently intoxicated*, and (b) the time since the patient's *last drink*.

Intoxication Syndromes

■ Alcohol Intoxication (DSM p. 214, 303.00)

Alcohol is a CNS depressant that initially disinhibits and then depresses. Early intoxication includes liveliness, a sense of well-being, and a smell of alcohol on the breath [blood alcohol levels (BALs) up to 100 mg/dl, 100 mg%, or 0.1%]; grading into irritability, emotional lability, and incoordination (0.1% to 0.15%); which grades into apathy, slurred speech, and ataxia (0.15% to 0.25%); which can become *alcoholic coma* (above 0.25% to 0.4%, an emergency—get blood alcohol level and check for presence of other drugs; treat with intubation, CPR, etc., if necessary). Blood alcohol levels vary with drinking history and thus are only approximate; behavior may vary from depressed and maudlin to agitated and aggressive. As intoxication wanes over a period of 6 to 12+ hours, a "hangover" usually supervenes (headache, malaise, dysphoria, nausea, shakes, diaphoresis), which can last the better part of a day.

Acute intoxication can mimic schizophrenia, mania, depression, hysteria, etc., so delay detailed interview and final diagnosis until the patient is sober. Evaluate *carefully* for medical problems (see later)—differential includes hypoglycemia, CNS infection, and toxic psychosis of other etiology. Intoxicated patients may be uncooperative, assaultive, and dangerous—be civil, nonthreatening, accepting, respectful, patient, but prepared with force. Attempt nonpharmacologic management (quiet room, support, coffee), but sedation may be necessary (e.g., diazepam, 5 to 20 mg i.m., erratically absorbed), but be cautious of oversedation. Decide if the patient just needs to "sleep it off" (most common), is at risk for withdrawal, or is becoming comatose. Should the patient go home with family, be observed overnight, be hospitalized, or go to jail? Be familiar with community resources.

Alcohol idiosyncratic intoxication or pathologic intoxication is an unusual and controversial condition (not currently in DSM-IV) of marked aggressiveness and emotional lability, occasionally of psychotic proportions, that follows ingestion of small quantities of alcohol in an otherwise normal person. Etiology is unknown.

Some patients retain this pattern for life. Episodes appear suddenly and may last for hours or a day or more, often with amnesia for the episode afterward. Sedate [benzodiazepines, haloperidol (Haldol)], and control until sober. Rule out temporal lobe epilepsy. *Alcoholic paranoia* (DSM p. 338, 291.5) has a similar presentation but with strong paranoid delusions, typically of jealousy: it usually occurs in chronic alcoholics who are actively drinking and who can become violent.

Alcohol-withdrawal Syndromes

These may occur in heavy drinkers or alcoholics who stop drinking *or* who *just reduce* their consumption. Do not overlook them in the "closet" alcoholic (e.g., the businessman or housewife who temporarily abstains while in the hospital for other reasons). If the patient is withdrawing, delay final diagnostic conclusions.

■ Alcohol Withdrawal (DSM p. 215, 291.81)

Tremulousness, hyperreflexia, weakness, nausea and vomiting, "dry heaves," anxiety, insomnia and bad dreams, mild illusions and hallucinations, hypervigilance, paresthesias, numbness, tinnitus, blurred vision, or a combination of these begin during the first 12 to 18 hours of reduced drinking and lead to a vicious cycle of worsening agitation. No EEG slowing is found; instead, the waves are normal or fast. Debilitated medically ill patients are at risk. *Alcoholic convulsions* (generalized, self-limited, single, or in small groups) occur in some (fewer than 10%), usually in the first 2 days of withdrawal but sometimes later. If the seizure is focal, suspect CNS pathology (e.g., subdural). Some patients experience marked hallucinations as part of the withdrawal, with intact reality testing: **A.W., with Perceptual Disturbance** (DSM p. 216).

■ Alcohol-induced Psychotic Disorder, with Hallucinations (DSM p. 338, 291.3)

The patient displays striking auditory hallucinations (voices, sounds), which the patient believes to be real, along with mixed other withdrawal symptoms (mild tremor, anger, apprehension), but the patient typically has a *clear sensorium* and is *oriented*. It usually occurs in the first 3 days after cessation of drinking in patients who have had years of heavy drinking. Patients may be dangerous or self-destructive while hallucinating. It may be self-limited (weeks to months), but occasional cases last for many months or become chronic, dependent in part on whether the patient continues drinking. Differential includes alcoholic paranoia and toxic psychosis (amphetamine, cocaine). Differentiation from paranoid schizophrenia is difficult in chronic cases (look for other signs of schizophrenia).

■ Alcohol-withdrawal Delirium (DSM p. 143, 291.0)

Alcohol-withdrawal delirium [*delirium tremens* (DTs)] is a life-threatening delirium that follows worsening withdrawal and is characterized by disorientation, agitation, memory disturbances, hallucinations (usually visual but also tactile, auditory, vestibular, etc.), delusions, powerful autonomic discharge (hypertension, tachycardia, sweating), tremor, ataxia, and fever beginning 2 to 8 days after reduced drinking. Tremulousness and seizures can precede, and often are mistaken for, the much less common DTs. Malnourishment and medical illness increase the risk of delirium. Mortality rate is 10% to 15% for the complete syndrome (often from secondary infection or acute heart failure). Perhaps 3%+ of alcoholics ever experience DTs.

COMPLICATIONS OF CHRONIC ALCOHOLISM

Medical

Gastritis, gastric ulcer, diarrhea, anemia, hypertension, acute pancreatitis (after 10 or more years of drinking), cirrhosis (in fewer than 10% of alcoholics: alcohol plus poor diet), vitamin malabsorption (particularly A, B_{12}, thiamine, and folate), persistent impotence, insomnia, results of accidents. (*Note*: Most alcoholics die 15 years early, but not of these diseases; rather they die of heart disease and cancer.)

Neurologic

1. Sensorimotor polyneuropathy (vitamin B deficiencies): 10% of alcoholics;
2. Alcoholic cerebellar degeneration: Perhaps half of very severe alcoholics;
3. Central pontine myelinolysis: Delirium and paralysis developing over days;
4. Marchiafava–Bignami disease: Primary degeneration of the corpus callosum;
5. Cerebral atrophy;
6. Alcoholic myopathy and cardiomyopathy: Mostly proximal limb muscles;

7. Wernicke encephalopathy [the *triad*: **delirium**, ataxia, eye-movement dysfunction (*vertical* and horizontal nystagmus and marked weakness of conjugate gaze and external rectus muscles)] develops over hours to days, because of thiamine deficiency (give 50 mg i.v. and 50 mg i.m., then 100 mg i.m. b.i.d. until patient is eating). This is an emergency—if treated early, it usually clears quickly and may prevent Korsakoff syndrome; untreated, 50% of patients die.

Psychiatric

1. **ALCOHOL-INDUCED PERSISTING AMNESTIC DISORDER** (*Korsakoff syndrome*) (DSM p. 177, 291.1) is a profound short-term memory loss (thus anterograde amnesia but may also lose decades retrograde) with confabulation, which often abruptly follows untreated Wernicke encephalopathy but may develop insidiously. Typically, events are remembered for several minutes and then are forgotten, yet this failing does not usually seem to bother the patient. Because of thiamine deficiency, lesions responsible for the anterograde amnesia are believed to be in the mammillary bodies, mammillo-thalamic tract, and anterior thalamus (previously thought to be in the dorsomedial thalamus). The retrograde amnesia and apathy found in many patients is believed to be due to diffuse frontal lobe damage. Treat as in Wernicke disease. Impairment is often incapacitating and lifelong, yet 75% improve somewhat with time.
2. **ALCOHOL-INDUCED PERSISTING DEMENTIA** (DSM p. 168, 291.2) refers to a dementia (i.e., all intellectual functions affected) that ranges from mild to severe and follows many years of alcohol abuse with no other obvious etiology. Personality changes dominate the clinical picture with varying cognitive impairments; cortical atrophy and ventricular enlargement by MRI appears; these are partially reversible if the patient stops drinking. Few alcoholics are affected, and the predisposition is unknown.
3. Suicide: Alcohol is involved in many/the majority of suicides.
4. Drug abuse: Assume the serious drug abuser is a drinker, until proven otherwise.

Other

1. *Fetal alcohol syndrome* describes small, hyperactive, retarded children with variable anatomic abnormalities, including pto-

sis, epicanthal folds, hypoplastic maxilla, cleft lip and palate, microcephaly, and hypospadias. Although not definite, it is thought to be due to a teratogenic effect on the fetus caused by alcohol consumed by the mother while pregnant. It is one of the most common causes of retardation (4).

TREATMENT OF WITHDRAWAL

Treatment varies with the severity of the symptoms. When in doubt, hospitalize temporarily; however, most patients manifesting mild withdrawal symptoms without medical complications can be treated in a supportive and *sober* environment, with daily clinic visits until stable and with good nutrition and occasionally little or no medication (social detoxification). The following apply to the more serious withdrawals; medication is used to ensure sleep, prevent exhaustion, reduce agitation, and control autonomic symptoms (monitor tremor). Serious withdrawal should be done in a hospital.

1. Be clear and unambiguous. Identify yourself. Explain procedures. Place patient in a lighted room. Include family and familiar people. Use restraints if needed. Keep under *constant observation.*

2. *Carefully* evaluate (PE, chest radiograph, chemistry, electrolytes including calcium and magnesium, CBC, CT, occult blood in stool, occasionally an LP). Incidence of complicating disorders is high (e.g., pneumonia, TB, UTIs, hypoglycemia, diabetic ketoacidosis, anemia, shock, gastritis with hematemesis, acute hemorrhagic pancreatitis, cirrhosis and hepatic failure, meningitis). Be particularly careful to exclude (a) a *subdural hematoma* due to a fall, and (b) withdrawal from other substances. Treat these conditions if present.

3. Benzodiazepines are currently the withdrawal medication of choice. Determine the starting dose by sedating until calm (e.g., control tremor; avoid oversedation), and address other symptoms, and then taper over a 4- to 8-day period (i.e., decrease by approximately 20% of total first day's dose each day). If a delirium is present, it often resolves within 1 day. Next best medication class is probably anticonvulsants [e.g., carbamazepine or valproate (5)]. Consider carbamazepine, 200 mg b.i.d. or t.i.d., or divalproex. 70 mg b.i.d. to start, and modify to control symptoms. Use a medium-acting benzodiazepine PRN to help with symptoms in the first several days if

necessary. Recognize, however, that the anticonvulsants do not seem to prevent alcohol-withdrawal seizures or DTs. Phenothiazines lower the seizure threshold but may be useful with psychosis and extreme agitation.

- *Tremulousness*: [e.g., chlordiazepoxide, 25 to 50 mg p.o. (or diazepam, 10 to 20 mg), every 4–6 hours until comfortable]. Lorazepam (6 to 12 mg/day) or oxazepam may be better choices in patients with liver disease or confusion. Moderate levels of benzodiazepines may be all that is necessary in most mild to moderate withdrawals.
- *Delirium*: [e.g., chlordiazepoxide, 50 to 100 mg, p.o. or i.m. every hour until calm (able to stay in bed) and then q4h]. Intramuscular doses are often poorly absorbed—can lead to early undersedation, and then cumulative oversedation. If condition is severe, give i.v. slowly. Benzodiazepines alone may not relieve delirium; consider low-dose haloperidol. Clonidine, a sympathetic inhibitor, may relieve sweating, tremor, and tachycardia but does not prevent DTs. β-Blockers (e.g., atenolol, 50 to 100 mg/day) used with benzodiazepines may shorten the course.

4. If withdrawal seizures persist or a primary seizure disorder exists, consider 5 to 10 mg of diazepam slowly by i.v., or oral diphenylhydantoin, carbamazepine, or depakote combined with a benzodiazepine.

5. Give thiamine, 100 mg i.m., and then 50 mg p.o. t.i.d. for 4 days. Also provide a high-carbohydrate diet and multivitamins daily (and for weeks/months).

6. Correct fluid and electrolyte imbalances, particularly hypokalemia (replace carefully over 24 hours or longer via i.v.) and significant hypomagnesemia (may exacerbate seizures—give magnesium sulfate, 2 to 4 ml of 50% solution i.m. q6h for 2 days).

7. Record pulse, BP, and temperature every half hour initially. Treat shock with fluids, whole blood, and vasopressors.

8. Check for and treat hypoglycemia, prolonged prothrombin time (PT; give vitamin K, 10 mg i.m.), and fever (aspirin, sponge baths—rule out superimposed infection).

9. Anxiety, irritability, depression, and insomnia may persist for weeks after the acute episode—a vulnerable period for the alcoholic. Even serious depression may spontaneously resolve after several weeks of sobriety; do not over (or under) treat. Antianxiety agents may be of use for several weeks but *do* discontinue.

TREATMENT OF ALCOHOLISM

Successful treatment of alcoholism is difficult but not hopeless. No definitive psychosocial treatment exists. Most alcoholics who become abstinent do so in addition to treatment, not because of it [see the classic *50-year* follow-up study of male alcoholics (6)].

1. Identify its presence. Get your facts straight (family drinking history, recent intake).
2. Develop a personal rapport with the patient—be warm and supportive but firm. Be open and matter-of-fact about the drinking, but insist on abstinence. Remember, you cannot really evaluate/work with a patient unless he is abstinent— wait until the patient is sober before investing time in treatment. Encourage the patient to maintain employment and social involvement. Help develop coping skills. Although it may seem cruel, allow the patient to experience the "natural consequences" of his behavior, but use good judgment in doing so.
3. Treat all medical complications of drinking.
4. Treat any complicating primary psychiatric illness (e.g., schizophrenia, affective disorder, anxiety disorder).
5. Enlist family members in treatment. Evaluate family's contribution to the problem. Consider family or marital therapy or both.
6. Consider disulfiram (Antabuse; a "sensitizing" agent) use in cooperative but backsliding patients (i.e., patients "who can't stop drinking") (7). It inhibits aldehyde dehydrogenase, leading to toxic acetaldehyde buildup 15 to 30 minutes after alcohol consumption, which leads to anxiety and apprehension, sweating, nausea and vomiting, tachycardia, headache, and hypotension. Give 500 mg p.o. qd for 1 week, and then maintain on 250 mg daily (range, 125 to 500 mg). Carefully inform patient of the possible reactions. Effects last up to 2 weeks after the last dose; however, not every patient shows an Antabuse reaction. Occasional adverse effects include sedation, a metallic taste, mild GI disturbances, mild ataxia, and a peripheral neuropathy. Question its use in irresponsible patients; hepatotoxicity and toxic psychoses can occur, and severe reactions (to a large alcohol challenge) can lead to hypotension and coma. It is contraindicated in patients with unstable medical conditions or histories of psychosis, brain trauma, MI, or heart failure. The biggest problem with disulfiram: patients stop taking it so they can drink. It is often only modestly effective.

7. *Naltrexone* (ReVia; 50 mg/day, p.o.), an opioid antagonist, is promising: It *decreases craving* (i.e., reduces the euphoria of alcohol and thus the drive to drink) in many alcoholics. It decreases relapse, decreases alcohol intake on relapse, and makes a remission more likely (8). It can be used with acamprosate (see later; 9). Compliance has been addressed with an effective, new, long-acting i.m. form (Vivitrol; give every 30 days) (10), which can be given to patients who are actively drinking. Typically used for 3 to 6 months in conjunction with intensive psychosocial interventions; may be needed over the long term if craving and relapse return. Another effective maintenance agent using a different neurobiologic mechanism is *acamprosate* (Campral; 666 mg p.o., give t.i.d.) (11). It reduces the elevated excitatory glutamatergic transmission and resultant NMDA-receptor stimulation that results from chronic alcohol use; the result seems to be a decreased alcohol use. Some patients respond well, others not at all; accurately predicting who will respond is not yet possible (12). Other (infrequently) effective drugs when used alone but better when used in special cases include anticonvulsants [e.g., divalproex, topiramate (13), lithium (with mania/depression), buspirone (in the anxious alcoholic), and antidepressants (definitely should be used when the patient is also depressed)].

8. *Group therapy* appears to be the most effective psychotherapy technique. In most cases, work with or refer patients to a specialized multidisciplinary treatment team. Make referral personally, with the patient present. Alcoholics Anonymous (AA) can help some (although it has a very high initial dropout rate)—encourage patients to give it a try. Alanon (spouses of alcoholics) also is useful. Hospitalize in an alcohol unit (milieu therapy) if even temporary sobriety cannot be achieved.

9. Be patient. Keep trying.

REFERENCES

1. Substance Abuse and Mental Health Services Administration. *Results from the 2002 National Survey on Drug Use and Health. National Findings* (DHHS Publ No SMA 03–3836). Rockville, MD: Substance Abuse and Mental Health Services Administration, 2003.

2. Sigvardsson S, Bohman M, Cloninger CR. Replication of the Stockholm Adoption Study of Alcoholism. *Arch Gen Psychiatry* 1996;53:681–687.

3. Ewing JA. Detecting alcoholism: the CAGE questionnaire. *JAMA* 1984;252:1905.

4. Steinhausen HC, Spohr HL. Long-term outcome of children with fetal alcohol syndrome: psychopathology, behavior, and intelligence. *Alcohol Clin Exp Res* 1998;22:334–338.

5. Reoux JP, Saxton AJ, Malte CA, et al. Divalproex sodium in alcohol withdrawal: a randomized, double-blind placebo-controlled trial. *Alcoholism, Clin Exp Res* 2001;25:1324–1329.

6. Vaillant GE. *The natural history of alcoholism revisited.* Boston, MA: Harvard University Press, 1995.

7. Fuller RK, Dranchey L, Brightwell DR, et al. Disulfiram treatment of alcoholism: a Veteran's Administration Cooperative study. *JAMA* 1986;256:1449–1455.

8. Kranzler HR, Armeli S, Tennen H, et al. Targeted naltrexone for early problem drinkers. *J Clin Psychopharm* 2003;23:294–304.

9. COMBINE Study Research Group. Testing combined pharmacotherapies and behavioral interventions for alcohol dependence (the COMBINE study): a pilot feasibility study. *Alcohol Clin Exp Res* 2003;27:1123–1137.

10. Garbutt JC, Kranzler HR, O'Malley SS, et al. Efficacy and tolerability of long-acting injectable naltrexone for alcohol dependence. *JAMA* 2005;293:1617–1625.

11. Bouza C, Magro A, Munoz A, et al. Efficacy and safety of naltrexone and acamprosate in the treatment of alcohol dependence: a systematic review. *Addiction* 2004;99:811–828.

12. Mann K, Lehert P, Morgan MY. The efficacy of acamprosate in the maintenance of abstinence in alcohol-dependent individuals: results of a meta-analysis. *Alcohol Clin Exp Res* 2004;28:51–63.

13. Johnson BA, Ait-Daoud N, Bowden CL, et al. Oral topiramate for treatment of alcohol dependence: a randomized controlled trial. *Lancet* 2003;361:1677–1685.

Psychiatry of Drug Abuse

Drug abusers are common (6% lifetime prevalence in the United States as a whole, but pockets exist with much higher prevalence; M > F for all age groups), often unrecognized, and poorly understood (1). Great variability is found in the degree of drug use from patient to patient; *multiple drug use* is common. **Abuse** occurs if the patient (a) uses drugs in a dangerous, self-defeating, self-destructive way; (b) has difficulty controlling his use, even though the use may be sporadic; and (c) has impaired social or occupational functioning or both because of that use, all within a 1-year period. Drug **dependence** requires the presence of tolerance, withdrawal, continuous, compulsive use, or a combination of these over a 1-year period. Patients may be classified by the type of drug abused (see later) or by the pattern and reason for abuse. Some recognized patterns of use (abuse) include the following:

- **Recreational use:** Patients take drugs "for fun" and are not physically or psychologically dependent on them. They may also take them "just to be part of the group" (e.g., adolescents) or because it is a countercultural requirement. This slowly may grade into compulsive use.
- **Iatrogenic addiction:** Patients addicted "by mistake." Patients (and physicians) may or may not recognize the addiction. Many of these patients are convinced that they must have the drug to function (e.g., to sleep, to interact with others) and may go to great lengths to talk their physician(s) into prescribing medication.
- **Chronic drug addiction:** These patients usually abuse "street" drugs (but not always; e.g., pain medications, sedative–hypnotics). Many have underlying depressions. Many have antisocial personalities. Some take drugs to self-medicate a chronic psychiatric disorder (e.g., major depression, schizophrenia).

Drug abusers are not "all alike," but they do have many common features, including the frequent presence of marked depression and anxiety, increased dependency needs (often hidden), low self-esteem, a familial association (genetic?) with antisocial personality disorder and alcoholism, a dysfunctional family, and a prolonged course resistant to treatment. Drug use to "self-medicate" specific psychiatric illnesses (anxiety, depression, panic disorder, schizophrenia) accounts for a modest amount of abuse. More commonly, however, it is the reverse: chronic drug abuse produces emotional problems.

Treatment of chronic drug abusers is difficult; frequently an inpatient setting is required. Whether as inpatients or outpatients, drug abusers should be treated firmly but with support and understanding. Set clear limits and stick to them. Deal with the patient only when he is not intoxicated (except for an acute crisis, of course). Be reasonably challenging. You will be tested and manipulated by many patients; do not respond with retribution. Follow many of the principles used in treating the alcoholic patient (see Chapter 16). Involve peers in a formal way, (e.g., group therapy). However, recognize that over time, 60% to 75% of drug-dependent people (of all types) stop by themselves. The most common drugs of abuse, their clinical presentations, and treatment follow.

OPIOIDS

Drugs Involved

- Opium (principal active ingredient, morphine)
- Morphine
- Diacetylmorphine (heroin, horse, smack)
- Methadone
- Codeine
- Oxycodone (e.g., Percodan, Percocet, Oxy Cotin)
- Hydromorphone (Dilaudid)
- Pentazocine (Talwin)
- Meperidine (Demerol)
- Propoxyphene (Darvon)
- Hydrocodone (Lortab, and others)

Some of these compounds are naturally occurring (opium and its constituents morphine and codeine), whereas the others are semisynthetic or wholly synthetic. Some of these drugs have legitimate uses (e.g., morphine, meperidine), whereas others are solely substances of abuse (e.g., heroin). Most are obtained illegally "on the street" and are used primarily by a young or middle-aged, lower socioeconomic population (although heroin is becoming "fashionable" among higher social classes currently), whereas others are abused more widely (e.g., Demerol, Dilaudid, and Percodan are commonly abused by professionals). Opioid drugs bind to *mu, kappa, delta,* and *lambda* **locus coeruleus** cell receptors (particularly **mu**) and inhibit norepinephrine release, producing the "high" of opioid abuse. After several weeks, the mu receptors have adjusted to the excess stimulus, and when the drug is stopped, the "mu agonist withdrawal syndrome" or norepinephrine hyperactivity of the locus coeruleus begins, producing the withdrawal syndrome. Typical routes of administration are i.v. (heroin, morphine, methadone: "mainlining"), s.c. (heroin, meperidine: "skin popping"), nasally (heroin: "snorting"), orally (methadone, Percodan), and smoked (opium). It is frequently very difficult to determine the daily dose used because (a) the abuser often consciously over- or underestimates the dose, and (b) the amount of active drug in a "bag" bought on the street is uncertain. A bag of heroin may be 95% adulterants (e.g., quinine, mannitol, lactose), although recently the purity of "street" heroin has increased (some bags being more than 50% heroin).

Abuse (**OPIOID ABUSE**, p. 271, 305.50) and dependency (**OPIOID DEPENDENCE**, p. 270, 304.00) are common in some populations, and the search for drugs or money for drugs accounts for the majority of the crime in some communities. Some people (fewer than 50%) are able to abuse opioids without becoming dependent (i.e., without progressing to tolerance or withdrawal or both), and they often use them recreationally without addiction. Those persons who become dependent represent a high-risk group. Recognize that we currently seem to be in a heroin epidemic similar to the "crack" epidemic of a decade ago: inexpensive, high-quality heroin is readily available and seems targeted at youth (e.g., heroin use has doubled among 8th graders over the past decade).

- 1%+ of all heroin addicts in the United States die each year; 25% die within 10 to 20 years from beginning their habit. The most common cause is an inadvertently fatal overdose (OD) (e.g., an addict using "bags" of 5% heroin accidentally buys a supply containing 15% heroin). Also common is death during violent crime or, increasingly, AIDS.
- 25%+ of addicts have a personality disorder, usually the antisocial type. They also have a high incidence of depression and anxiety. The suicide rate is elevated.
- Heroin addicts are at markedly increased risk (dirty needles, poor nutrition, etc.) for developing certain medical illnesses such as:
  - HIV/AIDS, but also
  - Serum or infectious hepatitis
  - Subacute bacterial endocarditis

- Pneumonia, TB; pulmonary edema, embolus, abscess
- Cellulitis, thrombophlebitis, septicemia
- UTIs, glomerulonephritis, nephrosis
- STDs
- Needle "tracks" on the arms (and legs)

Always carefully evaluate hospitalized addicts medically. Recognize that the analgesic properties of opioids may obscure acute medical problems. After several weeks of use, addicts lose the rush and are left with chronic anxiety and dysphoria; still the craving and hope for euphoria is so strong, and withdrawal so unpleasant, that they continue to abuse. The majority of addicts "grow out of" their habit over the years (or die); thus relatively few old abusers are alive.

Treatment of the opioid addict usually means treatment of the acute episodes (e.g., intoxication and withdrawal; see later). "Cure" of the addiction does occur in some well-motivated patients [and is particularly possible in new, young (e.g., teen) addicts], yet most addicts continue their abuse over many years. The three major forms of **maintenance** treatment (all with controversial results) are as follows:

Agonist Maintenance: (a) Patients are maintained as outpatients on daily doses of *methadone* of 40 to 120 mg (60 mg daily is sufficient for most patients). This level controls the craving for (and eliminates the euphoria from) heroin. The patient can then develop some skills, hold a job, go to school, etc.: psychotherapy can help some, but treatment demands careful limit setting (20% to 50% of patients abuse cocaine or alcohol or both while taking methadone). Moderately motivated patients *may* succeed by this route. Patients remain on methadone for 1 to 20+ years (or life); (b) *LAAM* (levo-α-acetylmethadol; ORLAAM, an oral solution), a chemical congener of methadone, has recently found use as a long-acting replacement for methadone (80 mg, 3×/wk) (2). Unfortunately, many of these patients as well continue to abuse other drugs while taking LAAM (cocaine and "crack" are common); (c) A new long-acting, sublingual, partial opioid agonist, *buprenorphine* (Subutex), appears safe [although some have concerns when given with benzodiazepines: deaths have occurred (3)], is given daily in a dose of 16 mg, and, perhaps most important, appears to decrease the patient's craving for cocaine as well (4).

Residential, drug-free, self-help programs are favored by some. Patients (usually highly motivated) stay 1 to 2 years (or more) in a close "therapeutic community," which insists on the drug-free state and on personal responsibility. Confrontation and behavior modification are frequently used. "Poor" candidates usually drop out. Similar outpatient programs are common.

The two major features of illicit opioid use that bring patients to medical attention are intoxication (and overdosage) and withdrawal.

OPIOID INTOXICATION (p. 271, 292.89). It develops rapidly after an i.v. dose (1 to 5 minutes). The time course of intoxication varies with the drug used (Table 17.1). The abstinence syndrome begins after this period in the dependent patient. It is because of these kinetics that many heroin addicts "shoot up" 3 to 4×/day, or more.

Intoxication symptoms are similar for most narcotics.

Psychological symptoms: A "rush" immediately follows i.v. administration (described as a "whole-body orgasm" with the focus in the abdomen). This is accompanied by euphoria and a sense of well-being or dysphoria (usually anxiety and fear), a drowsiness and "nodding off," apathy, psychomotor retardation, and difficulty concentrating.

Physical symptoms: Miosis (pupillary constriction), slurred speech, respiratory depression, hypotension, hypothermia, bradycardia, constipation, and nausea and vomiting. Skin ulcers are common with meperidine injection. Seizures may occur in the patient tolerant to meperidine.

An OD (either accidental or intentional) is a medical emergency; these patients may die of respiratory depression and pulmonary edema. Look for needle tracks and pinpoint pupils in the unconscious patient, but recognize that if the patient already has experienced significant CNS anoxia, the pupils may be dilated. Seizures occasionally occur (particularly with meperidine). Treat the OD with intensive medical care (ICU) and the narcotic antagonist naloxone (Narcan). Give 0.4 mg i.v. and repeat ×5 at 3-minute intervals. Expect a rapid response (i.e., clearing in 1 to 2 minutes), and if this does not occur after four doses, suspect another etiology for the coma. If the patient improves, continue monitoring; the patient probably will need additional doses of naloxone because it has a much shorter half-life than heroin and certainly methadone and LAAM. Excessive naloxone may throw

Table 17.1 ■ Time Course for Opioid Intoxication	
Drug	**Duration of action (hr)**
Heroin	4–6
Methadone	12–24
Meperidine	2–4

a dependent patient directly from coma into withdrawal; do not be confused. Multiple drugs may have been taken; be alert to the possibility of a more slowly developing coma from a second agent. Of course, get a STAT urine drug screen.

OPIOID WITHDRAWAL (p. 272, 292.0). In spite of its reputation as a dramatic and traumatic withdrawal syndrome, opioid withdrawal is uncomfortable but usually not life-threatening in healthy young adults and is not as dangerous or as difficult to manage as the withdrawal from sedative–hypnotic drugs. Symptoms are similar for each of the narcotics, but the time course varies (dependent partly on the "size of the habit") (Table 17.2).

Psychological symptoms: Early, often intense drug craving followed by severe anxiety, restlessness, irritability, insomnia, and decreased appetite. In this state, the hospitalized patient is frequently extremely demanding and manipulative.

Physical symptoms: Yawning, diaphoresis, tearing, rhinorrhea, *pupillary dilation, piloerection* (hard to "fake" so look for it), muscle twitching, and hot flashes. Later nausea and vomiting, fever, hypertension, tachycardia, tachypnea, diarrhea, and abdominal cramps appear. Seizures occur with meperidine withdrawal.

Newborn addicts: Babies born to addicted mothers, including those on methadone maintenance, often experience an abstinence syndrome, including a high-pitched cry, irritability, tremor, fever, decreased food intake, vomiting, yawning, and hyperbilirubinemia.

Be aware that successful withdrawal is only the beginning of the treatment of opiate dependence. **Withdraw** the opioid gradually by using oral methadone (chosen because of long half-life) to lessen the symptom severity. After a complete history and physical (including urine screen for opioids and other drugs), wait for signs of withdrawal, and then give methadone 10 mg p.o. Establish the stabilization dose over the first 1 to 2 days by adding 5 to 10 mg of methadone on a q.i.d. schedule as the

Table 17.2 ■ Time Course for Opioid Withdrawal			
Drug	Time after last dose that symptoms began (hr)	Symptoms peak	Symptoms disappear (days)
Heroin	4–8	1–3 days	7–10
Methadone	12–48	4–6 days	10–21
Meperidine	2–4	8–12 hr	4–5

patient continues to show *signs* of abstinence (recognize that some patients will vigorously demand more drugs even while they are sedated by their current dose). Once stabilized, give the methadone on a qd or b.i.d. schedule, and reduce the total daily amount by 5 mg/day (or 10% to 20% of the stabilization dose, but more slowly with outpatients). Most withdrawals from heroin addiction take 7 to 10 days; methadone-addiction withdrawals should be done more slowly (e.g., 2 to 3 weeks). An alternate method of opiate withdrawal is to use **clonidine** (Catapres), which reduces withdrawal symptoms (nausea, vomiting, diarrhea, cramps but not muscle aches, insomnia, or craving) by stimulating the α_2-adrenergic receptors on the locus coeruleus (0.1 mg q4 to 6h until stable to maximum of 1.2 mg/day, and then taper 0.1 to 0.2 mg/day) (5). (Withdraw Talwin from patients by using decreasing doses of Talwin.) Many patients who become free of their drug find the craving irresistible and need to be maintained on methadone to stay "clean." Naltrexone (ReVia) seems to block the euphoric effects of the opioids (50 mg daily), as it does with alcohol, and can be used in patients taking clonidine who are (temporarily) free of opioids. Given daily or 3 times weekly; it blocks the positive effects of opioids but may produce dysphoria, anxiety, and GI distress initially. Of course, the biggest problem is that the patient still craves the opioid and may become noncompliant with the naltrexone.

If a patient is withdrawing from both opioids and sedative–hypnotics (not uncommon), concentrate on a safe sedative–hypnotic withdrawal by maintaining the patient on the stabilization dose of methadone until the first withdrawal has been completed.

SEDATIVE–HYPNOTICS

- **Benzodiazepines:** Alprazolam (Xanax), chlordiazepoxide (Librium), clonazepam (Klonopin), clorazepate (Tranxene), diazepam (Valium), estazolam (ProSom), flurazepam (Dalmane), halazepam (Paxipam), lorazepam (Ativan), oxazepam (Serax), prazepam (Centrax), quazepam (Doral), temazepam (Restoril), triazolam (Halcion)
- **Benzodiazepine-like drugs:** Zolpidem (Ambien), eszopiclone (Lunesta)
- **Barbiturates:** Amobarbital (Amytal; *blues*), butabarbital (Butisol), butalbital (Fiorinal), pentobarbital (Nembutal; *yellow jackets*), phenobarbital (Luminal), secobarbital (Seconal; *reds*)

- **Older Sedative–hypnotics:** Much higher abuse potential; some discontinued (e.g., Quaalude)
- Chloral hydrate, ethchlorvynol (Placidyl), ethinamate (Valmid), glutethimide (Doriden; *blues*), meprobamate (Equanil, Miltown), methyprylon (Noludar)
- **Others:** γ-Hydroxybutyrate (GHB, "date rape" drug)

All of these sedative–hypnotic drugs are abusable and can produce dependency, even the safest of the classes, such as long–half-life benzodiazepines and zolpidem. Among this group of drugs, the benzodiazepines (and zolpidem) dominate clinical use: most of the older drugs are highly addictive but fortunately are becoming increasingly uncommon. Any "minimum addictive dose" should be considered very approximate; marked individual differences exist. Recognize that some patients can become dependent on benzodiazepines when the drugs are used *in therapeutic doses*: the signs are often very subtle but very real. The risk for addiction increases with factors such as (a) short-acting drugs, (b) rapid onset of action, (c) high doses, (d) increased chronicity of use [1 to 2 months is usually safe, but not always (particularly high-potency drugs)], whereas 8 to 12 months poses a great risk for withdrawal, even by using benzodiazepines (perhaps 90%+ at therapeutic doses (6)], (e) long-term PRN use (rather than continuous use; curious), (f) nonbenzodiazepine drugs, (g) concurrent alcoholism and polydrug abuse, (h) chronic anxiety or dysphoria, and (i) severe withdrawal effects (i.e., discomfort *and* a belief that the drug is required to treat the underlying condition).

Clinical Syndromes

The same variety of syndromes occurs with sedative–hypnotic abuse as occurs with alcohol. There is cross-tolerance between alcohol and the sedative–hypnotics as well as among the various drugs themselves. The clinical picture varies little from drug to drug (although withdrawal phenomena are more severe, but often briefer, with the shorter-acting drugs).

SEDATIVE, HYPNOTIC, OR ANXIOLYTIC INTOXICATION (p. 286, 292.89). Symptoms of intoxication are dose related. Mild intoxication includes a sense of well-being, talkativeness, irritability, and emotional disinhibition (uncommon; unpredictable). Increased doses produce apathy, confusion, stupor, and coma. Physical signs of intoxication include slurred speech, ataxic gait, incoordination, reduced DTRs, lateral nystagmus, and constricted pupils. Look for fast activity on the EEG. Fatalities are frequent with nonbenzodiazepine sedative–hypnotic ODs, usually due to respiratory depression. Benzodiazepine ODs generally are safe unless combined with another drug such as alcohol or an opiate.

Always evaluate sedative–hypnotic-abusing patients with intoxication for an overt or covert OD. If they are becoming increasingly lethargic, treat as a medical emergency with hospitalization and intensive medical care. Obtain blood and urine levels.

SEDATIVE, HYPNOTIC, OR ANXIOLYTIC ABUSE (p. 286, 305.40). This condition results from the pathologic use of one or more of this class of drugs for more than 1 month. These patients frequently cannot abstain from use, once started—a psychological addiction. Abuse of sedative–hypnotics is common. General cognitive impairment, anterograde amnesia, subtle psychomotor failings of which the patient is unaware, and mild to moderate depression become increasingly common the longer the drug is used, even at subintoxication doses. At least two distinct populations and patterns of abuse are recognized.

1. Male and female patients in their teens or 20s who obtain these drugs illegally and use them (as well as many other kinds) "for fun" and to get high or to block things out and "get away from the hassle."
2. Middle-aged women (and men) who are frequently chronically anxious or depressed and who obtain legal prescriptions from (one or more) physicians for complaints of anxiety and insomnia, gradually increase the dosage themselves in an effort to cope, and often become physiologically addicted. Although these patients are common, they are seen most commonly by general physicians because they ultimately have to "doctor shop" to obtain drugs. Recognize them. Recognize also that these patients frequently vigorously deny their illness, both to their physicians and, sometimes, to themselves.

Without exception, if the patient takes enough drug long enough, tolerance to it will develop and/or signs of physiologic withdrawal when it is stopped. If he or she *also* displays drug-seeking behavior and alters normal life activities to take the drug, then he has **SEDATIVE, HYPNOTIC, OR ANXIOLYTIC DEPENDENCE** (p. 285, 304.10). Most people are not "reinforced" by benzodiazepines and thus do not become dependent; alcoholics are the major exception. Some evidence suggests that a familial pattern exists for the abuse of these substances (e.g., family members also abuse sedative–hypnotics and *alcohol*). Once detoxified, the sedative–hypnotic addict is more likely to "stay clean" if treated with an antidepressant or an anticonvulsant (such as carbamazepine, but not phenobarbital).

SEDATIVE, HYPNOTIC, OR ANXIOLYTIC WITHDRAWAL (p. 287, 292.0). This may be the most dangerous of the drug-withdrawal syndromes and can occur both in the dependent person who abstains and also in the person who merely reduces his dose. Its severity depends on the particular drug abused, the duration of use, the speed of discontinuation, and the daily dose used (degree of tolerance). Keep a high index of suspicion. It is often difficult to differentiate withdrawal from a marked worsening of symptoms due to *rebound anxiety*. Drugs such as alprazolam (used in high doses for panic disorder), lorazepam, and triazolam are particular offenders. Recognize withdrawal (a) by a history of significant drug use (*often* denied by the patient), (b) by characteristic abstinence symptoms (see later), and (c) by a Tolerance Test. The patients are typically very uncomfortable.

Withdrawal Symptoms

Psychological: A subjective sense of severe anxiety, restlessness, apprehension, irritability, insomnia, and anorexia that has developed gradually over the past 24 hours (1 to 7 days with the longer acting sedative–hypnotics) and is worsening hour by hour. Delirium may occur (**SEDATIVE, HYPNOTIC, OR ANXIOLYTIC WITHDRAWAL DELIRIUM**, p. 143, 292.81) with visual hallucinations and formication (sense of insects crawling on the skin).

Physical: Tremulousness (coarse tremor, primarily the upper extremities), weakness, nausea and vomiting, hypertension, tachycardia, hyperreflexia, diaphoresis. After several days, this may progress to delirium, hyperpyrexia, and coma. Seizures may occur (typically after 2 to 5 days), usually generalized and single or in a short series, but occasionally status epilepticus.

Tolerance Test

Several methods are used for determining the degree of dependence (and thus the probable severity and length of withdrawal). One method is given here. It can be used regardless of the particular sedative–hypnotic drug of abuse (i.e., they are all cross-tolerant).
1. Hospitalize the patient for the test if possible.
2. Administer test to a patient who is comfortable or only mildly anxious (*not* to a patient who is intoxicated or presently withdrawing; the test would be invalid).
3. Give 200 mg of pentobarbital orally.

4. At 1 hour, evaluate the patient. If he is
   - asleep but can be aroused, patient has no tolerance.
   - grossly ataxic, with coarse tremor and nystagmus, the daily tolerance is 400 to 500 mg of pentobarbital.
   - mildly ataxic, with mild nystagmus, the daily tolerance is 600 mg.
   - comfortable, with slight lateral nystagmus, the daily tolerance is 800 mg.
   - asymptomatic or has continuing signs of mild withdrawal, the daily tolerance is 1,000 mg, *or more*. Wait 3 to 4 hours, and then give an oral dose of 300 mg of pentobarbital. Failure to become symptomatic at this larger dose suggests a daily tolerance of greater than 1,600 mg.

Treat withdrawal vigorously and carefully. Usually hospitalize unless the addiction is mild and the patient reliable. Evaluate for medical illness. Withdrawal can be accomplished safely by using several different sedative–hypnotics (reliable, iatrogenically addicted patients often are withdrawn with decreasing doses of their drug of abuse), although the most commonly used are diazepam, chlordiazepoxide, clonazepam, pentobarbital, and phenobarbital.

To withdraw with pentobarbital, give the estimated daily tolerance dose (obtained either by reliable history of all cross-tolerant drugs and alcohol used or by a tolerance test) equally divided on a q6h schedule for the first and second days, and then reduce 10% of the initial dose each day. Expect the patient to be somewhat uncomfortable, but if signs of serious withdrawal (or intoxication) appear, slow (or quicken) the decrease slightly. Also expect a waxing and waning course as the detoxification proceeds. If the patient is showing serious withdrawal symptoms before treatment, give enough pentobarbital over several hours to make him or her comfortable, and then begin the withdrawal procedure. The duration of the withdrawal may be as brief as 5 to 7 days for short-acting drugs and as long as a month or more for long-acting benzodiazepines.

SEDATIVE, HYPNOTIC, OR ANXIOLYTIC-INDUCED PERSISTING AMNESTIC DISORDER (p. 177, 292.83). This profound, short-term, anterograde and retrograde memory loss (Korsakoff syndrome) is usually reversible.

GHB (γ-hydroxybutyrate)

GHB is a dangerous drug currently used by young adults as a "club drug." In low doses (10 to 20 mg/kg), it usually produces euphoria, relaxation, and sexual disinhibition, grading into sedation and amnesia. At moderately higher doses, it produces anesthesia, coma, vomiting, respiratory depression, and death; treat with supportive care; the patient usually rouses after several hours, but may be variously combative. A narrow window exists between "normal" doses and a lethal dose.

Because it is odorless and almost tasteless (slight salty taste) and produces sleepiness, increased sexual drive, and amnesia, it has become known and used as a "date-rape drug"; it is slipped into someone's drink without their knowledge. It has a low likelihood of addiction but if taken numerous times daily (short half-life; gone by 3 to 6 hours), tolerance does develop. Withdrawal begins within 5 hours after a dose with tremor, nausea, anxiety, and tachycardia progressing to agitation, impaired cognition, delirium, and autonomic dysregulation in severe users lasting as long as several weeks (7). Treat with high to very high doses of benzodiazepines, often i.v.

HALLUCINOGENS

Drugs Involved (8)

LSD-like:
Lysergic acid diethylamide (LSD-25, *acid*)
Dimethyltryptamine (DMT)
Dimethoxymethylamphetamine (DOM, *peace, STP*)
5-Methoxy-3, 4-methylenedioxyamphetamine (MDMA, *ecstasy, XTC, X, Adam*)
3, 4-Methylenedioxyamphetamine (MDA)
Psilocybin
Mescaline (*peyote, tops, cactus*)
Salvinorin A (from *Salvia divinorum*; Salvia, Sally D)

Others:
Phencyclidine (PCP, *angel dust, crystal, hog*)
Thiocyclidine (TCP)
Ketamine (Ketalar)
Cannabis (marijuana, *hashish, pot, weed, grass, reefer*)
delta-9-Tetrahydrocannabinol (THC)

LSD, Mescaline, and Others:
Patients take these drugs orally (or smoked, e.g., salvinorin A), develop symptoms in 5 to 45 minutes, and are back to normal in several hours (e.g., LSD) to 1 to 2 days. New synthetic drugs, with different characteristics, are created and "hit the streets" regularly,

both in this class and among the stimulants: the world of *designer drugs*. The typical consequence of ingestion (**HALLUCINOGEN INTOXICATION**, p. 252, 292.89) is as follows.

Psychological symptoms: Marked perceptual distortions (changing object shapes, changing body image), illusions and hallucinations (mostly visual geometric designs, but also auditory and tactile), depersonalization, derealization, and synesthesias (stimuli in one modality produce sensations in another; e.g., sounds become colors)—all occurring in a clear sensorium. The patient is usually aware that what he or she is experiencing is due to drugs (i.e., has insight, unlike the patient with amphetamine psychosis). Occasionally the patient experiences strong depressive or anxious feelings (e.g., panic; a "bad trip"), but more typically, the mood is euphoric, and the patient feels that he or she is receiving profound, staggering insights (a "claim to fame" of *ecstasy*).

Physical symptoms: Tachycardia, palpitations, diaphoresis, pupillary dilation (responsive to light), blurred vision, tremor, incoordination, hyperreflexia, hyperthermia, piloerection.

The psychological symptoms are particularly sensitive to the "set" or expectations of the patient before drug use. Occasionally the patient will experience brief hallucinations weeks, months, or even years after the period of drug use: **HALLUCINOGEN PERSISTING PERCEPTION DISORDER**, p. 252, 292.89 (*flashbacks*). Flashback frequency generally decreases with time but may continue for years, even in the absence of additional hallucinogen use, if marijuana is used regularly. Although these are primarily recreational drugs, a few patients disrupt their lives with drug use (**HALLUCINOGEN ABUSE**, p. 252, 305.30). No withdrawal symptoms are experienced, although slight tolerance does develop.

Two clinical syndromes that may (infrequently) follow the use of these drugs by one or more days are

1. **HALLUCINOGEN-INDUCED PSYCHOTIC DISORDER, WITH DELUSIONS** (p. 338, 292.11). These delusions that occur with drug use may persist for a variable length of time after the drug is out of the body; and
2. **HALLUCINOGEN-INDUCED MOOD DISORDER** (p. 405, 292.84). Persistence of depression or anxiety lasts for days, weeks, or longer after taking the drug. The presentation may be identical to or gradually develop into a major mood disorder.

Treatment for "bad trips" usually consists of support ("talking down"); patient usually clears within hours. Benzodiazepines and phenothiazines may be used briefly (e.g., diazepam, 10 to 15 mg; haloperidol, 4 to 5 mg) if patient is "wild."

Phencyclidine (PCP)

PCP abuse (**PHENCYCLIDINE ABUSE**, p. 279, 305.90; **PCP DEPENDENCE**, p. 279, 304.90) is most common among young adult men. PCP typically is eaten, taken i.v., or (more recently) smoked. Symptoms begin in several minutes (smoked) or an hour or more (orally) and are dose dependent. Symptoms and side effects of **ketamine** are very similar but usually milder and with a shorter half-life (9).

Psychological symptoms: Low doses produce euphoria, grandiosity, a feeling of "numbness," and emotional lability. Higher doses cause symptoms that range from perceptual distortions, anxiety, excitation, confusion, and synesthesias to a paranoid psychosis, rigidity, and a catatonic-like state to convulsions, coma, and death. Violent (and self-destructive) behavior is probably rare (in spite of its reputation) either when intoxicated or perhaps several hours later during withdrawal.

Physical symptoms: Tachycardia, hypertension, vertical and horizontal nystagmus, ataxia, dysarthria, myoclonus, decreased pain sensitivity, diaphoresis, seizures.

The patient usually clears in 3 to 6 hours, but waxing and waning symptoms may last for days or longer with high doses. The symptom picture can be quite variable and can include a delirium lasting days but that may last weeks (**PHENCYCLIDINE INTOXICATION DELIRIUM**, p. 143, 292.81), delusions (**PCP-INDUCED PSYCHOTIC DISORDER, WITH DELUSIONS**, p. 338, 292.11), or a varying organic mood disorder (**PCP-INDUCED MOOD DISORDER**, p. 405, 292.84). Long-term organic symptoms may occur (memory loss, word-finding difficulty), perhaps because of massive fat storage. Diagnosis is based on the clinical picture, a history of PCP use, the presence of PCP in urine, and (possibly) hair analysis (11). Chronic, denied PCP use can easily be misdiagnosed as "atypical psychosis," so be wary. Infants from addicted mothers often show hyperirritability, hypertonia, and delayed development that may last for months or even years.

Treatment is controversial. ODs can be fatal. Hospitalize and use gastric suction, urine acidification (ascorbic acid), fluids and diuretics, and symptomatic medical maintenance. If agitation must be controlled, consider diazepam or haloperidol. Decrease external stimulation.

MDMA (ecstasy)

The role of MDMA, although illegal, is currently uncertain. It is the classic "club drug" used by teens and those in their early 20s at "raves," where frantic dancing may last all night and is considered by participants as safe, because it produces a sense of well-being, of emotional warmth and closeness to others, and of sharp mental clarity, all without apparently being addictive. However, a "hangover" can last for a day or two, and a few individuals may experience weeks or more of depression, anxiety, confusion and lack of mental clarity, and paranoia (11). An open question exists as to whether ecstasy produces permanent loss of serotonergic neurons to the hippocampus and amygdala with consequent impairment in cognition and memory. Moreover, deaths have occurred at "raves" from dehydration, hyperpyrexia, and hypertension. It is not an entirely "safe" recreational drug.

Cannabis

The active ingredient of cannabis is delta-9-tetra-hydrocannabinol (THC). The various forms (e.g., marijuana, hashish) are all either smoked or eaten, and the differences in the effects they produce depend primarily on their concentrations of THC. Cannabis is used widely (daily alcohol and marijuana use are about equal among high school seniors; in a recent study, 20% of 8th grade students have used marijuana), and a single dose usually produces mild physical and psychological alterations (**CANNABIS INTOX-ICATION**, p. 237, 292.89), which occur shortly after intake and last 2 to 4 hours.

Psychological symptoms: The primary effect is a sense of well-being, mild euphoria, and relaxation. Mild alterations and intensifications of perceptions occur (greater with the more-concentrated forms), as does a sense of indifference and slowed time. A few persons find the use of cannabis dysphoric, and depression, anxiety, panic, dissociation, or even a delusional syndrome develops (usually paranoid, often with depersonalization) (**CANNABIS-INDUCED PSYCHOTIC DISORDER, WITH DELUSIONS**, p. 338, 292.11). Impaired psychomotor perform-ance, attention, time sense, and memory (ability to learn) during and shortly after use is common (expected); driving is dangerous. Prolonged, frequent use produces broad cognitive and resulting social/occupational impairment (12).

Physical symptoms: Tachycardia, hypertension, *conjunctival injection*, dry mouth, hunger. Prolonged, heavy use is carcinogenic.

Toxic psychoses have been reported with high-dose use. Some persons are socially and occupationally handicapped by prolonged drug use (look for morning hangover) (**CANNABIS ABUSE**, p. 236, 305.20). These patients are frequently apathetic and "amotivational," but this may be more a reflection of their personality structure than an effect of cannabis. If a significant degree of tolerance occurs (often develops quickly with heavy use), coupled with continued use despite impaired life functioning, the patient has **CANNABIS DEPENDENCE** (p. 236, 304.30). Dependence is more common than previously believed and occurs in about 10% of users (13). Withdrawal symptoms tend to be mild: irritability, anxiety, "flu-like."

Treat "bad trips" with support. Surreptitious use of marijuana can be detected up to several weeks after use by a urine screen for delta-9-THC-11-oic acid (THCA).

STIMULANTS

Drugs Involved

- Amphetamine (Adderall, Benzedrine)
- Dextroamphetamine (Dexedrine)
- Methamphetamine [Desoxyn, Methedrine; snorted or swallowed (*speed, crystal*), smoked (*ice, glass*), i.v. (*crank*)]
- Methylphenidate (Ritalin)
- Phenmetrazine (Preludin)
- Cocaine (including "crack")

These are effective orally (except cocaine) and nasally (cocaine), but produce a more rapid and intense effect by smoking [cocaine ("crack"); crystal methamphetamine ("ice")] and i.v. (an orgasm-like "rush"). Street terms for amphetamines include speed, bennies, uppers, diet pills, crystal, double crosses, crosstops, and ice; for cocaine, they include coke, snow, and crack (rock); and "speedball" for amphetamine or cocaine with an opioid. *Crack*, the alkaloidal, free-base form of cocaine HCl, is inexpensive, widely available, and extremely addicting. Use of a new, smokable form of methamphetamine (ice), which produces a crack-like effect, has recently become the most popular and serious drug of abuse in the United States (and Asia) (14).

Clinical Syndromes

The effects of **AMPHETAMINE INTOXICATION** (p. 226, 292.89) and **COCAINE INTOXICATION** (p. 244, 292.89) occur within minutes (depending on route).

Psychological symptoms: Hyperalertness, restlessness, psychomotor agitation, pacing, talkativeness and pressure of speech, sense of well-being, elation. Frequently aggressiveness, agitation, violent behavior, and poor judgment occur as well. As use increases, look for paranoia, homicidal impulses, psychosis, and cognitive deterioration.

Physical symptoms: Tachycardia, hypertension, pupillary dilation, chills and diaphoresis, anorexia, nausea and vomiting, and insomnia. Occasionally stereotyped repetitive movements occur (e.g., endlessly taking something apart and then reassembling it). Prolonged smoking of methamphetamine reduces all the user's teeth to black rotting stumps (*meth mouth*).

With brief use, symptoms usually disappear within hours of stopping the drug. All these symptoms may disappear as tolerance develops.

If drug use becomes a consuming pattern that lasts for at least 1 month and interferes with social and occupational functioning, the patient has **AMPHETAMINE ABUSE** (p. 225, 305.70) or **COCAINE ABUSE** (p. 236, 305.60). Abuse usually develops over months and may include a pattern of "runs" of frequent, large-dose i.v. administration (crank), or smoking (ice, crack) over days or weeks. After a run, the person frequently sleeps for 12 to 18 hours, and then may begin another run. High-dose amphetamine use places the patient at risk for the following:

- **AMPHETAMINE DEPENDENCE** (p. 224, 304.40): Tolerance or withdrawal or both coupled with major life changes.
- **AMPHETAMINE INTOXICATION DELIRIUM** (p. 143, 292.81): A characteristic organic delirium (see Chapter 5) develops shortly after taking the drug and disappears as the blood level decreases. Violence is common during these episodes.
- **AMPHETAMINE-INDUCED PSYCHOTIC DISORDER, WITH DELUSIONS** (p. 338, 292.11): Patient becomes markedly paranoid, and persecutory delusions develop within a setting of clear consciousness, often accompanied by hostility, anxiety, ideas of reference, and psychomotor agitation. This condition may last for 1 week or longer than 1 year. It easily can be mistaken for paranoid schizophrenia, which it *closely* resembles.
- **AMPHETAMINE WITHDRAWAL** (p. 227, 292.0) (15): Cessation of drug in a heavy user may be followed by mild-to-severe

depression (watch for suicide), profound fatigue, irritability, anxiety, fearfulness, nightmares, and insomnia or hypersomnia. Severe symptoms seldom last more than 1 week but may be followed by chronic low-level depression or anxiety or both. Abnormal EEG patterns may last for weeks.

Cocaine produces similar syndromes. Serious medical complications occur with cocaine (particularly crack), and several can be fatal: myocardial infarction (MI; secondary to coronary artery constriction; an MI in a young person is "due to cocaine until proven otherwise"), *crack lung* (acute "pneumonia" with normal radiograph and no response to routine meds), and anoxia secondary to seizures. Depression, paranoia and paranoid psychosis, marked anxiety, malnutrition, and pneumonia may follow use. Crack, when smoked, typically produces a high within seconds, followed by a dysphoric crash several minutes later, leading to rapidly repeated administrations and addiction. Infants of crack mothers are *jittery babies* who take weeks to gain weight, develop an appetite, and settle down, but who then develop fairly normally, except that many seem to become "hyperactive kids." It is a very bad drug. "Ice" (methamphetamine) is smoked similarly but produces a high lasting for 4 to 6 hours and so is much more rewarding than crack—well on its way to becoming the new crack!

Make the diagnosis by the clinical picture and history of drug use. Most sympathomimetics and cocaine can be identified by a urine drug screen (cocaine is difficult; check with your laboratory).

Treatment

Stop the drug. If the patient is mildly or moderately excited, try to "talk him down," and use benzodiazepines (e.g., diazepam, 10 to 20 mg p.o.). The patient may be agitated and violent; take appropriate precautions (e.g., restraints). Treat severe intoxication, delirium, and delusional symptoms with an antipsychotic (e.g., haloperidol, 10 mg p.o. or 5 to 10 mg i.m.). Acidify the urine with ascorbic acid or ammonium chloride (maintain pH at 4 to 5). Be alert to potential suicide and to medical complications (e.g., MI, stroke, intracranial hemorrhage). Severe withdrawal depressions may respond to antidepressants.

Cure is difficult—crack and ice are *powerfully* addictive. Consider hospitalization if symptoms or habit are severe or if life is severely disrupted. Group therapy (in- or outpatient) should be tried at some point. Desipramine (200 to 250 mg/d), bupropion, or amantadine (Symmetrel, 200 to 300 mg/d) may (?) decrease cocaine-withdrawal cravings in a few, particularly depressed patients, yet neither medications nor formal psychotherapy has demonstrated prolonged effectiveness. Finally, some promising results have been achieved with disulfiram (Antabuse, 250 mg/day), even without comorbid alcohol dependence.

INHALANTS

The types of glues, solvents, and cleaners "sniffed" for their psychic effects are numerous and include gasoline, kerosene, plastic and rubber cements, airplane and household glues, paints, lacquers, enamels, paint thinners, solvents, aerosols, furniture polishes, fingernail polish removers, nitrous oxide, cleaning fluids, etc. Several active constituents are probably involved in most substances. This is a major abuse problem, particularly among young adolescents (begins at age 8 to 9, peaks at 14 to 15, disappears in most by age 20), and particularly among lower socioeconomic groups. It is often a group activity. Youth typically "grow out of it" (often moving to other drugs); addiction is very uncommon.

The effects of this variety of substances are usually quite similar—typically mild euphoria, giddiness, dizziness, slurred speech, confusion, disorientation, impulsivity, and ataxia—all of which may progress in the unusual case to a toxic psychosis, seizures, and coma (**INHALANT INTOXICATION**, p. 259, 292.89). Repeated and prolonged abuse is common (**INHALANT ABUSE**, p. 259, 305.90), but dependence is rare, and withdrawal symptoms (irritability, tremor, aches, nausea) seem to be mild. More severe withdrawal symptoms (seizures, delirium) occur in very severe abusers and are rare. Death has occurred from asphyxiation (e.g., confused child cannot remove a bag from the head), aspiration (usually vomit), dangerous behavior while intoxicated, and perhaps, most commonly, *sudden sniffing death syndrome* (child stimulated when high causes an outpouring of epinephrine, which produces ventricular fibrillation in the inhalant-sensitized myocardium). An acute brain syndrome (delirium) often occurs, but only in the unusual or very severe case does a degree of chronic CNS damage develop. Toluene produces the greatest physical damage, including general CNS damage, hearing loss, and renal tubular necrosis. Chronic abuse, particularly of toluene, can result in CNS atrophy.

Physical restraint and medical support may be needed in the acute situation, but the patient usually clears over hours or days. The nonintoxicated abuser often smells of solvent. Evaluate carefully for liver, kidney, and pulmonary damage. Encourage these children and their families to enter therapy.

NICOTINE

Nicotine in any form is highly addictive, producing both dependence (**NICOTINE DEPENDENCE**, p. 264, 305.10—slightly more than 20% of Americans smoke; most are dependent; a significant male > female gender gap is found. It is particularly addictive because of increased alertness and decreased anxiety immediately on smoking), and withdrawal (**NICOTINE WITHDRAWAL**, p. 265, 292.0; characterized by impaired concentration, irritability, restlessness, insomnia, hunger, anxiety, and depression). On abrupt discontinuation, craving will begin within hours and then will continue for months to years (lifetime?). Abusers of multiple drugs typically report that nicotine is the most difficult drug to stop permanently. Treatment should be aimed at withdrawal and discontinuation, if the patient will allow it. When best done, this is a three-part process: (a) a behavioral smoking-cessation program, (b) nicotine replacement and gradual dose decrease to keep craving tolerable, and (c) use of a drug specifically designed to decrease craving. A smoking-cessation program (relapse prevention and skills training; individual or group) seems to be essential for most patients. Nicotine replacement and a downward titration over 6+ weeks is most commonly accomplished by nicotine gum (Nicorette; may need 25+ pieces/day to start) or a transdermal skin patch (Habitrol, NicoDerm, Nicotrol, ProStep), or a carefully monitored combination of the two. Finally, anticraving drugs show promise, with the best evidence suggesting usefulness for sustained-release bupropion (Zyban SR) or possibly nortriptyline. For greatest effectiveness, combine a patch with 150 to 300 mg of bupropion/day; approximately 30% of patients will be smoking free at 1 year (16).

ANABOLIC STEROIDS

Not a problem in the "normal" doses used by patients with conditions like hypogonadism, anabolic steroids (e.g., testosterone and nandrolone i.m. weekly; methandienone, oxandrolone, etc., p.o. daily) used in supraphysiologic doses (up to 10 or even 100 times therapeutic doses) by athletes can produce euphoria, irritability, aggressiveness (*roid rage*), hypomania, and mania and psychosis in

10%+ of individuals on use (17). These effects are dose dependent: mood symptoms are unusual at less than the equivalent of 300 mg of testosterone weekly but may occur in up to 50% of people taking more than 1,000 mg weekly. Dependency may occur in 25% to 50%+ of abusers. On withdrawal, self-limited depression of several weeks occurs in many, whereas a few individuals may become seriously suicidal and require aggressive treatment of their depression. An association may exist between steroid abuse and either antisocial or narcissistic personality disorder in some individuals (a worrisome combination in regard to aggression).

REFERENCES

1. Lowinson JH, Ruiz P, Millman RB, et al., eds. *Substance abuse: a comprehensive textbook*. Philadelphia: Lippincott Williams & Wilkins, 2005.
2. Ling W, Charuvastra VC, Kaim SC, et al. Methadyl acetate and methadone as maintenance treatments for heroin addicts. *Arch Gen Psychiatry* 1976;3:709–720.
3. Reynaud M, Petit G, Potard D, et al. Six deaths linked to concomitant use of buprenorphine and benzodiazepines. *Addiction* 1998;93:1385–1392.
4. Schottenfeld RS, Pakes J, Ziedonis D, et al. Buprenorphine: dose-related effects on cocaine-abusing opioid dependent humans. *Biol Psychiatry* 1993;34:66–74.
5. Washton AM, Resnick RB. Clonidine for opiate detoxification: outpatient clinical trials. *Am J Psychiatry* 1980;137:1121–1122.
6. Rickels K, Schweizer E, Case G, et al. Long-term therapeutic use of benzodiazepines, I: effects of abrupt discontinuation. *Arch Gen Psychiatry* 1990;47:899–907.
7. Dyer JE, Roth B, Hyma BA. Gamma-hydroxybutyrate withdrawal syndrome. *Ann Emerg Med* 2001;37:147–53.
8. Nichols DE: Hallucinogens. *Pharmacol Ther* 2004; 101:131–191.
9. Weiner AL, Vieira L, McKay CA, et al. Ketamine abusers presenting to the emergency department: a case series. *J Emerg Med* 2000;18:447–51.
10. Sramek JJ, Baumgartner WA, Tallos JA, et al. Hair analysis for detection of phencyclidine in newly admitted psychiatric patients. *Am J Psychiatry* 1985;142:950–53.
11. Back-Madruga C, Boone KB, Chang L, et al. Neuropsychological effects of 3,4-methyldioxymethampheta-mine (MDMA or ecstasy) in recreational users. *Clin Neuropsychol* 2003;17:446–59.
12. Pope HG, Todd-Yurgelun D. The residual cognitive effects of heavy marijuana use in college students. *JAMA* 1996;275:521–7.
13. Warner LA, Kessler RC, Hughes M, et al. Prevalence and correlates of drug use and dependence in the United States. *Arch Gen Psychiatry* 1995;52:219–29.

14. Ahmad K. Asia grapples with spreading amphetamine abuse. *Lancet* 2003;361:1878–9.
15. McGregor C, Srisurapanont M, Jittiwutikarn J, et al. The nature, time course and severity of methamphetamine withdrawal. *Addiction* 2005;100:1320–9.
16. Jorenby DE, Leischow SJ, Nides MA, et al. A controlled trial of sustained-release bupropion, a nicotine patch, or both for smoking cessation. *N Eng J Med* 1999;340:685–91.
17. Pope HG, Kouri EM, Hudson JI. The effects of supraphysiologic doses of testosterone on mood and aggression in normal men: a randomized controlled trial. *Arch Gen Psychiatry* 2000; 57:133–40.

Chapter 18

Psychosexual Disorders

These disorders are often first brought to the attention of the general physician. The three distinct categories are the following:

- Psychosexual dysfunction: Inhibition in sexual desire or psychophysiologic performance or both;
- Paraphilia: Sexual arousal to deviant stimuli;
- Gender-identity disorders: Patient feels like the opposite sex.

PSYCHOSEXUAL DYSFUNCTION

Clinically observable features of the normal human *sexual response cycle* consist of four stages:

1. *Stage I: Excitement* (minutes to hours)
   - Males: Psychological arousal and penile erection.
   - Females: Psychological arousal, vaginal lubrication, nipple erection, and vasocongestion of the external genitalia.
2. *Stage II: Plateau* (seconds to 3 minutes)
   - Males: Several drops of fluid appear at head of penis (from the Cowper gland).
   - Females: Tightening of outer third of vagina, breast engorgement.
3. *Stage III: Orgasm* (5 to 15 seconds)
   - Males: ejaculation, involuntary muscular contraction (e.g., pelvis) followed by a refractory period.
   - Females: Contractions of outer third of vagina, some involuntary pelvic thrusting; may be multiple.
4. *Stage IV: Resolution*
   - Males: Relaxation, detumescence, sense of well-being.
   - Females: Relaxation, detumescence, sense of well-being.

Patients (or their partners) may complain of decreased sexual desire or of one or more specific abnormalities of the response cycle or both. The dysfunctions may be situational, partial rather than complete, and primary or acquired. The phases usually occur in a stepwise fashion, but that is not mandatory—identify the stage involved. Often marital problems, unrealistic expectations, long-standing personal "hangups," and chronic difficulty establishing and maintaining intimate interpersonal relations are found. Identify these through history and psychiatric evaluation. *Always* evaluate carefully for organic causes (particularly with impotence and dyspareunia). Organic conditions tend to be chronic and independent of the situation.

Treatment should be global with an emphasis on intimacy and relationship, not just technique (1). Identify and treat psychosocial causes with dynamic psychotherapy, marital therapy, hypnotherapy, and group therapy. Sedatives may help temporarily if anxiety is prominent. Even purely physical causes often have significant associated secondary interpersonal problems that must be addressed once the medical condition has been corrected. A good prognosis is associated with acute recent dysfunction in a psychologically healthy patient with good past sexual functioning and strong sexual interests. Some relationships between partners are sufficiently hostile and destructive that unless other matters are resolved, prognosis is very poor for a correction of the psychosexual dysfunction.

The "new sex therapy" (Masters and Johnson) uses individual psychotherapy, couples therapy, education, behavior-modification techniques, and often a male–female therapist pair (dual-sex therapy). Their numerous techniques have wide applicability with sexual dysfunctions and should be considered for use. Many of these methods center on decreasing a patient's (or couple's) anxiety about making love. Essential principles include the following.

- Good communication with full exploration of sexual feelings;
- Training in specific stimulation and coital techniques (through "pleasuring sessions");
- Emphasis on the couple as a pleasure-giving team;
- Prohibition of intercourse early in therapy (to reduce performance anxiety);
- Emphasis on multimodal sensory pleasure (touch, sight, sound) and sensory-awareness exercises;
- Insistence that physiologic responses be ignored (erection, etc.—"Don't worry about it; it will happen").

MALE ERECTILE DISORDER; FEMALE SEXUAL AROUSAL DISORDER (DSM, PP. 543 AND 545, 302.72)

Men have *impotence:* a persistent or recurrent failure to reach or maintain a complete erection (2). Two psychogenic forms exist: in *primary impotence*, the patient has never maintained an erection, and in *secondary impotence*, the patient has lost the ability—this may be person or situation specific (selective impotence). Moreover, biologically induced erectile disorder is the most common sexual dysfunction caused by **SEXUAL DYSFUNCTION DUE TO A GENERAL MEDICAL CONDITION** (DSM, p. 558) or **SUBSTANCE-INDUCED SEXUAL DYSFUNCTION** (DSM, p. 562), although several other sexual problems can have an organic etiology as well.

Impotence is a common sexual complaint of men, predominantly the secondary form. It is not a "natural consequence" of aging but does increase with age (6% to 8% of men in their 20s; 50%+ in men older than 70). Perhaps 50% are psychogenic, with an organic etiology more common with age. Organic causes include these:

- Disorders of the hypothalamic–pituitary–gonadal axis: low serum testosterone level due to primary testicular hypofunction, pituitary tumors, etc. Endocrine disorders: hyperthyroidism (may have elevated testosterone), hypothyroidism, hyperprolactinemia, diabetes mellitus, acromegaly, Addison disease, Cushing syndrome.
- Medication: Tricyclc antidepressants (TCAs), selective serotonin reuptake inhibitors (SSRIs; one third or more of patients), monoamine oxidase inhibitors (MAOIs), major tranquilizers (particularly thioridazine), cholinergic blockers, antihypertensive drugs (particularly adrenergic blockers and false sympathetic neurotransmitters), estrogens, exogenous steroids, ethyl alcohol (alcoholism), addictive drugs (particularly narcotics and amphetamines), and anticholinergic drugs, among others.
- Illness: Any illness may cause impotence temporarily but particularly chronic debilitating disease, chronic renal disease, peripheral vascular disease, obstructive sleep apnea, multiple sclerosis (MS), stroke, spinal cord trauma, lower abdominal surgery, and local physical and neurologic disorders.

Psychogenic causes include *depression*, anxiety (over cardiac status, performance, etc.), schizophrenia, hostility and marital conflict, etc.

First identify any physical cause. Do a complete medical evaluation (look for physical illness, absent beard and body hair, small testes, gynecomastia), and get serum testosterone (then further hormonal studies if low). Early morning sleeping erection or occasional successful intercourse *does not rule out* an organic etiology, nor does a normal pattern of nocturnal penile tumescence (NPT; erections during REM sleep) *rule in* a psychogenic etiology, although most psychogenic cases have normal NPT. Treat medical causes (often curative). Follow with couples or global therapy or both, if needed.

Therapy includes allowing the female to play the dominant role and insisting on a gradual shift from foreplay to intercourse.

Effective pharmacologic therapy has recently become available. The erect penis depends on the increased blood flow in the corpus cavernosum that is encouraged by increased local levels of cGMP elevated in response to sexual arousal. A new class of medication, the phosphodiesterase type 5 (PDE5) inhibitors, slows the degradation of cGMP by PDE5 in the penis and thus encourages blood flow to that organ. The first of the three such active drugs available was sildenafil (Viagra). Begin with 50 mg of sildenafil p.o. 1 hour before sexual activity. It starts working in about 30 minutes and lasts for about 4 hours. Use a maximum of 100 mg in 1 day. Side effects include primarily flushing (face), headache, and dyspepsia. Do not take with nitrates (i.e., be careful with the elderly heart patient who wants help with his impotence), and take care with any medications that inhibit the cytochrome P-450 isoenzyme 3A4 (primary metabolizer of sildenafil). Two other similar medications are vardenafil (Levitra; also lasts 4 hours) and tadalafil (Cialis; lasts for 24 to 36 hours). What advantages they may have, if any, over sildenafil is not yet clear.

In **women**, an inadequate genital sexual response (failure to reach the excitement or plateau stages) is seen, although the woman *may* find sexual activity pleasurable. It often reflects personality or marital problems, but other specific causes include poor physical health, alcoholism, fatigue, depression, fear of pregnancy, a postpartum state, and various medications such as some antidepressants and anticholinergics. Sex therapy is often helpful; also treat the couple. Sildenafil (25 to 50 mg) should be tried (3).

Premature Ejaculation (DSM, p. 552, 302.75)

The ejaculation occurs before the patient wishes it to and usually before his partner reaches orgasm (40% of all patients with sexual complaints; 30% of all males). Cause is often functional and secondary to anxiety (determine the source of the anxiety). It is much more common in stressful marriages. The "squeeze technique" can be effective: Just before ejaculation, the woman squeezes the head of glans. This is coupled with the man practicing imagery control. The young and vigorous male may benefit from 1% Nupercaine ointment applied to the coronal ridge and frenulum. PRN use of SSRIs (particularly paroxetine, 20 mg, but also sertraline, 50 mg, or clomipramine, 50 mg) taken several hours before intercourse or sildenafil PRN are often effective (4).

Male Orgasmic Disorder (DSM, p. 550, 302.74)

In spite of adequate erection, the patient fails to ejaculate. Differentiate from *retrograde ejaculation* ["ejaculation" into the bladder—due to organic factors (e.g., anticholinergic drugs, prostatectomy)]. Some patients can have an orgasm only under certain conditions (e.g., with masturbation, with a stranger). Identify the circumstances in which orgasm can take place. Other psychological causes include lack of interest (e.g., primary sexual deviation), anxiety, compulsive personality, marriage stresses, and sexual "hangups." Physical causes are more common and include medication [guanethidine, methyldopa, antipsychotics (e.g., risperidone and particularly thioridazine), MAOIs, and one third or more of patients taking SSRIs or clomipramine], genitourinary (GU) surgery, and lower spinal cord impairment (e.g., parkinsonism, syringomyelia). If the cause is psychological, try training the patient to ejaculate by himself, and then treat the interpersonal relationship—individual psychotherapy is often needed. The technique of the female self-inserting her partner's penis may be effective.

Female Orgasmic Disorder (DSM, p. 547, 302.73)

The patient persistently fails to reach orgasm during intercourse despite evidence of adequate arousal (e.g., lubrication, strong libido). Primary (the majority; 30% of women) and secondary forms occur, although be aware that many women become orgasmic as they get older (peak at age 35). A biologic basis may exist in some (e.g., clitoral injury, antihypertensives, antipsychotics, common with SSRIs), but most causes are psychological. This condition is very situation specific: some women never have orgasm despite ample excitement; others have orgasm only with masturbation; still others require clitoral manipulation digitally or orally during intercourse; and some women can have an orgasm with intercourse alone. Psychotherapy often involves first training the woman to have an orgasm by herself and then treating the couple. Bupropion (150 to 300 mg/day) may help some.

Dyspareunia (DSM, p. 554, 302.76)

Pain with intercourse. Most often it is related to a physical condition (50%+): cervical or vaginal infection or anatomic abnormality, endometriosis, tumor, or other pelvic pathology. Anxiety about sexual activity (for a variety of reasons) can produce pelvic muscle tightening and pain, but remember, pain from organic causes can produce anxiety, which exacerbates the pain. Dyspareunia can produce vaginismus, and vaginismus can produce dyspareunia.

Vaginismus (DSM, p. 556, 306.51)

During coitus, the patient has an involuntary spasm of the muscles surrounding the outer third of the vagina and may prevent penile entrance. It may be related to physical causes producing pain—dyspareunia. Psychological causes include past sexual trauma (e.g., rape), a hostile marital relationship (perhaps from a vicious cycle), or sexual "hangups." Individual therapy and relaxation techniques are usually required. Hegar dilators (size increased over 3 to 5 days) may be useful.

Hypoactive Sexual Desire Disorder (DSM, p. 539, 302.71)

Common (lifetime prevalence: $\male$ = 15%, $\female$ = 30%) and difficult to treat (5). It may first be seen as inhibited excitement or inhibited orgasm—do not be misled. Causes often are functional (e.g., troubled relationship, previous sexual trauma). It varies with time, the sexual partner, depression, anxiety, a fear of intimacy or pregnancy, a passive–aggressive personality style, strong religious orthodoxy, or homosexuality, among others. Medical causes include various drugs (e.g., antidepressants, anabolic steroids) and medical conditions (e.g., menopause, low testosterone, hypothyroidism). Individual or couple therapy is useful. Testosterone replacement may be useful (e.g., methyltestosterone, p.o. 0.25 to 1.0 mg/day), as may bupropion.

Sexual Aversion Disorder (DSM, p. 541, 302.79)

This is similar to hypoactive sexual desire disorder but represents an *active* avoidance of sexual activity. Patient has often been sensitized by past (unpleasant) experiences.

PARAPHILIA (SEXUAL DEVIATION)

These patients become sexually excited only by unusual or bizarre stimuli (practices or fantasies). The particular type of arousing stimulus or fantasy determines the diagnosis. Orgasmic release usually occurs by masturbation during or after the event. Etiology is uncertain but is possibly biologic, learned, dynamic–instinctual, or a combination of these. Most types are rare (courts see them most frequently), although physicians will occasionally encounter them. Men vastly predominate, although women may display sadomasochism, voyeurism, and exhibitionism.

These patients may not be troubled by their desires (ego syntonic) but only by the consequences of acting on them, and thus are difficult to treat, although depression, anxiety, and guilt do occur. These conditions frequently coexist with personality disorders, alcohol and drug abuse, and other psychiatric disorders—treat them. The patients often have impaired interpersonal relationships, particularly heterosexual relations.

Psychotherapy is frequently unsuccessful. Specific behavior-modification and cognitive–behavioral techniques to eliminate the deviation may be useful (e.g., aversion, covert conditioning), although these must be paired with a more global retraining program. Relapse is common. Hypersexual states and some other sexual deviations may benefit from medroxyprogesterone acetate (Depo-Provera) or cyproterone acetate. Early work suggests that paraphilias with a high degree of obsessive urges may respond somewhat to SSRIs.

Pedophilia (DSM, p. 571, 302.2)

These patients repeatedly approach prepubertal children sexually (touch, explore, mutually masturbate; occasionally intercourse). They are usually anxious, depressed, inadequate men who know the child involved (a neighbor, relative). Three general types are recognized: *heterosexual pedophilia* (prefers preadolescent girls), *homosexual pedophilia* (prefers early teenage boys—very resistant to therapy; usually has by far the greatest number of victims), and mixed pedophilia (younger children, either sex). Pedophiliacs derive sexual arousal primarily from children: do not confuse with child molestation due to decreased impulse control (e.g., organic conditions, intoxication, retardation, psychosis) or a one-time event (e.g., due to loneliness or after a marital crisis). Biologic, familial roots may be present. Behavior modification is very modestly useful.

Exhibitionism (DSM, p. 569, 302.4)

Usually timid men (onset usually in teen years) who become sexually aroused by exposing their genitals to an unsuspecting female (adult or child). They are only rarely aggressive. They may masturbate during the exposure and need a shock reaction from the female for satisfaction. Very resistant to treatment, although "compulsive" exhibitionism may respond to SSRIs.

Less frequent paraphilias include the following:

- **FETISHISM** (DSM, p. 569, 302.81): Sexual arousal to inanimate objects. May be combined with other sexual preferences.
- **FROTTEURISM** (DSM, p. 570, 302.89): Arousal from touching or fondling a nonconsenting person, usually in a crowded place where escape is possible. Usually teenage or young adult men.
- **TRANSVESTIC FETISHISM** (DSM, p. 574, 302.3): Aroused by female clothing and cross-dressing. Do not confuse with transsexualism (the wish to *become* a female) or effeminate homosexuality (cross-dressing to attract others, not to produce arousal itself).
- **VOYEURISM** (DSM, p. 575, 302.82): Sexual arousal by watching unsuspecting people who are naked or sexually active. Masturbation usually takes place concurrently.
- **SEXUAL MASOCHISM** (DSM, p. 572, 302.83): Arousal from being sexually bound, beaten, humiliated, etc. This is chronic.
- **SEXUAL SADISM** (DSM, p. 573, 302.84): Sexual excitement after inflicting psychological or physical (sexual or nonsexual) harm on a consenting or nonconsenting partner. The severity of the harm required to produce excitement may increase with time, making the person a potential killer. Some rapists deserve this diagnosis.

GENDER IDENTITY DISORDER (DSM, P. 576)

These adults have experienced prolonged discomfort about their anatomic sex and identify with and wish they were the opposite sex. A few actively want to change their sex (transsexuals). Men predominate (M:F, 3:1), and their clinical characteristics are more variable. They may have experienced the discomfort since childhood or only recently. They may be homosexual, heterosexual, or have little sexual interest. Many have an effeminate appearance and cross-dress. Women with this disorder are usually homosexual and masculine appearing. Cross-dressing is common; *no* desire for a sex change is found; and a diversity of additional psychiatric symptoms are seen.

Etiology is unclear; it may be predominantly biologic or psychological or both, although the mother–child bond usually appears disturbed (often too close). Check karyotype and sex hormone levels. These patients are very likely to have personality disorders, particularly of the borderline type. The course is chronic, with significant risk for depression, suicide, anxiety, and genital self-mutilation. Rule out effeminate homosexuality (patient does *not* want to be the other sex), schizophrenia, and hermaphroditism.

Treat with supportive psychotherapy and feminizing–masculinizing hormones. Sex-change surgery (castration, penectomy, vaginoplasty, phalloplasty), although still done after extensive preparation, may be falling out of fashion (6). It is irreversible, and the results may be no better than psychotherapy alone. Isolated reports exist of gender identity changes with intensive behavior modification.

Homosexuality

Homosexuality (an arousal to and preference for sexual relations with adults of the same sex) is not currently considered to be a mental disorder, unless the patient is "persistently and markedly" distressed by it (classed as **SEXUAL DISORDER NOT OTHERWISE SPECIFIED,** DSM, p. 582, 302.9). It may be a temporary phase during adolescence.

Homosexuality is common in the United States, with possibly 5% to 10% of males and 2% to 4% of females. Despite numerous theoretic explanations, the cause(s) is unknown. Congenital, prenatal, familial, biologic, or genetic [e.g., a gene on the X chromosome (7) are debated by others (8)] etiologies may exist for some; environmental factors may dominate in the choice of sexual orientation in others. We are still a long way from understanding the biologic etiology of this human characteristic (9).

These distressed homosexuals often have internalized a negative attitude toward homosexual behavior and consistently want to change. They have depression, anxiety, and shame. Psychotherapy for these symptoms may be helpful, but efforts at the patient's request to change sexual orientation has shown very limited long-term success.

REFERENCES

1. Cole M. Sex therapy: a critical appraisal. *Br J Psychiatry* 1985;147:337–351.
2. Shabsigh R, Anastasiadis AG. Erectile dysfunction. *Annu Rev Med* 2003;54:153–168.
3. Caruso S, Intelisano G, Lupo L, et al. Premenopausal women affected by sexual arousal disorder treated with sildenafil: a

double-blind, cross-over, placebo-controlled study. *Int J Obstet Gynecol* 2001;108:623–628.

4. Waldinger MD, Zwinderman AH, Olivier B. SSRIs and ejaculation: a double-blind, randomized, fixed-dose study with paroxetine and citalopram. *J Clin Psychopharm* 2001;21:556–560.

5. Warnock JJ. Female hypoactive sexual desire disorder: epidemiology, diagnosis and treatment. *CNS Drugs* 2002;16:745–753.

6. Snaith P, Tarsh MJ, Reid R. Sex reassignment surgery. *Br J Psychiatry* 1993;162:681–685.

7. Hamer DH, Hu S, Magnuson VS, et al. A linkage between DNA markers on the X chromosome and male sexual orientation. *Science* 1993;261:321–327.

8. Rice G, Anderson C, Risch N, et al. Male homosexuality: absence of linkage to microsatellite markers at Xq28. *Science* 1999;284:665–667.

9. Rahman Q. The neurodevelopment of human sexual orientation. *Neurosci Biobehav Rev* 2005;29:1057–1066.

Chapter 19

Sleep Disturbances

Sleep disorders are extremely common: 40% of the population have had trouble sleeping within the past year, 10% have had diagnosable insomnia, and 3% to 4% have had hypersomnia (1–3).

Current understanding and classification of sleep problems rests on knowledge of normal sleep. Much of this has been obtained through *polysomnography* (4), that is, electrophysiologic measures (EEG, EMG, EOG), as well as airflow, O_2 saturation, etc., of patients in sleep laboratories. The two major categories are the **dyssomnias** (poor sleep, excessive sleep) and the **parasomnias** (peculiar events associated with sleep).

NORMAL SLEEP

Normal sleep is cyclical (four to five cycles/night) and active, *not* passive. Distinct stages [rapid-eye-movement (REM) and non-REM sleep], measured by EEG, occur each night. From *waking* (beta waves; alpha waves, 8 to 12 cps), sleep is initiated by melatonin release from the pineal gland and passes stepwise through discrete stages during the night:

NREM Sleep

Low level of activity: reduced blood pressure (BP), heart rate, temperature, and respiratory rate. Good muscle tone and slow, drifting eye movements.

Stage 1: (**5%** of sleep), lightest sleep, a transition stage; low-voltage, desynchronized waves.

Stage 2: (**50%**), mostly theta waves (low voltage, 5 to 7 cps) but with some bursts of *sleep spindles* (13 to 15 cps for 2 to 3 seconds) and high spikes (*K complexes*); awakens easily.

Stage 3: Theta with some delta waves (high voltage at 0.5 to 2.5 cps).

Stage 4: Deepest sleep (hard to awake), mostly in first half of night; mostly delta waves.

REM Sleep

Active sleep (**20% to 25%** of sleep), characterized by *rapid synchronous eye movement*, twitching of facial and extremity muscles, penile erections, and variation in pulse, BP, and respiratory rate. Muscles appear *paralyzed* (no tone). Depth is similar to stage 2; theta waves, sleep spindles, and K-complexes reappear. *Dreaming* can occur in several stages but is most common in REM sleep. Brain activity is quite elevated.

Patients enter lightest sleep (stage 1), descend by steps over approximately 30 minutes to deepest sleep (stage 4), plateau there for 30 to 40 minutes, and then ascend to lighter stages (1 to 2) to enter REM sleep 90 to 100 minutes after falling asleep. Then the cycle repeats. As the night progresses, the REM periods lengthen, stage 4 disappears, and the sleep is generally lighter. The length of time spent in any one stage varies in a characteristic fashion with age (e.g., longer stages 3 and 4 in youth, shorter and fewer in old age). The significance of each stage is not known. Serum cortisol is low initially during the night but peaks just before awakening.

For clinical purposes, patients can be divided into those complaining of insomnia or hypersomnia. In each category, distinct syndromes must be ruled in or out.

INSOMNIA

Primary Insomnia (DSM, p. 599, 307.42)

Primary insomnia is persistent insomnia that has been present for at least 1 month and has no obvious cause. Explore the differential diagnosis. Take a good history of the sleep problem; include the 24-hour sleep–wake cycle (sleep laboratory studies usually are not needed). Identify the pattern: trouble falling asleep (onset insomnia), trouble staying asleep (frequent awakenings), early morning awakenings (terminal insomnia). Inquire about life stresses, drug and alcohol use, and marital and family problems. Rule out the following:
- Is the insomnia simply normal sleep?
  a. Some "insomniacs" get ample sleep (*sleep-state misperception syndrome* or *pseudoinsomnia*); they just believe they sleep poorly. Use reassurance and psychotherapy.
  b. Sleep time lessens with age—explain to concerned elderly. Help them avoid a "worry over sleeplessness" cycle.

　　c. Some patients are substance abusers seeking drugs; do not be fooled.

- Is the insomnia transient (*situational insomnia*)? This is the most common form of insomnia: usually trouble falling asleep, due to worry. Identify the stress. Help the patient deal with it. Consider time-limited (1 to 2 weeks) use of sleeping medication (e.g., zolpidem, 5 to 10 mg p.o., hs; temazepam, 15 to 30 mg p.o., hs). Differentiate from *psychophysiologic* or *conditioned insomnia:* The patient has inadvertently *trained* him or herself to stay awake at bedtime, usually by worrying about not falling asleep (a type of primary insomnia).

- Is a *chronic minor psychiatric illness* present? Prolonged insomnia (usually sleep-onset problems with decreased stage 4 sleep) is common with chronic depression or anxiety or both (and obsessive–compulsive patients). They may self-medicate, producing more insomnia. Such patients may have trouble expressing distressed or aggressive feelings and thus internalize their problems.

- Is a major psychiatric illness present (**INSOMNIA RELATED TO ANOTHER MENTAL DISORDER;** DSM, p. 645, 307.42)?
　　a. *Acute psychosis:* Often produces major sleep disruption—use antipsychotics.
　　b. *Mania or hypomania:* Very short sleep time—use anticonvulsants or lithium.
　　c. *Major depression:* Typically early morning awakening, but frequent awakenings during the night are also common. REM sleep begins very quickly after sleep onset (*short REM latency*). Treat the depression with SSRIs, etc.

- Is a medical problem present (**SLEEP DISORDER DUE TO A GENERAL MEDICAL CONDITION, INSOMNIA TYPE,** DSM, p. 651, 780.52)?
　　a. Nighttime pain or distress, often with related anxiety and depression [e.g., back pain, headache, arthritis, asthma, nocturnal angina (increased chest pains during REM sleep), duodenal ulcer].
　　b. Hyperthyroidism, epilepsy, parkinsonism, chronic renal failure.
　　c. Is the patient simply worried about a medical problem?

- Is substance use or abuse present (**SUBSTANCE-INDUCED SLEEP DISORDER,** DSM, p. 655)? It is very common, so always inquire.
　　a. Alcohol: The most common self-prescribed hypnotic. Intoxication yields heavy sleep for 2 to 4 hours and then restless dream-filled sleep. Prolonged use produces increasingly fragmented sleep after initial sedation. Withdrawal generates intense REM sleep with vivid dreams.

b. Hypnotic medication: Often prescribed for insomnia, it produces decreased REM sleep. Tolerance develops to each type with, ironically, sleep disruption ("sleeping-pill insomnia"). Severe rebound insomnia usually occurs with withdrawal. Treatment *must* begin with medication withdrawal.

c. Amphetamines, methylphenidate, cocaine, caffeine (patients often overlook; insomnia *particularly* in the elderly; ask), hallucinogens, aminophylline, ephedrine, thyroid, and steroids all can interrupt sleep. Usually hypersomnia with withdrawal.

d. Cigarettes (nicotine) can stimulate; a commonly overlooked explanation.

- Is there *sleep cycle disruption* (**CIRCADIAN RHYTHM SLEEP DISORDER,** DSM, p. 622, 307.45)? Sleepiness slips out of phase if there is "jet lag" or night-shift work; most commonly patients fall asleep (finally) in early morning and waken around noon or early afternoon. Usually self-limited, but improved sleep can be hastened by forced awakening and exposure to bright light increasingly earlier in the morning. Bright morning light on the retina sends a signal through the retinohypothalamic tract to the ventrolateral parts of the suprachiasmatic nuclei (SCN, the brain's circadian "pacemaker," in the anterior hypothalamus). The impulse from this light causes the SCN to stimulate the pineal gland to *decrease* output of **melatonin,** causing alertness. With darkness, melatonin increases, causing sleepiness and feeding back to the SCN, which has melatonin receptors. Thus bright light every morning uses this SCN–melatonin feedback loop to reset our brain's automatic internal clock located in the SCN. Melatonin *may* become a help with jet lag and other sleep rhythm disorders (5).

- Is there **DYSSOMNIA NOS** (DSM, p. 629, 307.47)? Could it be *periodic limb movement of sleep* (nocturnal myoclonus): restless sleep with frequent awakenings secondary to rhythmic (every 20 to 60 seconds) muscle jerks in the legs? Ask the bed partner. However, recent evidence suggests that nocturnal myoclonus rarely awakens the patient (only the partner). Onset is early adult to elderly; it is autosomal dominant. The best treatment at this point seems to be pergolide (0.05 to 2.0 mg) (6), clonazepam (0.5 to 2.0 mg), and others. Or could insomnia be caused by the *restless legs syndrome?* Legs feel "uncomfortable," with a strong urge to move the legs; the feeling is relieved by moving. This is found in about 5% of population; it is more common in elderly. Treat with ropinirole (Requip— approved by the FDA for RLS), pramipexole (Mirapex) (7) (0.125 to 0.75 mg, 1 to 2 hours before bed), pergolide (8) (0.05 to 1.0 mg, 1 to 2 hours before bed), carbidopa/levodopa (9), and others.

- Are there **parasomnias** [e.g., frequent *nightmares* (**NIGHT-MARE DISORDER,** DSM, p. 631, 307.47), *night terrors* (*pavor nocturnus*; **SLEEP TERROR DISORDER,** DSM, p. 634, 307.46), or *sleepwalking* (*somnambulism*; **SLEEPWALKING DISORDER,** DSM, p. 639, 307.46)?

  a. Nightmares (REM sleep) can be chronic and disruptive. They are common in children (25% to 50%) but often disappear by adulthood; F/M ratio is 2 to 4:1. Psychotherapy *may* help.

  b. Night terrors (stage 4 sleep) occur early in the night in children, are terrifying to observers, but are not remembered by the patient. They usually disappear with adulthood. Some respond to low doses of minor tranquilizers or SSRIs (10).

  c. Somnambulism (stage 4 sleep) can persist into adulthood. The patient's behavior appears strange to an observer, with marked clouding of consciousness. Protect the patient from his or her actions. Diazepam, 15 mg hs, imipramine, 50 mg hs, or SSRIs may help.

General Treatment of Insomnia

1. Rule out, or treat, specific syndromes.
2. Practice good **sleep hygiene**. Maintain a regular bedtime; use bedroom for sleeping only. Keep room dark, quiet, and cool. Develop a "sleeping ritual" for the hour before going to bed. Arise about the same time every morning (*very* important). Regular exercise during the day helps, but not after dinner. Avoid vigorous mental activities late in the evening. Try a bedtime snack (yes, warm milk helps—tryptophan) but *do not* drink alcohol after supper or caffeine after mid-afternoon.** If not asleep after 30 minutes, get up and read or watch television until sleepy again, but still rise at the regular time in the morning, even if it produces daytime sleepiness for a few days (sleep restriction).**
3. Provide support and reassurance. Use psychotherapy, if there are issues. Try relaxation techniques: progressive relaxation, biofeedback, self-hypnosis, meditation, etc. Emphasize a sense of self-control.
4. Use sedative-hypnotics for a limited time only (see Chapter 23). Most hypnotic medications become ineffective within 2 weeks if used nightly. Try initially for 1 week in an effort to

establish a successful sleep pattern (e.g., zolpidem, 10 mg HS; zaleplon 10 mg HS; trazodone 25–100 mg HS). If used longer than several weeks, introduce drug holidays or use 2–3 times/week and do not exceed recommended dosages.

HYPERSOMNIA

Primary Hypersomnia (DSM p. 604, 307.44)

Patients with *primary hypersomnia* sleep 10–12 hours at night and typically are sleepy and nap during the day. Their hypersomnia often starts in later teens; polygraph tracings are normal. They may make up 1%–2% of the population. Sleep often provides an escape from stress. Depression also occurs but is not typical, unlike its common presence in **HYPERSOMNIA RELATED TO ANOTHER MENTAL DISORDER,** DSM p. 645, 307.44. Key differential conditions include the following.

■ Narcolepsy (DSM p. 609, 347)

Narcolepsy is a lifelong disorder (minimum requirement for diagnosis is 3 months) of brief, frequent, *refreshing* episodes of daytime sleep that usually begins near or shortly after puberty, has a genetic component [10% of 1° relatives; 90%–100% have a specific histocompatibility (HLA) antigen], occurs with a frequency of about 1 in 2,000 (0.05%), and requires (a) below as well as one or more of (b) through (d). About 15% of patients experience the whole **narcoleptic tetrad** (number of symptoms increase with middle age):

a. Daytime *sleep attacks*—The patient falls asleep in seconds or minutes (REM activity on EEG) during the day despite efforts to stay awake. The patient usually sleeps for 10–30 minutes and wakes refreshed, typically experiencing a single to a dozen episodes a day. Attacks occur most often during "slow times" but can happen while the patient is active and engaged (during a speech, driving a car) and can be embarrassing or dangerous.

b. *Cataplexy* (70% of patients)—A sudden loss of muscle tone, usually in the face and neck, but occasionally a complete physical collapse, typically precipitated by a strong emotion (e.g., anger, laughter). Attacks usually last for seconds and may be weeks apart. The patient is conscious throughout.

c. *Hypnagogic hallucinations* (30% of patients)—Dreamlike and often frightening auditory and/or visual hallucinations (REM on EEG) that occur as the patient falls asleep (or awakens—*hypnopompic*).

d. **Sleep paralysis** (25% of patients)— A flaccid, generalized, terrifying paralysis lasting for several seconds in a fully conscious patient, either while waking or falling asleep. It may resolve spontaneously or when the patient is touched or his name is called.

Many patients with narcolepsy also have disturbed nighttime sleep with frequent awakenings and nightmares. Diagnosis usually is not hard: Along with the classic tetrad, there is a remarkably short latency between falling asleep and REM sleep.

Treatment

- Train the patient to avoid dangerous occupations and precipitating stimuli. Planned daytime naps (15–30 minutes) can help.
- Sleep attacks—methylphenidate (Ritalin), 5–15 mg PO tid; dextroamphetamine (Dexedrine), 5–15 mg PO tid; a new medication modafinil (Provigil), 200 mg q A.M. Try occasional drug holidays. Medication advances are on the horizon (11).
- Cataplexy—imipramine, 10–25 mg PO tid, or fluoxetine, 20 mg/day (suppresses REM sleep).
- Consider sedation for nighttime insomnia (i.e., benzodiazepines); use sparingly.

■ Sleep Apnea (BREATHING-RELATED SLEEP DISORDER, DSM p. 615, 780.59)

This set of serious nighttime respiratory abnormalities can cause long-standing daytime sleepiness, particularly during quiet times (not during stimulation, like narcolepsy). It occurs in three types:

1. A few patients, usually elderly, briefly cease nighttime breathing efforts due to abnormal chemoreceptors and develop repeated air hunger and *insomnia* (*Central Sleep Apnea*).
2. Most considered to have sleep apnea struggle to draw air through relaxed, flaccid nose and mouth passageways that have markedly increased sleep-induced resistance (*Obstructive Sleep Apnea*). From 30 to several hundred episodes may occur each night, lasting from 10 seconds to more than 2 minutes. Males are affected 10:1 [look for obese men (majority of these patients) older than 50 with short, thick necks]. The patients may experience a variety of symptoms, including *loud snoring, morning headaches, restless sleep*, frequent awakenings, impaired libido, sleepwalking, hypertension, depression, and intellectual and personality changes. Only a few cases will demonstrate

fixed anatomic abnormalities of upper airway structures, but in many with weight gain and thickened necks, abnormalities appear during sleep. In serious chronic cases, pulmonary hypertension (12), right heart failure, cardiac arrhythmias, or a combination of these may occur. The polysomnograph shows fragmented sleep with frequent awakenings.

3. *Mixed Sleep Apnea*, with both phenomena.

No treatment has been clearly effective for central sleep apnea. A permanent tracheotomy or other surgical procedure (13) may be dramatically successful in obstructive sleep apnea, but first try weight loss or continuous positive airway pressure (CPAP) or both. Hypnotics and alcohol can further compromise nighttime breathing, so avoid them. This important diagnosis is significantly underrecognized (14) and can mimic depression, anxiety, panic disorder, and early dementia.

■ Other Causes

Rule out current chronic overuse of sedative drugs and alcohol, or rebound in chronic stimulant users. Rule out medical conditions **(SLEEP DISORDER DUE TO A GENERAL MEDICAL CONDITION, HYPERSOMNIA TYPE, DSM, p. 651, 780.54)**, e.g., myxedema, hypercapnia, any brain tumor but particularly those involving the mesencephalon and walls of the third ventricle, seizures, cerebrovascular disease, and hypoglycemia. Severe hypersomnia with marked postawakening confusion occurs with both the pickwickian syndrome (obesity and respiratory insufficiency) and the Kleine–Levin syndrome (attacks of hyperphagia, hypersomnia, and hypersexuality).

REFERENCES

1. Chokroverty S. *Sleep disorders medicine: basic science, technical considerations, and clinical aspects.* Boston: Butterworth, 1999.
2. Kryger MH, Roth T, Dement WC. *Principles and practice of sleep medicine.* Philadelphia: WB Saunders, 1994.
3. Reite M, Ruddy J, Nagel K. *Evaluation and management of sleep disorders.* Washington, DC: American Psychiatric Press, 1997.
4. Reite M, Buysse D, Reynolds C, et al. The use of polysomnography in the evaluation of insomnia. *Sleep* 1995;18:58–70.
5. Silver R, LeSauter J, Tresco P, et al. A diffusible coupling signal from the transplanted suprachiasmatic nucleus controlling circadian locomotor rhythms. *Nature* 1996;382:810–814.
6. Silber MH. Restless legs syndrome. *Mayo Clin Proc* 1997;72:261–264.

7. Montplaisir J, Nicolas A, Denesle R, et al. Restless legs syndrome improved by pramipexole. *Neurology* 1999;52:938–943.

8. Wetter TC, Stiasny K, Winkelmann J, et al. A randomized controlled study of pergolide in patients with restless legs syndrome. *Neurology* 1999;52:944–950.

9. Earley CJ, Allen RP. Pergolide and carbidopa/levodopa treatment of the restless legs syndrome and periodic leg movements in sleep in a consecutive series of patients. *Sleep* 1996;19:801–810.

10. Lillywhite AR, Wilson SJ, Nutt DJ. Successful treatment of night terrors and somnambulism with paroxetine. *Br J Psychiatry* 1994;164:551–554.

11. Mitler MM, Aldrich MS, Koob GF, et al. ASDA standards of practice: practice parameters for the use of stimulants in the treatment of narcolepsy. *Sleep* 1994;17:348–351.

12. Chaouat A, Weitzenblum E, Krieger J, et al. Pulmonary hemodynamics in the obstructive sleep apnea syndrome. *Chest* 1996;109:380–386.

13. ASDA Standards of Practice Committee. Practice parameters for the treatment of obstructive sleep apnea in adults: the efficacy of surgical modifications of the upper airway. *Sleep* 1996;19:152–155.

14. Reite M. Sleep disorders presenting as psychiatric disorders. *Psychiatric Clin North Am* 1998;21:591–607.

Personality Disorders

Personality is a consistent style of behavior uniquely recognizable in each individual. ***Personality disorders*** (Axis II of DSM, p. 685) refers to personality characteristics of a form or magnitude that are stable, chronic, pervasive across settings, deviate significantly from cultural norms, and are maladaptive and cause poor life functioning (1). Many patients display a mixture of several different maladaptive traits. These *long-term* traits feel "natural" (ego syntonic), even though a person may be bothered by the results of his or her behavior. Elements of the personality disorders exist in all of us, and the difference between health and pathology may be one of degree. Moreover, some patients display their pathology clearly only when under stress. The diagnoses of personality disorders have the poorest reliability of any DSM conditions, in part because their symptoms overlap extensively with one another.

Most personality disorders begin to form in childhood and become fixed by the early 20s, yet some occur after organic insults to the brain. Some may have a biologic, genetic (2,3) component (e.g., schizotypal and borderline personality disorders). Psychological testing may facilitate diagnosis (i.e., WAIS, MMPI, Bender–Gestalt, and Rorschach). Atypical and mixed types are common, and some may grade into or be confused with similar-appearing Axis I disorders (e.g., paranoid personality disorders look like delusional disorder). These patients often resist treatment and change slowly but occasionally respond to a variety of treatment modalities, including individual or group therapy and short-term use of antianxiety agents or low doses of major tranquilizers (4,5). Some may require inpatient treatment during periods of decompensation. Adolescents (younger than 18), and even children, may receive a personality disorder diagnosis (except antisocial personality disorder) if the pattern is stable, clear, and incompatible with an Axis I childhood disorder.

The 10 personality disorders are divided into three distinct groups ("clusters") based on their clinical patterns: the *odd eccentric* cluster, the *dramatic, emotional, and erratic* cluster, and the *anxious, fearful* cluster. They are as their names suggest.

ODD ECCENTRIC CLUSTER (CLUSTER "A")

Paranoid Personality Disorder (DSM, p. 690, 301.0)

These aloof, emotionally cold people (1% to 2%$^+$ of population; $\male > > \female$) typically display unjustified suspiciousness, hostility, hypersensitivity to slights, jealousy, and an inability for intimacy. They tend to be grandiose, rigid, unforgiving, sarcastic, contentious, and litigious and are thus isolated, disliked, and have few friends. They accept criticism poorly, blaming others instead. This disorder may be associated with chronic central nervous system (CNS) impairment, drug use (e.g., amphetamines), depression, obsessive–compulsive states, and a family history of schizophrenia. Psychotic decompensation sometimes occurs, requiring low-dose antipsychotics. Although 1% of the population, they rarely seek treatment. Therapy is of little value, but low-dose, limited side effect antipsychotics (e.g., risperidone) may help.

Schizoid Personality Disorder (DSM, p. 694, 301.20)

These people are seclusive, with little wish or capacity to form interpersonal relations, are indifferent to and derive little pleasure from social and sexual contacts, and yet prefer and can perform well at solitary activities (e.g., night watchman). They have a limited emotional range, experience little pleasure, daydream excessively, and are humorless and detached. They "may" have a family history of schizophrenia but do *not* seem to have an increased risk of developing schizophrenia themselves (6). "Loners" are not necessarily schizoid unless they have impaired functioning; be alert for mild PDD, Asperger syndrome, and schizotypal personality disorder. Treatment seems of little help.

Schizotypal Personality Disorder (DSM, p. 697, 301.22)

In addition to having features of the schizoid (isolated, anhedonic, aloof), these people are "peculiar." They relate strange intrapsychic experiences, display odd and magical beliefs as well as strange speech, reason in odd ways (e.g., ideas of reference), are frequently anxious, and are difficult to "get to know," yet these features rarely and briefly reach psychotic proportions. It is found in 3% of the population ($\male > \female$), commonly occurs with major depression, and is associated with an increased incidence of schizophrenia in family members (suggesting that this condition is part of the "schizophrenic spectrum" of disorders) (7). Biologic measures found in schizophrenia also occur (e.g., impaired eye tracking and atrophy of left superior temporal gyrus). Low-dose antipsychotic medication may reduce the more flamboyant symptoms.

DRAMATIC, EMOTIONAL, AND ERRATIC CLUSTER (CLUSTER "B")

Antisocial Personality Disorder (DSM, p. 701, 301.7)

Antisocial behavior begins in childhood or early adolescence (must have Conduct Disorder before age 15 years): aggressiveness, fighting, "hyperactivity," poor peer relationships, irresponsibility, lying, theft, truancy, poor school performance, runaway, inappropriate sexual activity, and drug and alcohol use. As adults, they show criminality, assaultiveness, self-defeating impulsivity, hedonism, promiscuity, unreliability, and crippling drug and alcohol abuse. They fail at work, change jobs frequently, go AWOL and receive dishonorable discharges from the service, are abusing parents and neglectful mates, cannot maintain intimate interpersonal relationships, and spend time in jails and prisons (50% or more of prisoners). These patients are frequently, if temporarily, anxious and depressed (suicide, often impulsive, in as many as 5%) and are second only to patients with hysteria in the production of conversion symptoms. The behavior peaks in late adolescence and the early 20s with improvement in the 30s; however, the patients usually continue their antisocial patterns, and they rarely recover from the "lost years." Men are involved more severely, earlier, and more frequently (3%+ of population); M:F = 3–5:1.

Their rearing is generally impaired by rejection, neglect, desertion, poverty, and inconsistent discipline; they are frequently illegitimate and unwanted. The parents are often criminals (30% of fathers), alcoholics (50% of fathers), and chronically unemployed. Male first-degree relatives have an increased incidence of antisocial personality disorder, alcoholism, and drug abuse, and female relatives have associated somatization disorder. A genetic component is likely.

No tests are diagnostic, although a 4–9 MMPI profile is common, and an increased incidence of nonspecific EEG abnormalities occur (increased slow-wave activity, etc.). It is necessary to rule out primary drug and alcohol abuse (difficult, look for normal childhood behavior), schizophrenia (thought disorder present), OBS (disorientation, memory impairment), ADHD (8), early mania, explosive disorder, and **ADULT ANTISOCIAL BEHAVIOR** (DSM, p. 740, V71.01). Several very specialized disorders of impulse control can also mimic this disorder: **PATHOLOGICAL GAMBLING** (DSM, p. 671, 312.31), **KLEP-TOMANIA** (DSM, p. 667, 612.32), and **PYROMANIA** (DSM, p. 669, 312.33). The patients are resistant and manipulative. Do not rely on the patient's report; check your data. They rarely seek help for personality change, and treatment is difficult and often unsuccessful. Best results follow closely supervised inpatient care: Use strong, frequent, and accurate confrontation of inter-personal behavior, particularly by peers. Individual outpatient psychotherapy is of little value. The terms antisocial personality disorder, sociopathy, and psychopathy generally (but not always) are used synonymously.

Borderline Personality Disorder (DSM, p. 706, 301.83)

These usually socially adapted patients have complex clinical presentations, including diverse combinations of anger and sarcasm, anxiety, intense and labile affect, brief disturbances in consciousness (e.g., depersonalization, dissociation), chronic loneliness, boredom, a chronic sense of emptiness, unstable and volatile interpersonal relations, identity confusion, impulsive behavior (including self-injury—cutting and self-mutilation; recurrent suicide attempts; and death by suicide in 8% or more), and a *hypersensitivity to abandonment*. Stress can precipitate a transient psychosis. Many other diagnoses are often suggested or can also be made: depression, brief psychotic disorder, other personality disorders, cyclothymic disorder, and substance-related disorders. Some of this common (2% in general popula-tion; F/M ratio, 3:1) heterogeneous group may be related genetically to affective disorders or schizophrenia and others to subtle organic deficits, whereas specific symptoms may be related to specific neurotransmitters (e.g., impulsivity and low CNS serotonin). Often, but *not* always, a history of early childhood abuse is found. Psychological testing is useful. Be sure to rule out organic states such as mild delirium, psychomotor epilepsy, or drug use in the acute presentation. Long-term, intermittent, supportive and psychodynamic psychotherapy is often beneficial (9), although *numerous* other psychotherapies have their supporters (*dialectical behavior therapy* has become recently popular) (10–12). Medication may be useful for specific symptoms (13). Psychotic-like symptoms may respond to low-dose antipsychotic agents (thioridazine, 100 to 300 mg hs, olanzapine) for short periods, mood disorders may respond to antidepressants (particularly SSRIs; fluoxetine for anger as well as depression), and affective lability and impulsivity may respond to mood stabilizers such as divalproex or lithium carbonate. Borderline patients tend to stabilize in their 40s and 50s (14).

Histrionic Personality Disorder (DSM, p. 711, 301.50)

Histrionic patients (♀ > ♂) initially seem charming, likable, lively, and seductive but gradually become seen as emotionally unstable, egocentric, immature, dependent, manipulative, excitement seeking, and shallow. They demand attention, are exhibitionistic and suggestible, and present a "caricature of femininity," yet have a limited ability to maintain stable, intimate, interpersonal relationships with either sex. This common disorder (2% or more in general population) is associated with depression, substance abuse, and conversion and (particularly) somatization disorders. Suicidal gestures and attempts are common. Lesser impaired patients respond to psychotherapy.

Narcissistic Personality Disorder (DSM, p. 714, 301.81)

Although often symptom free and well functioning, these patients (♂ > ♀) are chronically dissatisfied because of a constant need for admiration and habitually unrealistic self-expectations. They are impulsive and anxious; are arrogant, envious, and lacking in empathy; have ideas of omnipotence and of being "a special person"; become quickly dissatisfied with others; and maintain superficial, exploitative interpersonal relationships. Under stress and when others are not adequately admiring, they may become depressed, develop somatic complaints, have brief psychotic episodes, or display extreme rage. Mixtures with other personality disorders such as antisocial (15) are common. Long-term psychotherapy only occasionally helps.

ANXIOUS FEARFUL CLUSTER (CLUSTER "C")

Avoidant Personality Disorder (DSM, p. 718, 301.82)

The classic presentation is of an exceedingly shy, lonely, socially awkward, hypersensitive individual with low self-esteem who would rather avoid personal contact than face any potential social disapproval, even though desperate for interpersonal involvement (as opposed to the schizoid person). They assume others will be critical: This affects performance in school, work, and life (16). These patients are troubled by anxiety (especially social phobia, which is a close mimic) and depression. Group therapy, assertiveness training, and social skills training may help. Consider a trial of an SSRI or an anxiolytic.

Dependent Personality Disorder (DSM, p. 721, 301.6)

These are excessively passive, unsure, pessimistic, isolated people who are hypersensitive to criticism and who become abnormally dependent on one or more people. Initially acceptable, the behavior can become subtly controlling of others. Anxiety and depression are common, particularly if the dependent relationship is threatened. Appropriate psychotherapy may be helpful.

Obsessive–Compulsive Personality Disorder (DSM, p. 725, 301.4)

These patients, frequently successful men (M:F = 2:1; 1% of population), are inhibited, stubborn, perfectionistic, judgmental, overly conscientious, rigid, and chronically anxious individuals who avoid intimacy and may experience little pleasure from life but, in selected situations, can do well occupationally. They are indecisive yet demanding and are often perceived as cold, reserved, and in need of control. They are at risk to develop depression. Psychotherapy can effect changes over time.

Attention-Deficit/Hyperactivity Disorder (DSM, p. 85, 314.01)

Attention-deficit/hyperactivity disorder (ADHD) is a disorder diagnosed in childhood that can continue to produce problems in adults and has many features of, and is frequently mistaken for, a personality disorder. These patients have been distractible, *disorganized*, inattentive, *impulsive*, unable to tolerate stress, restless, quick tempered, and display *affective lability* (often hour by hour) since childhood. They may have learning disabilities. Their lability impairs interpersonal relations and job stability and often produces depression. They are at serious risk for drug abuse and alcoholism. Frequently, with age, the full criteria cannot be met (often the hyperactivity disappears), and the diagnosis becomes *ADHD, In Partial Remission* (commonly referred to as attention-deficit disorder or ADD). Differentiate from personality disorders, cyclothymic disorder (more recent onset), intermittent explosive disorder (normal between episodes), and primary depression. ADHD is most effectively treated with stimulants [methylphenidate and dextroamphetamine, in short-acting form or a variety of new longer-acting drugs; dextroamphetamine (Adderall & Adderall-XR, Dexedrine Spansule); methylphenidate (Concerta, Ritalin-SR, Ritalin-LA, Metadate CD, Focalin); other forms are being developed, including skin patches], but use them very cautiously due to abuse potential. Useful, alternative, nonstimulant medications include TCAs such as desipramine, bupropion, modafinil (?), and atomoxetine, none of which seems as effective as the stimulants, with the possible exception of bupropion. Combine medication with supportive psychotherapy.

REFERENCES

1. Millon T. *Disorders of personality: DSM-IV and beyond*. New York: Wiley, 1996.
2. McGuffin P, Thapar A. The genetics of personality disorder. *Br J Psychiatry* 1992;160:12–23.
3. Livesley WJ, Jang KL, Vernon PA. Phenotypic and genetic structure of traits delineating personality disorder. *Arch Gen Psychiatry* 1998;55:941–948.
4. Stone MH. Long-term outcome in personality disorders. *Br J Psychiatry* 1993;162:299–313.
5. Davis JM, Janicak PG, Ayd FJ. Psychopharmacotherapy of the personality-disordered patient. *Psychiatr Ann* 1995;25:614–620.
6. Tienari P, Wynne LC, Laksy K, et al. Genetic boundaries of the schizophrenia spectrum: evidence from the Finnish Adoptive Family Study of Schizophrenia. *Am J Psychiatry* 2003;160:1587–1594.
7. Bedwell JS, Donnelly RS. Schizotypal personality disorder or symptoms of schizophrenia? *Schizophr Res* 2005;80:263–269.
8. Biederman J, Monuteaux MC, Mick E, et al. Young adult outcome of attention deficit hyperactivity disorder: a controlled 10-year follow-up study. *Psychol Med* 2006;36:167–179.

9. Bateman A, Fonagy P. Effectiveness of partial hospitalization in the treatment of borderline personality disorder: a randomized controlled trial. *Am J Psychiatry*, 1999;156:1563–1569.

10. Binks CA, Fenton M, McCarthy L, et al. Psychological therapies for people with borderline personality disorder. *Cochrane Database Syst Rev* 2006;CD005652.

11. Lynch TR, Chapman AL, Rosenthal MZ, et al. Mechanism of change in dialectical behavior therapy: theoretical and empirical observations. *J Clin Psychol* 2006;62:459–489.

12. American Psychiatric Association. Practice guideline for the treatment of patients with borderline personality disorder. *Am J Psychiatry* 2001;158:1–52.

13. Binks CA, Fenton M, McCarthy L, et al. Pharmacological interventions for people with borderline personality disorder. *Cochrane Database Syst Rev* 2006;1:CD005653.

14. Stevenson J, Meares R, Comerford A. Diminished impulsivity in older patients with borderline personality disorder. *Am J Psychiatry* 2003;160:165–166.

15. Gunderson JG, Ronningstam E. Differentiating narcissistic and antisocial personality disorders. *J Person Dis* 2001;15:103–109.

16. Alden LE, Laposa JM, Taylor CT, et al. Avoidant personality disorder: current status and future directions. *J Person Dis* 2002;16:1–29.

21

Mental Retardation

There are 2 to 4 million mentally retarded persons in the United States (1% to 2% or more of population, depending on upper cutoff; M:F = 1.5:1; coded on Axis II in DSM), of whom 80% to 85% are only mildly retarded (1). The diagnosis of mental retardation requires decreased intellectual functioning (measured by standard IQ tests—two standard deviations below the mean IQ of 100) and impaired general functioning. Its presentation is modified by age, experience, and the environmental and cultural setting. When mild, it is most commonly first identified in grade-school children. Most mildly retarded adults, when no longer in school, are indistinguishable from the lowest socioeconomic segment of the general population and may no longer receive the diagnosis of mental retardation [i.e., they develop skills, adapt, and "grow out of it" (2)], but, although self-sufficient, they tend to be poor and to experience stress and emotional problems (3). Adults with intellectual impairment that developed before age 18 have (usually nonprogressive) *retardation,* and those developing it after age 18 (i.e., regressing from a higher level) have *dementia.*

CLASSIFICATION

- **MILD MENTAL RETARDATION** (DSM, p. 43, 317): IQ 50 to 70; considered *"educable."* Usually recognized when they enter school (and are tested) and require special education. Constitutes **85%** of the retarded (but this is the group that decreases markedly with adulthood). Many become self-supporting, with help, although they have limited judgment, social sensitivity, and insight.
- **MODERATE MENTAL RETARDATION** (DSM, p. 43, 318.0): IQ 35 to 50; **10%** of all retarded. Usually recognized during preschool years. They are *"trainable,"* can learn simple work skills, can read at a 2nd grade level and speak simply, and can be partly self-supporting in sheltered settings. They tend to be clumsy and uncoordinated.

- **SEVERE MENTAL RETARDATION** (DSM, p. 43, 318.1): IQ 20 to 35; **3% to 4%** of all retarded. These are the *dependent retarded*: They are capable of simple speech but require institutional or other intensely supportive care. Malformations and severe physical handicaps are frequent.
- **PROFOUND MENTAL RETARDATION** (DSM, p. 44, 318.2): IQ below 20; **1%** of all retarded. They are totally dependent on others for survival and usually have significant neurologic damage; cannot walk or talk.

A presumably retarded patient who is untestable is considered to have **MENTAL RETARDATION, SEVERITY UNSPECIFIED** (DSM, p. 44, 319).

CAUSES

Distinct causes (usually biologic) are identified in fewer than 50% of patients; these are most of the moderately-to-profoundly retarded patients. Other causes include environmental factors (e.g., pre- and perinatal problems, infant illness, psychosocial neglect, malnutrition), with an uncertain polygenic contribution in some cases. Moderate-to-profound retardation is distributed uniformly across social classes, whereas mild retardation (usually from sociocultural etiology) is weighted toward the lower classes. Retardation is a familial disorder (genetics or environment or both); the risk of retardation in a child with normal parents and siblings is less than **2%**, whereas the risk if both parents and one sibling are afflicted may be as great as **40% to 70%** (4).

Biological causes include

- Chromosomal abnormalities: Numerous types including *Down syndrome* (5) [mongolism, trisomy 21; the most common abnormality; more typical among older mothers; 10% to 16% of all retarded; most develop *Alzheimer disease* in their 30s or 40s (6)], *fragile X syndrome* (7) (2% to 7% of retardation among males; 1 in 2,000 live births; second most common abnormality), Klinefelter syndrome (XXY; 1% to 2% of retarded), Cri-du-chat syndrome, and Turner syndrome (XO/XX).
- Dominant genetic inheritance: Neurofibromatosis (Von Recklinghausen disease), Huntington chorea (with childhood onset), Sturge–Weber syndrome, tuberous sclerosis.
- Metabolic disorders: Phenylketonuria (PKU; early detection essential), Hartnup disease, fructose intolerance, galactosemia, Wilson disease, a variety of lipid disorders, hypothyroidism, hypoglycemia.

- Prenatal disorders: Maternal rubella (particularly in the first trimester), syphilis, toxoplasmosis, or diabetes; maternal alcohol abuse [fetal alcohol syndrome (8)] and use of some drugs (e.g., thalidomide); toxemia of pregnancy; erythroblastosis fetalis; maternal malnutrition.
- Birth trauma: Difficult delivery with physical trauma or anoxia or both, prematurity.
- Brain trauma: Tumors, infection (particularly encephalitis, neonatal meningitis), accidents, toxins (e.g., **lead**, mercury), hydrocephalus, numerous types of cranial abnormalities.

Social causes produce *many of the mild retardations* and include substandard education, environmental deprivation, childhood abuse and neglect, and restricted activity.

Rule out pervasive developmental disorders, dementia, and residual schizophrenia. Rule out **BORDERLINE INTELLECTUAL FUNCTIONING** (DSM, p. 740, V62.89; IQ 70–85). Look for associated psychiatric or neurologic syndromes.

TREATMENT AND PROGNOSIS

Formal cognitive testing at 1 to 2 years of age often is predictive of global outcome in many cases (9). However, mildly retarded individuals do develop further, often at an unpredictable but slower rate, with education (particularly with careful *mainstreaming*) and a supportive enironment. They are at risk for adjustment reaction, hyperactivity, and depression [50% or so demonstrate aggression and self-injury (10), psychotic reactions, and behavioral disturbances secondary to a negative self-image at some time]. Treat the patient with supportive reality-oriented psychotherapy. Determine the patient's coping style and temperamental strengths and encourage them but do not demand too much (11). Simple behavior-modification techniques may be very effective and should be part of any treatment program.

Severely retarded persons may require some form of institutionalization, yet training in sheltered settings should be considered if possible. If the patient lives with his or her family, treat the family. Parents and siblings frequently display anger, rejection, overprotection and overcontrol, denial, guilt, or a combination of these—all of which should be recognized and dealt with by the physician. Provide genetic counseling. Coordinate with outside agencies and specialists, when available.

Psychiatric syndromes are 3–4 times more common among the retarded. Consider psychopharmacology in patients with typical syndromes (12). Low doses of minor or major tranquilizers (e.g., risperidone, 0.5 to 2 mg/day) may help disruptive behavior problems (e.g., aggressiveness): do not overuse (it is easy to do). Lithium or propranolol may moderate self-abuse and aggression in some cases. Self-mutilation may respond better to clomipramine.

REFERENCES

1. Burack JA, Hodapp RM, Zigler E. *Handbook of mental retardation and development.* New York: Cambridge University Press, 1998.
2. Torrey WC. Psychiatric care of adults with developmental disabilities and mental illness in the community. *Community Ment Health J* 1993;29:461–481.
3. Maughan B, Collishaw S, Pickles A. Mild mental retardation: psycho-social functioning in adulthood. *Psychol Med* 1999;29:351–366.
4. Thapar A, Gottesman II, Owen MJ, et al. The genetics of mental retardation. *Br J Psychiatry* 1994;164:747–758.
5. Collacott RA, Cooper SA, Branford D, et al. Behavior phenotype for Down's syndrome. *Br J Psychiatry* 1998;172:85–89.
6. Holland AJ, Oliver C. Down's syndrome and the links with Alzheimer's disease. *J Neurol Neurosurg Psychiatry* 1995;59:111–114.
7. de Vries BB, Halley DJ, Oostra BA, et al. The fragile X syndrome. *J Med Genet* 1998;35:579–589.
8. Olney JW, Wozniak DF, Farber NB, et al. The enigma of fetal alcohol neurotoxicity. *Ann Med* 2002;34:109–119.
9. Largo RH, Graf S, Kundu S, et al. Predicting developmental outcome at school age from infant tests of normal, at-risk and retarded infants. *Dev Med Child Neurol* 1990;32:30–45.
10. Charlot LR. Irritability, aggression, and depression in adults with mental retardation. *Psychiatr Ann* 1997;27:190–197.
11. Siperstein GN, Leffert JS. Comparison of socially accepted and rejected children with mental retardation. *Am J Ment Retard* 1997;101:339–351.
12. Aman MG, Collier-Crespin A, Lindsay RL. Pharmacotherapy of disorders seen in mental retardation. *Eur Child Adolesc Psychiatry* 2000;9:98–107.

The Psychotherapies

Dozens of different psychotherapies address innumerable different patient problems (1). With the possible exception of a few specific behavioral and cognitive–behavioral methods applied to several discrete problems, rigorous proof of psychotherapy's effectiveness does not exist. However, much nonrigorous but very compelling experience indicates that various psychotherapies can help many patients—almost every therapist educates, gets patients to voice their concerns, encourages them to try out new behaviors, etc. Unfortunately, specific indications for specific therapies generally are not available. Some experts argue that many supposedly different psychotherapeutic methods are actually quite similar in practice (2). Other experts suggest that trained therapists using specific techniques may be less important for the patient's improvement than the therapist's personal characteristics of *accurate empathy*, *nonpossessive warmth*, and *genuineness*. Studies comparing the effectiveness of empathic trainees with that of experienced therapists have often found only modest differences in outcome (3).

Psychotherapy is a field without a high level of scientific objectivity. However, it is clear that some patients benefit from such care and that an essential ingredient to that care is a good patient–therapist relationship built on trust and genuine interest. Psychotherapy is an art, and a good therapist does make a difference. In general, one needs to find a therapy that is a "good fit" for the patient (i.e., the patient is comfortable with the therapist and the type of therapy). Patients resist psychotherapy unless they feel that it is both tolerable and likely to be of benefit; the dropout rate from therapy can be quite high. Individual treatment is the most common form of psychotherapy and comes in endless variations; group, family, and marital therapy are in widespread use as well (4).

INDIVIDUAL THERAPY

Supportive Therapy

Supportive therapy is probably the most common form of individual therapy (5). Therapists skilled in this method include psychiatrists, clinical psychologists, and social workers, although some approximation of supportive therapy is used by just about anyone who tries to help a person in emotional distress. The goal is to evaluate the patient's current life situation and his strengths and weaknesses and then to help him make whatever realistic changes will allow him to be more functional. Patients usually are seen weekly (or more often) for several weeks or months (although some patients are followed up infrequently for years). Also included is brief (1–3 session) crisis intervention.

The therapist deals with the patient's symptoms but works very little with the patient's unconscious processes and does not attempt major personality change. Psychological defenses are reinforced; techniques used include *reassurance*, suggestion, ventilation, abreaction, and environmental manipulation. The therapist must be active, interested, empathic, and warm—listen to the patient, understand his concerns, and help him find direction. Medication may be used.

Patients who are failing to cope successfully with present stress are good candidates, whether or not they have underlying psychiatric problems. Patients with serious psychiatric illnesses (e.g., schizophrenia, major affective disorder) often benefit from concurrent use of biologic methods and supportive psychotherapy.

Psychoanalytic Psychotherapy

Psychoanalysis is the classic, long-term insight-oriented therapy. The goal is to make major personality changes by identifying and modifying ("working through") unconscious conflicts by means of free association, analysis of transference and resistance, and dream interpretation. An "analysis" typically takes several hundred hours. "Neurotics" and those with personality disorders are the preferred patients. It is lengthy, expensive, and of uncertain effectiveness and so is infrequently used.

Psychoanalytic psychotherapy is similar to supportive therapy in that the goal is removal of symptoms, yet is similar to psychoanalysis in requiring a dynamic understanding of the patient's unconscious conflicts (insight) and in using analysis of the transference and dream interpretation. It is briefer than psychoanalysis and is used much more often.

Recently, **brief psychotherapy** has been explored as a way to affect a patient's problems while limiting both the number of therapy sessions (12 to 25+) and the number of issues addressed.

Usually a single conflict or interpersonal issue is chosen for therapy and explored in depth, most commonly from a psychodynamic perspective. Early results appear promising (6). Recognize that brief therapy can be approached from numerous different theoretical perspectives as well (e.g., using *humanistic principles* such as a belief that we all share an innate need for acceptance, love, and respect and that given proper support and help, we all have an innate drive toward psychological growth and health).

Interpersonal Therapy

A recent, reasonably well-controlled study (the New Haven–Boston Collaborative Depression Project) compared the effectiveness of various forms of psychotherapy with, and without, medication in the treatment of mild to moderate depression (7,8). **Interpersonal therapy** (ITP) was found effective. The combination of ITP and drugs improved most depressions, and maintenance medication or ITP or both seemed to prevent relapse.

ITP focuses on the patient's interpersonal relationships, their nature and their failings, and on improving those relationships. The idea is that if a person has vigorous, healthy, rewarding relations with other people, the person is less likely to become, be, or stay depressed (or anxious, etc.), and more likely to be happy. Evidence suggests this to be true. Treatment consists of:

1. **Education** (e.g., about depression; how common it is, its biologic nature, the risk that we all share of becoming depressed under stress). An effort is made to **destigmatize** the patient's mental problem.

2. **Information collection** about the patient's interpersonal relationships in an effort to determine which one(s) is not working. Such an inventory of the important interpersonal relationships in a person's life usually identifies, interestingly enough, a relationship that is poor or failing. Treatment begins with concentration on that relationship.

3. Several classical types of problems are found within relationships. Identify the most important one present, and attempt to repair it. Sample problems include

   INTERPERSONAL ROLE DISPUTES: Is the patient "hopelessly" at odds with someone of vital importance to him (e.g., spouse, parent, child, boss)? *SOLUTION:* You help the patient (a) determine what the dispute is about so he or she can see *both* sides, (b) clarify his or her own position in the dispute and also bring a degree of objectivity to his or her view of the problem, (c) form a reasonable plan of action to resolve the dispute, (d) identify any ways in which he may have been *miscommunicating with* or *misperceiving* the other person, and (e) modify his expectations for the relationship, if they seem unrealistic.

ROLE TRANSITIONS: Has a change in a relationship already occurred, and is the patient failing to cope with the new situation? *SOLUTION*: "Mourning" is going on here, too—grieving over a loss of an old role—and you must help facilitate that mourning as well and encourage the patient to see his new life situation as positive and as a "growth opportunity."

GRIEF AND LOSS: Has a relationship been lost and the patient been grieving? *SOLUTION*: (a) You facilitate the mourning process; and (b) You help the patient reestablish interests and develop new relationships to substitute for that which was lost.

4. This is meant to be brief therapy, lasting no more than 12 sessions of about 1 hour each. (That worked in the depression study.)

Cognitive–Behavioral Therapy

Cognitive-behavioral therapy (9,10) is a mixture of cognitive therapy and behavior therapy. It attributes emotional difficulties to faulty thinking or beliefs (**cognition**) that lead to counterproductive **behavior**. Psychiatric conditions presumably improve when the patient's thinking is more accurate and when the behavior is more appropriate. Thus the therapist works with the patient to identify and correct misperceptions (one by one) and (mis)behaviors. Therapy is very reality based and emphasizes the "here and now" (what is the patient thinking now; how is the patient behaving now). The patient is encouraged to think about his thinking. Cognitive–behavioral therapy has been used most successfully in the treatment of mild to moderate depression, panic disorder, OCD, and eating disorders, but seems to be even more widely useful.

■ Behavior Therapy

Behavior therapy is based on *learning theory*, which postulates that problem behaviors (i.e., almost any of the manifestations of psychiatric conditions) are involuntarily acquired because of inappropriate learning. Therapy concentrates on changing *behavior* (behavior modification) rather than on changing unconscious or conscious thought patterns, and to that end, it is very directive (i.e., patient receives much instruction and direction). Specific techniques to facilitate those changes include the following:

OPERANT CONDITIONING: These therapeutic techniques are based on careful evaluation and modification of the antecedents and consequences of a patient's behavior. Desired behavior is encouraged by *positive reinforcement* and discouraged by *negative reinforcement*. These new ways of responding to the patient can be taught to the people who live with the patient or, for inpatients, may take the form of a *token economy*.

AVERSION THERAPY: A patient is given an unpleasant, aversive stimulus (e.g., electric shock, loud sound) when his or her behavior is undesirable. Some of these procedures have been legally discouraged. An alternate technique, *covert sensitization*, is less objectionable because it uses unpleasant thoughts as the aversive stimulus.

IMPLOSIVE THERAPY: The patient with a situation-caused anxiety is directly exposed for a length of time to that situation (*flooding*) or exposed in imagination (*implosion*).

SYSTEMATIC DESENSITIZATION: The anxious or phobic patient is exposed to a gradual hierarchy of frightening situations or objects, beginning with the least worrisome. He eventually learns to handle the more frightening ones. If this is paired with relaxation (i.e., an antagonistic response pattern; relaxation is incompatible with anxiety), the technique is *reciprocal inhibition*.

Common to these methods (and numerous others) is rigorous data collection. Behavior therapy relies on careful measurement of behavior. A technique is considered useful only if it is successful, and its success is determined by whether it eliminates measurable undesired behavior or increases desired behavior.

■ Cognitive Therapy

(1) The way a person interprets his life experiences on a day-to-day basis determines how he feels day in and day out. (2) People with emotional distress tend to interpret their experiences in a dysfunctional, distorted way: these become the **core beliefs** of the person. (3) Over time, these distortions become "habitual errors in thinking." Common logical errors include, among others, *overgeneralization* [generalizes from a single event to all situations (e.g., if something went wrong once, a similar event is likely to go equally wrong)]; *magnification* (blowing an event out of proportion); *selective abstraction* (drawing conclusions from a detail taken out of context); and *personalization* (relating an event to yourself when no reason exists to do so). (4) Layered on top of these dysfunctional core beliefs and logical errors are **automatic thoughts**. These are "reflex thoughts" that we have in many situations; they are quick, and we are barely aware of them, yet they determine to

a large extent how we react emotionally to events. Automatic thoughts are typically followed by emotions such as sadness, anxiety, or anger. (5) Treatment involves identifying the core beliefs, habitual errors in thinking, and automatic thoughts and correcting them.

Cognitive therapy has been shown to be effective for a number of common psychiatric conditions (particularly depression, panic disorder, and generalized anxiety disorder). Sufficient, double-blind evidence suggests that cognitive therapy really works, particularly when coupled with behavioral approaches.

GROUP THERAPY

Group therapy (11) comes in many different forms, most of them derived from types of individual therapy.

INTERPERSONAL EXPLORATION GROUPS: The goal is to develop self-awareness of interpersonal styles through corrective feedback from other group members. The patient is accepted and supported, thus promoting self-esteem. It is the most common type of group therapy.

GUIDANCE-INSPIRATIONAL GROUPS: Highly structured, cohesive, supportive groups that minimize the importance of insight and maximize the value of ventilation and camaraderie. Groups may be large [e.g., Alcoholics Anonymous (AA)]. Members often are chosen because they "have the same problem."

PSYCHOANALYTICALLY ORIENTED THERAPY: A loosely structured group technique in which the therapist makes interpretations about a patient's unconscious conflicts and processes from observed group interactions.

Numerous other types of group therapies include behavioral therapy, Gestalt, encounter, psychodrama, transactional analysis (TA), marathon, EST, etc. Groups may run for weeks, months, or years, and usually meet weekly. They usually have five to 12 members (depending on type). Therapists from many different disciplines conduct groups; many groups run with co-therapists.

Some groups have patients with only one diagnosis (e.g., schizophrenia, alcoholism), whereas others are mixed. It is not clear which patients will benefit (or will be harmed) by group therapy, but most patients can be treated safely in groups. Most of the success of a group appears to depend more on the experience, sensitivity, warmth, and charisma of the leader than on the group's theoretic orientation.

A group experience that is too intense or confrontive can produce anxiety, depression, or psychotic reactions in susceptible patients. Acutely psychotic patients should not be included, and paranoid individuals make poor group members.

FAMILY THERAPY

Family therapy (12) can be conceptualized as a variant of group therapy. Numerous types of family therapy exist, but no one "right way." Although a family often enters therapy because one of the family members is "having problems," it is the implicit or explicit assumption of many family therapists that the family system is sick, not the patient. The expectation is that improvement in unhealthy interpersonal interactions and communications will result in improvement of the identified patient.

Most (but not all) family therapists recognize that some patients bring problems to family therapy that are not due to family malfunctioning, but most therapists argue that those problems are frequently worsened by any untreated malfunctioning.

MARITAL THERAPY

Therapy for a married couple is often called for if that relationship is at risk. It is particularly common if a psychosexual problem is present. Theoretic orientations and treatment techniques are diverse; none has been clearly shown to be superior. No clear guidelines exist for choosing couples likely to improve with marital therapy. Therapists may come from one of several professional disciplines (e.g., psychiatry, psychology, social work, marriage and family counseling).

MILIEU THERAPY

Milieu therapy usually takes place in an inpatient "therapeutic community." Often the entire community is geared toward support for the patient and toward helping him develop more adaptive coping skills. In a sense, all the staff members are therapists, and all the patients are likewise concerned with facilitating each other's well-being. It is a useful adjunct to other forms of therapy (e.g., pharmacotherapy).

REFERENCES

1. Tillett R. Psychotherapy assessment and treatment selection. *Br J Psychiatry* 1996;168:10–15.
2. Kovitz B. To a beginning psychotherapist: how to conduct individual psychotherapy. *Am J Psychother* 1998;52:103–115.
3. Krupnick JL, Sotsky SM, Simmens S, et al. The role of the therapeutic alliance in psychotherapy and pharmacotherapy outcome. *J Consul Clin Psychol* 1996;64:532–539.
4. Gabbard GO, Lazar SG, Hornberger J, et al. The economic impact of psychotherapy: a review. *Am J Psychiatry* 1997;154:147–155.
5. Winston A, Rosenthal RN, Pinsker H. *Introduction to supportive psychotherapy*. Washington, DC: American Psychiatric Publishing, 2004.
6. Levenson H. *Time-limited dynamic psychotherapy: A guide to clinical practice*. New York: Basic Books, 1995.
7. Elkin I, Shea T, Watkins JT, et al. NIMH Treatment of Depression Collaborative Research Program. *Arch Gen Psychiatry* 1989;46:971–982.
8. Elkin I, Gibbons RD, Shea MT, et al. Science is not a trial (but it can sometimes be a tribulation). *J Consult Clin Psychol* 1996;64:92–103.
9. Beck AT. *Cognitive therapy and the emotional disorders*. New York: International University Press, 1976.
10. Beck AT, Emery G. *Anxiety disorders and phobias: A cognitive perspective*. New York: Basic Books, 1985.
11. Yalom ID. *The theory and practice of group psychotherapy*. New York: Basic Books, 1995.
12. Pittman FS. *Turning points: treating families in transition and crisis*. New York: WW Norton, 1987.

Biologic Therapy

ANTIPSYCHOTICS

These are the "major tranquilizers" that revolutionized psychiatry by providing an effective treatment for large numbers of psychotic patients (1). Their antipsychotic effect is due not to sedation but to a specific action on the thought and mood disorder.

Drugs Available

Many different available antipsychotics are divided into two major categories: (a) for the first 30 years, we have used the *traditional antipsychotics*, drugs that acted through powerful D_2 receptor blockade; and (b) since the early 1990s, we have added the *atypical antipsychotics*, drugs that affect the D_2 receptor to a lesser degree while providing significant blockade of the $5\text{-}HT_{2A}$ receptor (2). Although both types of drugs are effective, the newer medications have several significant advantages that have caused them rapidly to become the "class of choice." Common examples of both classes are listed in Table 23.1.

TRADITIONAL ANTIPSYCHOTICS

Indications for Use

Recommended for
1. Acute schizophrenia and other acute psychoses (e.g., amphetamine psychosis, organic psychoses). They should be used in conjunction with lithium in the acute manic attacks of bipolar disorder.
2. Chronic schizophrenia.
3. Major depression with significant psychotic features; used in conjunction with an antidepressant.
4. Tourette syndrome: haloperidol is the drug most commonly used.

TABLE 23.1 ■ The Antipsychotics

TRADITIONAL ANTIPSYCHOTICS

Equivalent doses (mg)

PHENOTHIAZINES

Dimethylamino-alkyl derivatives

Chlorpromazine (Thorazine)	100

Piperidine-alkyl derivatives

Thioridazine (Mellaril)	100
Mesoridazine (Serentil)	50

Piperazine-alkyl derivatives

Fluphenazine (Prolixin)	1–2
Fluphenazine decanoate (long-acting)	
Trifluoperazine (Stelazine)	8
Perphenazine (Trilafon)	10

THIOXANTHENES

Thiothixene (Navane)	4

DIBENZOXAZEPINES

Loxapine (Loxitane)	15

DIHYDROINDOLONES

Molindone (Moban)	15

BUTYROPHENONES

Haloperidol (Haldol)	1–2
Haloperidol decanoate (long-acting)	

DIPHENYLBUTYLPIPERIDINES

Pimozide (Orap)	1–2

ATYPICAL ANTIPSYCHOTICS

Therapeutic dose (mg/day)

Clozapine (Clozaril)	200–600
Olanzapine (Zyprexa)	10–25
Quetiapine fumarate (Seroquel)	100–800
Risperidone (Risperdal)	4–6
Ziprasidone (Geodon)	80–160
Aripiprazole (Abilify)	10–30

Other uses:

- Antipsychotics can be of temporary use in several conditions (e.g., acute agitation of a nonpsychotic nature, antiemesis).

Mechanisms of Action

The dopamine hypothesis postulates that schizophrenia is secondary to increased central dopamine activity. Traditional antipsychotics are thought to act primarily by a broad and powerful postsynaptic blockade of the D_2 receptors. The three major CNS dopamine pathways affected by these medications, with their putative activities, are

- Nigrostriatal: Extrapyramidal actions
- Tuberoinfundibular: Endocrine actions (increased prolactin)
- Mesolimbic: Antipsychotic actions (probably)

The different side-effect patterns of the various antipsychotic drugs are thought to be due to their different locations of primary activity. However, traditional antipsychotics also block central noradrenergic (norepinephrine; NE) receptors, thus we cannot be certain whether dopamine (DA) or NE blockage (or another mechanism entirely) is responsible for the antipsychotic effect of these drugs.

Pharmacokinetics

Chlorpromazine (as a classic example) is variably absorbed from the intestine and is probably partly degraded in the mucosal wall. It is approximately 95% protein bound. Much higher blood levels are attained after i.m. or i.v. than p.o. administration. The half-life is 1 to 2+ days, but variable, with the majority of the drug stored in body fat. _Marked_ interindividual differences are found in blood levels (reasons are unclear).

Metabolism is complex (e.g., chlorpromazine is degraded by sulfoxidation, hydroxylation, deamination, and demethylation to form well over 100 metabolites). Some of the metabolites are active, and some are inactive; it is not completely worked out. In part because of this complexity, measured plasma levels of many antipsychotics are not clinically useful. In contrast, certain other antipsychotics (e.g., haloperidol, thiothixene) have a simple metabolism; however, their plasma measurement as a guide to outcome is of uncertain value.

Side Effects

Side effects are common and are almost unavoidable at higher drug dosages. Fewer side-effect problems is a major reasons for the superiority of the newer antipsychotics. The particular pattern of

TABLE 23.2	Most Common Side Effects of the Traditional Antipsychotics		
Drug	Sedation	Extrapyramidal	Hypotension
Phenothiazines			
Aliphatic	3+	2+	3+
Piperidine	2+	1+	2+
Piperazine	1+	3+	1+
Dibenzoxazepines	2+	3+	2+
Butyrophenones	2+	3+	1+
Dihydroindolones	1+	2+	1+

side effects is in part determined by the chemical class of any given antipsychotic. These side effects also have marked interindividual variability. The most common side effects (Table 23.2) of these medications include sedation, extrapyramidal and anticholinergic symptoms, hypotension, weight gain, and reduced libido, but many other side effects occur as well.

- Sedation: Common; use a qd schedule, if possible.

- **Anticholinergic symptoms:**
  Dry mouth: Common. May lead to moniliasis, parotitis, and an increase in cavities. Consider treatment with oral water and ice, sugarless gum; also neostigmine, 7.5 to 15 mg p.o.; pilocarpine, 2.5 mg p.o. q.i.d.; or bethanechol, 75 mg daily.
  Constipation: Treat with stool softeners.
  Blurred vision: Near vision. Treat with physostigmine drops, 0.25% solution, 1 drop q6h, if it is a major problem.
  Urinary hesitancy and retention: Consider using urecholine, 10 to 25 mg p.o. t.i.d.
  Exacerbation of glaucoma
  Central anticholinergic syndrome: Occurs particularly in those patients simultaneously taking several drugs with anticholinergic properties [e.g., an overdose (OD) or a patient taking an antipsychotic, an antidepressant, and an antiparkinsonian]. The syndrome can vary from mild anxiety and vasodilatation to a toxic delirium or even coma. It is much more common in the elderly. Symptoms and signs to be looked for include:
      Anxiety, restlessness, agitation—grading into confusion, incoherence, disorientation, memory impairment, visual and auditory hallucinations—grading into seizures, stupor, and coma.

Warm and dry skin, flushed face, dry mouth, hyper-pyrexia.

Blurred vision, dilated pupils.

Absent bowel sounds.

Treat an acute delirium with withdrawal of the causative agent, close medical supervision (e.g., cardiac monitor), and physostigmine, 1 to 2 mg i.m. or slowly i.v. (e.g., 1 mg/min). Repeat in 15 to 30 minutes and then every 1 to 2 hours, if needed. Avoid physostigmine in patients with bowel or bladder obstruction, peptic ulcer, asthma, glaucoma, heart disease, diabetes, or hypothyroidism. Watch for cholinergic overdose (salivation, sweating, etc.), and treat with atropine (0.5 mg for each milligram of physostigmine).

- **Extrapyramidal symptoms:** These reactions are common, get worse with stress, disappear during sleep, and wax and wane over time.

  Acute dystonic reaction: An involuntary sustained contraction of a skeletal muscle that usually appears suddenly (over 5 to 60 minutes). The jaw muscles are most frequently involved (i.e., "lock-jaw"), but other muscle systems may also be disturbed (e.g., torticollis, carpopedal spasm, ocu-logyric crisis, even opisthotonos). Usually occurs during the first 2 days of treatment (in 2% to 10% of patients, more common in younger patients).

  Parkinson-like syndrome: The three primary symptoms occur individually or together, usually during weeks 1 to 4 of treatment. They are more common in older patients.

  "Tremor": An irregular tremor of the upper extremities, tongue, and jaw. It occurs with both movement and rest and is slower than the tremors produced by tricyclic antidepressants (TCAs) and lithium.

  "Rigidity": A cogwheel rigidity that starts with the shoulders and spreads to the upper extremities and then throughout the body.

  "Akinesia": A "zombie-like" effect with slowness, fatigue, micrographia, and little facial expression. It may occur alone and at any time during the course of treatment and is easily mistaken for social withdrawal or depression.

  Akathisia: Common. Patients are fidgety, constantly move their hands and feet, rock from the waist, and shift from foot to foot. Easily mistaken for anxiety or agitation. The patients are typically dysphoric. Treat with anticholinergics, propranolol (10 mg t.i.d., 30 to 120 mg/day), or lorazepam.

  Rabbit syndrome: Involuntary chewing movements.

Tardive dyskinesia: Slow choreiform or tic-like movements, usually of the tongue and facial muscles, but occasionally of the upper extremities or the whole body. Risk is increased in the aged, those with organic brain syndrome (OBS), females, high doses of medication, simultaneous use of several antipsychotics, and possibly long duration of treatment. Develops over months or years of antipsychotic use; a few severe cases may be irreversible, but it usually follows a stable, benign, long-term course. Symptoms disappear with an increased dosage of antipsychotic: do not "misread" the movements as a worsening psychosis, raise the dose of medication, remove the symptom, and thus begin a vicious cycle. "Drug holidays" do not seem to prevent, and may even worsen, the development of TD. No acceptable treatment is known. Try to discontinue the antipsychotic, if possible.

Treatment of Extrapyramidal Symptoms

Treat with the anticholinergic *antiparkinsonism drugs* (Table 23.3):

TABLE 23.3 ■ Antiparkinsonism Drugs	
Drug	**Typical dosage**
Benztropine (Cogentin)	1–4 mg, q.d.-b.i.d., p.o.
Biperdin (Akineton)	1–2 mg, t.i.d., q.i.d., p.o.
Procyclidine (Kemadrin)	2–5 mg, t.i.d.-q.i.d., p.o.
Trihexyphenidyl (Artane, Tremin)	2–5 mg, t.i.d.-q.i.d., p.o.
Diphenhydramine (Benadryl)	25–50 mg, t.i.d.-q.i.d., p.o.
Amantadine (Symmetral)	100 mg, q.d.-t.i.d., p.o.

Begin at a lower dosage and increase over a several-day period. Use for several weeks, and then discontinue if possible. Try not to use for more than 2 to 3 months (although they may be necessary over the long term in a few patients). They probably should not be used prophylactically (begun when antipsychotics are started), except in those patients very likely to be resistant to taking medications. Treat acute dystonic reactions immediately (i.m. or i.v.) with (for example) benztropine (Cogentin), 1 mg; diphenhydramine (Benadryl), 25 to 50 mg; or diazepam (Valium), 5 to 10 mg; and then begin regular oral dose for several weeks. These drugs often worsen side effects of TD; they may also be abused.

- α-Adrenergic blocking symptoms: Orthostatic hypotension, inhibition of ejaculation (particularly thioridazine).
- Cholestatic jaundice: Probably a sensitivity reaction. Fever and eosinophilia, usually during the first 2 months of treatment

(in 1% of patients taking chlorpromazine). Little cross-sensitivity with other antipsychotics.

- Agranulocytosis: Usually in elderly women during the first 4 months of treatment but can occur any time. Train patients to report persistent sore throats, infections, or fever. Rare.
- Neuroleptic malignant syndrome (NMS): Rapidly developing (hours to 1 to 2 days) muscular rigidity and cogwheeling, fever, confusion, hypertension, sweating, tachycardia. Look for rhabdomyolysis with myoglobinemia and *very* elevated CPK. In 1%+ of pts, particularly (but not exclusively) after high-dose, high-potency depot medications, but not strongly dose related. Often fatal if untreated. Stop medications immediately; provide medical support; "possibly" helpful are dantrolene (muscle relaxant; blocks intracellular Ca^{2+} release; 400 mg/day) and bromocriptine (dopamine agonist; 7.5 to 45 mg/day, t.i.d.). Patient may recover over a 5- to 15-day period. It typically does *not* recur on later reexposure to antipsychotics.
- Hypothermia; hyperthermia: Watch out for hot seclusion rooms.
- Weight gain, obesity.
- Pigmentary changes in skin: Particularly with chlorpromazine. A tan, gray, or blue color.
- Retinitis pigmentosa: Possible blindness. Occurs with dosages of thioridazine greater than 800 mg/day.
- Photosensitivity: Bad sunburns with chlorpromazine (Thorazine).
- Grand mal seizures: Particularly with rapid increases in dose.
- Nonspecific skin rashes: In 5%.
- Reduced libido in men and women.
- Increased prolactin levels: Produces galactorrhea, amenorrhea, and lactation.
- ECG changes: Particularly with thioridazine: T-wave inversions, occasionally arrhythmias.
- Appears safe during pregnancy: no known congenital abnormalities. Slight hypertonicity among newborns, but little effect on a nursing infant.

Suicide is difficult but possible with the antipsychotics; it requires very large doses.

Drug Interactions

Antacids: May inhibit absorption of oral antipsychotics.

Tricyclic and selective serotonin reuptake inhibitors (SSRI) antidepressants: May inhibit antipsychotic metabolism and increase plasma levels, and vice versa.

Treatment Principles

- Drug choice: The primary reason to choose one drug over another is the side-effect spectrum. They are all equally capable of controlling psychosis when used appropriately. If a patient or a similarly affected family member has responded well to one medication, try it. If a patient has a seizure disorder, use a high potency drug (e.g., fluphenazine, haloperidol).
- Treatment of acute psychosis: Sedating antipsychotics that can be given i.m. usually provide the best control initially (e.g., haloperidol, chlorpromazine), although they have no long-term advantages. Give orally if the patient is cooperative, but i.m. if he or she is not.
  1. If possible, give a small test dose (e.g., haloperidol, 5 mg) and wait 1 hour to see if it is tolerated.
  2. Then begin haloperidol, 10 to 15 mg/day; chlorpromazine, 300 to 400 mg/day; or the equivalent. Use t.i.d. or q.i.d. schedule initially, and then switch to b.i.d. or qd after 1 to 2 weeks. A HS schedule is usually well tolerated and helps insomnia. It may be necessary to increase to 500 mg/day of chlorpromazine, 15 to 20 mg/day of haloperidol, or the equivalent. Rarely go higher. If side effects become a problem, begin antiparkinsonism drugs or reduce the dosage and increase more slowly, or both.
  3. If the patient is wild and needs immediate control and effective physical control is not readily available, consider more rapid tranquilization [e.g., haloperidol, 5 mg i.m. every hour x3 to 4 (or, perhaps more effective, haloperidol, 5 mg + lorazepam, 2 to 4 mg, i.m., in the same syringe)]. Monitor carefully for hypotension or oversedation. Once the patient is under control, switch to the preceding daily schedule.
- Disease control is cognitive as well as behavioral: The goal is not just to "quiet" the patient. Improvement is slow and often partial. Increasing socialization is an early sign of a drug response. Agitated, disruptive behavior usually improves in the first several days. The thought disorder disappears over weeks or months. Traditional antipsychotics improve the *positive symptoms* of psychosis (e.g., hallucinations, delusions, bizarre behavior), but, unfortunately, they usually do not change the *negative symptoms* (e.g., flat affect, social impairment)—a major problem (addition of a low-dose SSRI occasionally helps). Patients who are "acutely crazy" are *most* likely to respond well, as are those with good premorbid functioning who are having their first psychotic episode. If significant obsessive–compulsive symptoms are present, consider a trial of clomipramine. If a

depression appears, consider switching to an atypical antipsychotic: antidepressants are of modest help at best.

- If a patient does not respond, switch to another drug of a different type. However, the unimproved patient needs at least one 2- to 3-week trial at a higher dose of an antipsychotic before you conclude that he does not respond to medication. Rarely is there any reason to use two different antipsychotics simultaneously. The most common cause for lack of response is underdosage (and noncompliance), but always be wary that the patient may have an organic psychosis.

- Once improvement has occurred, maintain drug levels over a 1- to 2-month period and then consider reducing to maintenance levels. If this is the first episode of an acute psychosis in a previously well-functioning patient, consider discontinuing the medication in 6 months to 1 year. If this episode is one of many, the patient may need maintenance medication for years.

- Antipsychotic maintenance therapy: Decrease dosage slowly (over weeks to months) to one third or one fourth of the immediate dose. If a relapse begins, increase the dose. About 90% of patients relapse (during first 24 months) without medications; 40%[+] relapse while taking them. Teach the patient to recognize his or her own developing relapse so it can be caught early.

Traditional antipsychotics are often unpleasant to take, so compliance is a major problem with outpatients (particularly those patients who are suspicious and paranoid). Pay attention to and work aggressively to control side effects (particularly akathisia). If the patient is reluctant to take daily medication, consider the long-acting depot forms of two very potent antipsychotics: fluphenazine decanoate and haloperidol decanoate. They can be given i.m. every 2 to 4 weeks in very low doses [e.g., fluphenazine decanoate (12.5 to 25 mg i.m. every 2 weeks) or haloperidol decanoate (50 to 100[+] mg i.m. every month)]. The relapse rate may be slightly increased at these doses, but side effects and compliance usually are improved. (Depot medications may be preferable, whether or not the patient is noncompliant, particularly in the medication-refractory patient.)

ATYPICAL ANTIPSYCHOTICS

Currently six new antipsychotics are available in the United States. Five of the six quickly have become the initial **treatment of choice** for schizophrenia and other psychotic conditions. Choose one of them first because

1. They have many fewer side effects than the traditional antipsychotics in low to moderate doses. Thus compliance is likely to be much improved. However, they do produce weight gain, hyperglycemia, and perhaps diabetes.
2. They are at least equally effective in treating the positive symptoms of schizophrenia and all "may" have greater effectiveness at treating the **negative symptoms** as well.
3. They may produce less **cognitive impairment** than the traditional medications.
4. They seem to allow the patient a higher quality of life than the traditional antipsychotics, and they improve **mood**.
5. With the exception of clozapine, they appear quite safe.
6. Early studies have found them to have a comparatively low relapse rate.

Although these medications seem to be a marked improvement over earlier antipsychotics, questions are being raised [e.g., the CATIE study (3)]. With the exception of clozapine, they appear to be no more effective than the traditional antipsychotics, although more free from side effects. However, it does appear that they all work through some variation of the same mechanism: they all have a modest to moderate effect at blocking the D_1 to D_4 receptors and, unlike the older drugs, a moderate ability to block the 5-HT_{2A} receptor, among others. Clozapine, the only one of the six medications that is not a first-line drug (because of an uncommon but very dangerous side effect of agranulocytosis), has been shown fairly clearly to be the drug of choice for treatment-resistant schizophrenia. Suggestive, but less complete and convincing, evidence is available that one or more of the other newer medications also are effective in patients in whom the older antipsychotics have failed (4). Too few comparison studies among these medications have been done to allow the clinician to decide which one is preferable for which patient. They all seem to be roughly equivalent. They currently also are being used fairly widely (and successfully) in conditions like bipolar disorder (mania), intermittent explosive disorder, and in geriatric patients with agitated behavior or dementia or both. The limits of their utility has not yet been reached. One negative feature (at this time) to these medications is that they all are quite expensive. Also, they may, as a group, require 2 to 3 weeks before significant improvement is seen. Finally, they have a "black box" warning for increased mortality when used in elderly patients with dementia-related psychosis.

Most of the general principles followed when treating patients with the older medications also apply here. For example, (a) a complete trial takes about 8 weeks, (b) a patient who smokes heavily generally requires a higher dose of medication because of increased clearance, and (c) if a patient is prone to relapse when taken off medication, any one of these drugs appears to be an appropriate choice for a maintenance regimen.

Specific New Medications

- **Clozapine** (Clozaril), a unique antipsychotic (modest D_2, receptor blockade; strong D_4 and 5-HT_{2a} receptor blockade) should be used with schizophrenic patients who cannot tolerate or are refractory to traditional and/or atypical medications (5). Marked improvement occurs in almost 30% of treatment-resistant patients with chronic illness; modest improvement in another 10% to 20%. Unlike other antipsychotics, clozapine may improve symptoms of apathy, withdrawal, anhedonia, and flat affect: a "significant cure" in a few patients. It also has mood-stabilizing properties; consider in schizoaffective, manic (6), and psychotically depressed patients.

  After a thorough medical (laboratory) examination, begin dosage at 25 mg and increase to 300 to 400 daily (b.i.d. to t.i.d. schedule) over a 2-to 3-week period. (It is very expensive, although a generic is available.) A response may take weeks or even months. Upper limit is 900 mg/day, but be very cautious above 600 mg, because some side effects are related to dose and speed of increase [e.g., *sedation, grand mal (GM) seizures* (unusual under 300 mg; 5% of patients over 600 mg; do not use in patients with a history of a seizure disorder)]. Other SEs include sialorrhea, *weight gain* (and very likely diabetes), tachycardia, hypotension, fever, and elevated liver enzymes. It produces almost no EPS or TD. Its blood level may increase if used with SSRIs (particularly fluvoxamine), and NMS may be a risk, particularly if lithium is used concurrently. Clozapine has a difficult withdrawal, so discontinue slowly.

  The life-threatening side effect is **agranulocytosis**: about 1% of patients; usually during months 1 to 6 (but possible anytime); requires *weekly* WBC with differential for the first 6 months, then every 2 weeks for 6 months, then monthly indefinitely (stop medications if the WBC is less than 3,000 or granulocytes less than 1,500); not dose related. If WBCs decrease below 2,000, never rechallenge the patient with clozapine. Do not start clozapine unless the WBC count is more than 3,500. Do not use in patients with known blood dyscrasias or who are taking drugs with similar effects on the WBCs (e.g., carbamazepine). TAKE THESE GUIDELINES SERIOUSLY.

- **Risperidone** (Risperdal) was the second new antipsychotic released in the United States. It has fewer side effects than previous antipsychotics, is safe in overdose, and seems to affect both positive and negative symptoms. Begin with 0.5 to 1 mg b.i.d. and increase slowly; the ideal final dose for most patients is 4 to 6 mg/day (usually b.i.d. or qd). It is usually effective and well tolerated at that level, although the risk for EPS, orthostatic hypotension, agitation, and elevated prolactin is real and increases significantly above 6 mg/day. TD has been seen with this medication; weight gain is minor. A long-acting injectable form is available (Risperdal Consta); the usual dose is 25 to 50 mg i.m. q2 weeks.

- **Olanzapine** (Zyprexa) is effective when taken in a once-daily dose of 10 to 20 mg (begin with 5 mg/day), and it is available in an i.m. form for immediate treatment. It seems to produce less EPS than risperidone but produces considerably more *weight gain* (and diabetes and hyperlipidemia) as well as *sedation* and postural hypotension. It might be slightly more effective than the other atypicals (except clozapine), but it presents very high metabolic risk if not monitored very closely.

- **Quetiapine** (Seroquel) appears the equal of the other new antipsychotics. Its side effects are similar to those of olanzapine, although perhaps not as severe, but weight gain, *sedation*, *dizziness* and orthostatic hypotension may be problems. The range of dosage is broad, with clinically similar patients requiring anywhere from 200 to 800 mg daily (b.i.d. recommended, short half-life).

- **Ziprasidone** (Geodon) seems to be a very effective medication, which has the advantage of very minimal EPS and weight gain (if any at all) and improvement in mood. Its side effects tend to be GI complaints: nausea, abdominal pain, dyspepsia, dizziness and constipation, although they are generally mild. Ziprasidone also has the advantage of being available in pill, liquid, and i.m. form. It appears to be effective for treating acute mania. Finally, it acts as a $5-HT_{1A}$ agonist and thus may be an effective antianxiety agent as well. Dosage should be 60 to 80 mg, p.o. b.i.d. or 10 mg 1m q 2hr as needed to a maximum of 40 mg.

- **Aripiprazole** (Abilify) possesses most of the characteristics of the atypical antipsychotics and, at a normal dose of 10 to 30 mg/day (once daily), may be particularly free of side effects. It can be too activating for some patients, so begin slowly. The most common side effects include agitation, nausea, akathisia, tremor, and headaches.

MOOD STABILIZERS

Lithium Carbonate

Lithium carbonate (Li$^+$, atomic number 3), is available in slow-release form: Eskalith CR, Lithobid Slow-Release Tablets.

Indications for Use

It is recommended for
1. *"Classic" acute bipolar disorder, manic.* Lithium is the drug of choice for stabilization of an acute manic attack (80% of patients normalize) although, because of the usual 7- to 10-day delay in clinical onset, an additional drug *may* be needed initially for control. Best for "classic" bipolar disorder; for "rapid cyclers," use anticonvulsants instead (only about one third respond to Li).
2. *Acute depression: bipolar* (good; up to 80% respond, but it is slow to act, takes 3 to 6 weeks), and *unipolar* (about one third respond, thus it is a second-choice drug). Definitely consider the addition of Li to augment a partial response to another (any other) antidepressant; 50% respond (usually quickly, in 1$^+$ weeks).
3. Long-term prophylaxis of mania in a bipolar patient: It is quite effective at preventing recurrences when coupled with an anticonvulsant. Be careful of chronic renal toxicity.

   Possible uses include
   - Prophylaxis for bipolar disorder, depressed, and for major depression.
   - May assist (usually) or replace antipsychotics in treatment of a few patients with schizoaffective disorder.
   - May help control mood swings, *impulsive aggression*, and *explosive outbursts*, regardless of cause, and retarded patients with aggressiveness or self-mutilation or both.
   - Curiously, it is effective in chronic prophylactic treatment of *cluster headaches*.

Mechanisms of Action

The reasons for the clinical effects are poorly understood, although Li does enhance presynaptic serotonergic neurotransmission, "seems" to reduce pre- and postsynaptic dopamine transmission, and increases plasma NE levels.

Pharmacokinetics

Lithium is quickly absorbed from the GI tract (completely absorbed in 8 hours) and develops a peak plasma level in 1 to 3 hours. It is *not* protein bound or metabolized and is excreted by the kidney. The cerebrospinal fluid (CSF) concentration is 30% to 60% of that in plasma and equivalent to that in red blood cells (RBCs). It is concentrated by bone and by thyroid (4 to 5 times that in plasma).

Lithium can be used safely *only* if blood concentrations are monitored carefully (oral dosage is *not* an adequate measure). To obtain consistent levels, draw blood 12 hours after the last dose (e.g., take evening dose, then draw before breakfast). The lithium half-life is 18 to 36 hours (fastest in youth, slowest in elderly); a constant oral dosage requires 5 to 8 days to reach steady state. Once a steady state is reached, the lithium level is proportional to the daily oral dose (and determined by the renal clearance).

Side Effects

The number and severity of side effects increase with elevated or rapidly changing/increasing Li blood levels. A slight change in blood level (0.1 to 0.2 mEq/L) may alter dramatically the number or intensity of the side effects. Minor side effects (tremor, impaired coordination, dysarthria, thirst, anorexia, and GI distress) commonly occur at therapeutic levels (0.8 to 1.5 mEq/L), and serious effects (nausea and vomiting, slurred speech, diarrhea, coarse tremors, severe ataxia, confusion, delirium, seizures, coma, death) may occur at only slightly higher levels (e.g., as low as 2.0 to 2.5 mEq/L but more commonly at 3 to 5 mEq/L). Some evidence suggests that mild side effects can be controlled with a daily dietary supplement of 20 to 40 mEq of K^+. Lithium has a very narrow margin of safety and is a dangerous drug in overdosage. It should be given cautiously (or not given at all) in patients who are dehydrated, febrile, have sodium depletion (kidney reabsorbs more lithium), or have major renal or cardiovascular disease. Brain-damaged patients and the elderly are at risk for side effects even at low blood levels: use with care.

Normal subjects administered lithium report irritability and emotional lability, anxiety, mild depression, tiredness and malaise, weakness, inability to concentrate, impaired memory, and slowed reaction time. Patients taking lithium often experience a "lithium-induced dysphoria"; 25% to 50% stop lithium against medical advice (AMA). Unlike other psychoactive medication, sedation is *not* a side effect.

■ **Neurologic**

EEG: Usually shows increased amplitude and generalized slowing (in 50% of patients at therapeutic blood levels).

Headaches, occasional slurred speech.

Toxicity: confusion, poor concentration, and clouding of consciousness; leads to delirium; leads to coma; leads to death.

Cerebellar effects: dysarthria, ataxia, nystagmus, severe incoordination.

Basal ganglia effects: Parkinsonian symptoms, choreiform movements.

Seizures: grand mal; status epilepticus.

■ **Neuromuscular**

Hand tremor (fine, fast) that does not respond to anticholinergics. Occurs in 50% of the patients started on lithium, but the incidence decreases with time (5% of long-term patients).

Treat with β-blockers (e.g., propranolol, p.o., 30 to 80 mg/day.

Muscular weakness: one third of patients during the first week of treatment; transient.

Neuromuscular toxicity: hyperactive reflexes, fasciculations, paralysis.

■ **Kidney**

Polyuria and polydipsia: secondary to a vasopressin-resistant, diabetes insipidus–like syndrome. Reversible and occurs in 50% of all new patients (5% of all with chronic disease).

Reversible oliguric renal failure with acute lithium intoxication.

Possible irreversible nephrotoxic effect in a few with chronic disease: focal interstitial cortical fibrosis with tubular atrophy and sclerotic glomeruli. Look for a gradually increasing blood lithium in patients taking a constant oral dose. Increased serum creatinine and an increased 24-hour urine volume are found. Poorly characterized currently, this serious effect of prolonged lithium administration may limit the ability to use lithium prophylactically in some.

■ **Blood**

Leukocytosis (10,000 to 14,000 WBCs: neutrophilia with lymphocytopenia). Common and reversible, it is persistent but periodic while the patient is taking lithium.

Occasional increased erythrocyte sedimentation rate (ESR).

■ Gastrointestinal

About 30% of patients have GI symptoms in the early weeks of treatment: gastric irritation, nausea, anorexia, diarrhea, bloating, abdominal pain (a switch to lithium citrate may relieve symptoms).

■ Heart

T-wave flattening or inversion (common but reversible).

Unusual: Myocarditis, SA block, primary AV block; ventricular irritability and perhaps sudden death (particularly in older men with cardiac pathology; more common at toxic levels).

■ Thyroid

Lithium may produce hypothyroidism with (10% of patients with chronic disease) or without a goiter. Measure thyroid-stimulating hormone (TSH). Low-dose thyroxine may help, but consult an endocrinologist.

■ Other

Impaired memory

Lithium accumulates in bone: no known harmful effects.

Occasional maculopapular rash, acne: Also (rarely) alopecia, ulceration, and exacerbation of psoriasis.

Weight gain in 10% of patients. Partly related to a Li-induced *reactive hypoglycemia.*

Occasional benign, reversible exophthalmos.

Hyperparathyroidism: increased serum calcium and parathyroid hormone, usually without other symptoms.

Most of the side effects disappear with chronic lithium administration. Persistent side effects include tremor, polyuria, leukocytosis, goiter, and elevated blood sugar.

In *pregnancy*:

1. Lithium crosses the placenta freely and can produce cardiac malformations (Ebstein anomaly and others), although they seem to be infrequent. Pregnant women should avoid lithium unless the risks of a "manic pregnancy" outweigh the small risk of fetal malformations. Such infants also are at risk for nephrogenic diabetes insipidus, hypoglycemia, and euthyroid goiter.

2. Lithium in milk is 30% to 100% of the maternal blood level; thus these mothers should not breast feed.

3. Lithium clearance increases 50% to 100% early in pregnancy and returns to normal at delivery; so a dosage that had been increased during pregnancy must be immediately reduced, or the mother will become toxic.

Drug Interactions

Diuretics: Thiazides decrease lithium clearance and increase blood levels; furosemide, ethacrynic acid, spironolactone, and triamterene may also. Mannitol, urea, and acetazolamide decrease blood levels. Tetracyclines, indomethacin, phenylbutazone, and methyldopa may increase lithium blood levels.

Haloperidol (and other high-potency neuroleptics): A (usually) reversible neurotoxicity may occur in some patients at higher doses of antipsychotic (confusion, disorientation, etc). Potentially life-threatening: watch for it.

Chlorpromazine may increase the rate of lithium excretion.

Tricyclic antidepressants may act *synergistically* with lithium.

Aminophylline increases lithium excretion.

Lithium probably prolongs the neuromuscular blocking effect of succinylcholine.

Treatment Principles

- Select appropriate patients. Screen for serious medical illness. Preadministration laboratory evaluation should include the following:

  CBC, BUN, UA

  Serum creatinine.

  T_3, T_4; examine thyroid.

  Serum Na^+ if reason occurs to question the patient's electrolyte status.

  ECG if the physical examination or history suggest cardiac disease.

  If prolonged use of lithium is expected, obtain 24-hour urine volume, creatinine clearance, and protein excretion.

- Treatment of acute mania: The goal is to produce a therapeutic blood level (1.2 to 1.4 mEq/L) and maintain it until a clinical effect is seen (usually 7 to 10 days after an appropriate level is attained). Begin lithium, 300 mg p.o. b.i.d. to t.i.d. Always give in divided doses (usually t.i.d. to q.i.d.; b.i.d. to t.i.d. with slow-release form). Increase by 300 mg every 2 to 3 days (typical effective oral dose is 1,200 to 2,400 mg/day). Slow-release total oral dosage should be the same as that of regular Li.

  Methods to determine the appropriate steady-state dose of Li based on blood levels after a single initial test dose of Li have been developed. As yet, none can be considered standard, but some appear promising; they would help speed the treatment of manic patients.

Because acute mania is not controlled by lithium for 2 to 3 weeks, it may be necessary on the first day of treatment to begin a benzodiazepine (e.g., lorazepam, 2 to 4 mg p.o./i.m. q2h, with an average of 20+ mg/day initially) or an antipsychotic (e.g., haloperidol, 5 to 20 mg/day, in divided doses) if the patient is excessively agitated. Both provide rapid control of the psychomotor activity, whereas the lithium acts more gradually but is more specific for control of the affect and ideation of mania.

Once the mania begins to remit, the *blood Li level may increase* (mechanism unknown); keep watch. Maintain a therapeutic level until the mania is completely controlled (measure blood levels every 1 to 2 weeks). Lithium is best for "classic," long-period bipolar disorder; if response is poor, consider adding an anticonvulsant (e.g., valproic acid).

- Maintenance treatment of mania: If a patient has a history of recurrent mania, continue lithium after the acute attack (drug of choice). An effective maintenance blood level is 0.8 mEq/L (range, 0.6–1.0). When the patient is stable, measure the blood level every 2 to 3 months (be aware, a crash diet or strenuous exercise program may change the patient's level). Unfortunately, noncompliance is common, so work with the patient. If you choose to discontinue the Li, taper *slowly* (7).

  Teach the patient to be alert to side effects that suggest toxicity: Measure lithium level if they occur. Lithium level increases with sodium loss, so advise the patient to be aware of changes in dietary salt intake, sweating, and hot climates (although Li *may* be lost more rapidly than sodium, causing the Li level to decrease).

  Concern about gradual lithium-induced renal toxicity is decreasing: Standard measures of serum creatinine, UA, BUN, protein excretion, and 24-hour urine volume every 6 to 12 months may not be necessary. Monitor thyroid function: T_3, T_4, and physical examination every 6 months.

- Lithium prophylaxis of mania/depression is only partial. If a patient on maintenance lithium shows signs of developing mania, increase the lithium to an acute therapeutic level (50%+ respond). If a severe depression develops, begin an antidepressant (although in a few patients, subclinical hypothyroidism will develop secondary to Li, so consider thyroid supplementation instead). However, equally effective medications for prophylaxis may include carbamazepine, valproate, other anticonvulsants, as well as clonazepam; Li and valproate may be the maintenance combination of choice in difficult patients.

OTHER MOOD STABILIZERS

A blossoming has occurred in the use of selected anticonvulsants as mood stabilizers (8). Carbamazepine, and then valproic acid, have been used for years for most of the same indications as lithium. Because of equal or superior efficacy and greater safety, particularly with valproic acid, these drugs have gradually been replacing Li as the first-line medication. More recently, several additional anticonvulsants have been considered as alternatives, most important, lamotrigine. Moreover, combinations of Li and one of the other mood stabilizers or combinations of different mood stabilizers seem to be particularly effective.

- **Carbamazepine** (Tegretol) is an anticonvulsant that seems to be as effective as lithium for treating acute mania (better than lithium for *rapid cyclers*) and bipolar depression, and for mania prophylaxis. Moreover, it may be of use in treating certain violent individuals. Doses are typically 800$^+$ mg/day (blood level, 6 to 8 mg/L); begin slowly, increase over a 2- to 3-week period, and check blood level 5 to 6 times during the first month because level changes as the drug induces its own metabolism. Side effects include fatigue, nausea, ataxia, and diplopia. Allergic rashes are common (5% to 15%), as are dose-related side effects like *sedation* and dizziness. Initial, mild, benign leukopenia is common (10%), but watch for more serious problems of aplastic anemia, *agranulocytosis*, and hepatic toxicity, which develop over months or years. Get a CBC and differential at least with every drug blood level. Because of side effects, carbamazepine has gradually been replaced by valproic acid and lamotrigine.
- **Valproic acid** (Depakene) has a similar spectrum of utility (rapid-cycling bipolars, particularly mania and mania prophylaxis, but also depression) but with a different and safer side-effect spectrum (*sedation*, weight gain, GI upset, rare hepatotoxicity and pancreatitis). Half-life is 12$^+$ hours: maintain a blood level modestly above 50 ng/ml (start at 250 mg b.i.d., but may require 2,000$^+$ mg/day). In most situations, valproic acid is a better choice than carbamazepine.
- **Lamotrigine (Lamictal)** is the third anticonvulsant currently shown to be of value in treating bipolar disorder. Bipolar depression may respond to 50 to 200 mg/day, and consider 100 to 500 mg/day for mania and rapid cycling. Moreover, lamotrigine has been found effective for bipolar maintenance. Take any rash seriously: Stevens–Johnson syndrome is a rare side effect but can be fatal. To minimize the risk of rash, headache,

dizziness, nausea, and sedation, start slowly. Consider using as an adjunct with other more proven mood stabilizers.

- Other mood stabilizers have been considered but as yet are without convincing evidence of effectiveness. **Gabapentin (Neurontin)** is useful with neuropathic pain and may be modestly useful with social phobia and panic disorder but has not as yet been shown to be useful for bipolar disorder or other serious conditions. Consider its use as an adjunct. Its strength is its relative lack of side effects. **Topiramate (Topamax)** has shown very modest effects on bipolar disorder, usually as an adjunct. Consider in rapid cycling if other medications fail. A primary side effect of weight loss allows it to be considered in combination with a primary medication that has produced weight gain. **Oxcarbazepine (Trileptal)** is being reviewed for bipolar disorder, but time will tell.

Finally, increasing evidence suggests that the majority of the new antipsychotic medications may, by themselves, be useful drugs for treating bipolar I disorder.

ANTIDEPRESSANT DRUGS

Three groups of antidepressant drugs are in common use: tricyclic antidepressants (TCAs), newer antidepressants, and monoamine oxidase inhibitors (MAOIs) (Table 23.4). Combinations of these drugs are also occasionally helpful. Until recently, the TCAs have been the first choice in treating depressions, but the newer antidepressants [the selective serotonin reuptake inhibitors (SSRIs), serotonin-norepinephrine reuptake inhibitors (SNRIs), and others] have shown themselves to be just as effective as the TCAs in treating dysthymia, major depression, and a number of other disorders, as well as causing fewer side effects. Thus these newer medications have supplanted the TCAs as the initial therapeutic choice for most situations. Lithium carbonate can improve some major depressions, as can the occasional atypical antipsychotic, and the antipsychotic drugs are essential in psychotic depression. The MAOIs remain effective, but generally are used only after more than three other medications have failed. The FDA has placed a recent "black box" warning on **all** antidepressants that children and adolescents are at potential increased risk for suicidal thinking and suicide during the first several months after being started on an antidepressant. Even more recently, that concern has been extended to young adults up to age 25 years. This warning remains debated.

TABLE 23.4 ■ Antidepressant Drugs in Common Use

Drugs available (in U.S.)	Anticholinergic	Sedation	Dose (mg/day)
TCAs			
imipramine (Tofranil)	4+	3+	75–300
amitriptyline (Elavil, Endep)	5+	5+	75–300
clomipramine (Anafranil)	4+	3+	75–250
doxepin (Sinequan, Adapin)	4+	5+	75–300
desipramine (Norpramin)	1+	1+	75–300
nortriptyline (Pamelor)	3+	2+	40–150
protriptyline (Vivactil)	3+	1+	20–60
trimipramine (Surmontil)	3+	4+	75–200
Newer antidepressants			
alprazolam (Xanax)	1+	5+	2–6
amoxapine (Asendin)	2+	3+	200–300
buprorion (Wellbutrin)	0–1+	0–1+	200–450
duloxetine (Cymbalta)	1+	1+	30–60
maprotiline (Ludiomil)	2+	2+	50–225
mirtazapine (Remeron)	2+	3+	30–45
nefazodone (Serzone)	0–1+	2+	300–600
trazodone (Desyrel)	1+	3+	100–600
venlafaxine (Effexor)	1+	1+	75–375
citalopram (Celexa)	0–1+	1+	30–60
escitalopram (Lexapro)	0–1+	0–1+	10–30
fluoxetine (Prozac)	0–1+	0–1+	10–40+
fluvoxamine (Luvox)	0–1+	0–1+	100–300
paroxetine (Paxil)	0–1+	0–1+	20–50
sertraline (Zoloft)	0–1+	0–1+	50–200
MAOIs			
phenelzine (Nardil)	1+	1+	30–90
isocarboxazid (Marplan)	1+	1+	10–30
Selegiline (Eldepryl)	1+	0	20–60
(Emsam)	0–1	0	20–40 by daily patch
tranylcypromine (Parnate)	1+	0	20–60

Tricyclic Antidepressants

■ Indications for Use

TCAs are recommended for
1. Major depression, particularly with vegetative symptoms and a diurnal variation (70% to 75% of patients respond).
2. Bipolar disorder, depressed or mixed, particularly if vegetative symptoms are present. Lithium may be useful as well.
3. Short-term maintenance therapy in patients with resolved major depression or bipolar disease.
4. Prophylaxis in patients with severe, recurrent major depression.
5. Psychotic depression (hallucinations, delusions, paranoia, etc.); must be combined with antipsychotics [although electroconvulsive therapy (ECT) may be preferable for some].
6. Severe postpartum depressions.

■ Other uses:

- Dysthymic disorder: Mild chronic depressions deserve a trial of TCAs.
- Atypical depression: Patients with significant anxiety, hypochondriasis, and "neurotic" complaints, as an alternative to MAOIs.
- Panic disorder: One among several choices.
- Agoraphobia: with panic attacks.
- Obsessive–compulsive disorder: Particularly those patients who also have a depressed mood. Clomipramine is uniquely effective with OCD.
  PTSD: One among several choices.
- Selected patients with chronic pain (with, and without, depression).
- Childhood conditions: Both enuresis and school phobia may respond to low doses of a TCA.

TCAs should *not* be used routinely in the various minor depressive syndromes.

■ Mechanisms of Action

The effects of TCAs on CNS neurotransmitters are complex and vary from one tricyclic to another. Therapeutic impact is *thought* to be related to some combination of CNS interneuronal norepinephrine increase due to presynaptic NE reuptake blockade and to the sensitization of postsynaptic neurons to serotonin. Although affecting both systems, *secondary amines* (desipramine, protriptyline, and nortriptyline) may preferentially increase NE levels, whereas *tertiary amines* (amitriptyline, imipramine, and doxepin) have a greater effect on serotonin, a fact used to account for some interpatient response differences. In summary, however, knowledge is incomplete, and rely on "clinical wisdom."

■ Pharmacokinetics

TCAs are absorbed rapidly and completely from the GI tract, undergo an enterohepatic cycle, and develop peak plasma levels in 2 to 8 hours. TCAs are highly bound to plasma and tissue proteins and are fat soluble. Free TCA is only about 1% of the total body load. They are metabolized by the liver and excreted by the kidney. The half-life ranges from several hours to more than 2 days.

Well-studied plasma blood levels are available for imipramine, nortriptyline, desipramine, and amitriptyline. Do not measure them routinely; indications include

1. Treatment failure: Interindividual plasma levels vary markedly after the same oral dose (up to 30-fold differences), so always consider an ineffective plasma level when explaining a treatment failure. Therapeutic range is 150 to 300 ng/ml for imipramine (+ its metabolite, desipramine), amitriptyline (+ nortriptyline), or desipramine, and 50 to 160 ng/ml for nortriptyline.
2. Therapeutic window: Some TCAs may have a *therapeutic window* (e.g., nortriptyline and possibly desipramine); the drugs are less effective outside this range, whereas others seem to have no therapeutic upper limit (e.g., imipramine; the range limited only by side effects).
3. Suspected patient noncompliance.
4. Patients with significant side effects on a usual oral dose: They may have an excessively high plasma level.
5. Patients with cardiac disease: Attempt to maintain a low (but effective) plasma level.
6. The medically unstable patient (particularly the elderly).
7. Overdose: Plasma levels are mandatory.

■ Side Effects

Side effects are frequent and usually mild, but they can be serious or fatal (particularly cardiac effects in TCA overdoses) and are more common in the elderly.

Anticholinergic:
- Dry mouth
- Blurred vision (near vision)
- Constipation, urinary hesitancy

Autonomic:
- Sweating
- Impotence, ejaculatory dysfunction

- Cardiac:
  In normal dosages:
  Tachycardia
  ECG changes (T-wave flattening, increased PR and QT interval)

  In overdose:
  PVCs, ventricular arrhythmias
  AV block and BBB
  CHF and cardiac arrest

Other:
- Orthostatic hypotension (can be severe)
- Sedation
- Restlessness, insomnia
- Rashes, allergic reactions
- Weight gain (a common cause of patient noncompliance)
- Anorexia, nausea and vomiting
- EEG changes
- Tremor (fine, rapid, usually hands and fingers)
- Confusion (in elderly)
- Seizures in patients who are predisposed

Tolerance usually develops to the anticholinergic and sedative side effects. Use cautiously in the elderly and in patients with benign prostate hyperplasia (BPH); avoid in patients with narrow-angle glaucoma. Pregnancy is not an absolute contraindication for TCA use, although suggestive (but not convincing) evidence exists of teratogenicity: avoid use in the first trimester if possible. Severe hypotension occasionally can limit drug use (it is least with nortriptyline and doxepin).

Most worrisome are the cardiac effects. A few reports exist of sudden death from presumed arrhythmias; patients with preexisting heart disease (particularly bundle-branch disease) or hypertension (e.g., the elderly) or both are at risk for any of the cardiac side effects. Do *not* use after an acute myocardial infarction (MI) or while in congestive heart failure (CHF). The danger is greatest with higher doses (e.g., after an OD with a TCA).

Wide differences exist between agents in their ability to produce some side effects, and these should be considered when choosing a drug. The presence of side effects is *not* a good indication that a therapeutic plasma level has been reached.

Certain psychiatric conditions may be adversely affected by TCAs.

- Schizophrenia may be made worse.
- A depressed bipolar patient may become manic (10%[+]; "may" be lower with other antidepressants).

A withdrawal syndrome occurs in some patients who have been taking high doses of TCAs (e.g., imipramine, 150 to 300 mg/day) for weeks or months. If medication is stopped abruptly, symptoms begin in 1 to 2 days and include anxiety, headache, myalgia, chills, malaise, and nausea. Withdraw the medication gradually (e.g., 25 to 50 mg/week).

■ Drug Interactions

- TCA plasma level is increased (at times dangerously) by methylphenidate, Antabuse, MAOIs, antipsychotics, SSRIs, exogenous thyroid, cimetidine, and guanethidine.
- TCA plasma level is decreased (*frequently* below therapeutic range) by barbiturates, alcohol, carbamazepine, phenytoin, doxycycline, and *smoking* (may need to monitor level in heavy smokers).
- CNS depression occurs with antipsychotics, anticonvulsants, hypnotic–sedatives, and alcohol.
- TCAs impair the antihypertensive effect of methyldopa, guanethidine, and bethanidine.
- A synergistic anticholinergic effect is found with other central anticholinergics; may produce a toxic psychosis.
- Marked hypertension can be caused by administration of TCAs with sympathomimetic drugs (e.g., isoproterenol, epinephrine, phenylephrine, amphetamines).
- TCAs may dangerously increase the half-life of anticoagulants (e.g., Dicumarol); monitor prothrombin time.

■ Treatment Principles

Identify the patient likely to benefit from a TCA (remember: for most patients, the starting drug of choice is likely to be one of the newer antidepressants).
1. Appropriate clinical presentation.
2. Personal history of good TCA response.
3. Family history of good TCA response.
   - Unless side effects are likely to be a problem, begin with a tertiary TCA. They are metabolized in the liver to secondary TCAs (imipramine to desipramine; amitriptyline to nortriptyline), and thus both the tertiary and secondary TCAs are present in the body.
   - Side effects may be useful (e.g., consider amitriptyline or doxepin in the agitated depressive, desipramine in the elderly

with anticholinergic intolerance, protriptyline if sedation is a problem, and nortriptyline if hypotension is excessive).
- One technique for treating depression with TCAs is:

Begin imipramine, 50 mg p.o. hs (or equivalent; less in elderly; more in the obese), and increase by 25 to 50 mg every 2 to 3 days until 150 mg is reached. If side effects interfere, slow down.

Hold dosage at 150 mg for 1 week. If depression remains, increase to 200 mg (50 mg during the day, 150 at hs).

Hold dosage at 200 mg for 1 week, and then increase in 50-mg steps to 300 mg (150 mg in divided doses during the day, 150 mg at hs). Consider hospitalizing the patient for trials above 200 mg/day. Maintain at 300 mg for 2 to 3 weeks. It is important to do complete trials, if side-effect problems allow. If depression remains,
1. Has patient been taking medication?
2. Has a therapeutic window been passed?
3. Measure plasma level.

If the patient is unimproved, consider
1. A newer antidepressant or a different TCA.
2. ECT.
3. An MAOI. Allow 1 to 2 weeks for transfer.
4. After two to three unsuccessful trials, reevaluate the diagnosis.

With a good response, sleep and appetite usually return first, and then an improved mood. Usually a 1- to 3-week delay occurs in the therapeutic effect, so do not stop medications prematurely.
- Never give a worrisomely depressed or seriously suicidal patient a prescription for more than 1,000 mg of imipramine (or equivalent).
- If treating a psychotic depression, use a TCA and an antipsychotic simultaneously.
- If treating a depression in a bipolar patient taking lithium, continue the lithium if it has been effective prophylactically. The lithium *may* help prevent a manic overshoot.
- If treating a phobic–anxiety disorder, expect improvement with a lower dosage (e.g., 100 mg).
- Simultaneous use of a TCA and an MAOI is currently discouraged by the FDA but may be useful.
- Maintenance care: In a successfully treated patient, maintain the medication at initial levels for 6 months. If the patient has had a recurrence of a major depression, consider long-term TCA maintenance at full dosage (reduces likelihood of a relapse by 50%). Consider lithium maintenance in a recurrent bipolar illness. If no previous history of illness is found, gradually withdraw the medication.

Recognize (a) as many as one fourth of the improved patients relapse during the first 4 months, and (b) a significant number of patients (30%⁺) maintain a chronic, low-level depression, even though treated successfully for the acute illness ("double depression"). Depression, all too often, is a chronic illness.

- Clomipramine (Anafranil) is a little special: approved for OCD but an effective TCA antidepressant with a significant serotonin effect. Range of effectiveness is closer to some of the new antidepressants (although it has all the TCA side effects).

- TCA overdose is life-threatening and should be treated in a medical inpatient unit. Dangerously high plasma levels may continue for more than 1 week.

- Although generally not considered drugs of abuse, illicit use of amitriptyline to produce anticholinergic intoxication has been reported. Watch for it.

NEWER ANTIDEPRESSANTS

The following medications have become the "drugs of first choice," to be used before the TCAs and MAOIs. The primary reason for using "newer antidepressants" is their different side-effect spectrums and toxicity: they differ little from TCAs in effectiveness, disorders treated, or speed of onset. Their mechanisms of action are diverse. The key drugs fall into three categories: (a) SSRIs (selective serotonin reuptake inhibitors), (b) SNRIs (serotonin and NE reuptake inhibitors), and (c) a mixture of other drugs with more complex mechanisms. These drugs include

Serotonin reuptake blockers: as a group these antidepressants are safe and effective. They have similar (modest) side effects (a common problem of all seems to be sexual dysfunction), but if one medication cannot be tolerated, another one might be fine. Moreover, subtle differences in mechanism of action occur among each of the drugs, and some will work better for a given patient than others. Usually begin treatment of a depression with one of the following.

- **Citalopram** (Celexa): An *almost pure* SSRI blocker (it is also slightly less expensive than similar medications), it is broadly effective: depression, OCD, panic disorder, social phobia, and others. Side effects are typical: nausea, headache, sweating, diarrhea, tremor, and sexual side effects. Discontinuation is a very modest problem when citalopram is used in the dose range of 20 to 60 mg daily.

- **Escitalopram** (Lexapro): Very similar to citalopram, only it causes even fewer and milder side effects. It can be used in lower doses: 10 to 30 mg/day. This is because citalopram is a racemic mixture, whereas escitalopram consists only of the active "S" stereoisomer. Thus it is an even cleaner drug than citalopram, working exclusively as a serotonin reuptake blocker.

- **Fluoxetine** (Prozac): Little sedation and few anticholinergic effects (perhaps daytime sedation in a few); it does produce GI upset, rashes, sexual inhibition, insomnia, and restlessness. Clearly effective in mild/moderate depressions, it also is effective in panic disorder, OCD, bulimia, and possibly other related conditions. Try 20 mg daily [one dose (long half-life, days); the active metabolite, norfluoxetine, has a half-life of ≤15 days], but remember it may take 1 week or more to get out of the system. Some patients require 40 mg, whereas a few are all right with 20 mg every other day. A taper is usually not needed on discontinuation.
- **Fluvoxamine** (Luvox): An SSRI similar to the others, although it is FDA approved for OCD, it is not for depression (however, it is used "off label" for depression, OCD, and other SSRI-responsive conditions). Discontinuation is a problem second only to that of paroxetine, so taper slowly.
- **Paroxetine** (Paxil): Undoubtedly effective, but it presents some problems. It has been found effective for some patients with unipolar and bipolar depression, OCD, GAD, social anxiety disorder, PTSD, and PMDD. Side effects are similar to those of sertraline. Unfortunately, paroxetine can be difficult to discontinue, with a substantial "SSRI discontinuation syndrome" consisting of nausea, headache, dizziness, insomnia, and nervousness. Patients are often reluctant to stop the medication. Finally, a recent study suggested that Paxil may increase birth defects if taken by the mother during pregnancy, so the manufacturer has included a warning to that effect. Whether this will hold up awaits future studies. Daily dose is 20 to 50 mg.
- **Sertraline** (Zoloft) is similar to fluoxetine and also is useful for panic disorder, OCD, PTSD, and PMDD; safe and mild side effects consist of nausea, diarrhea, tremor, insomnia, somnolence, dry mouth, ejaculatory delay, and rarely the syndrome of inappropriate antidiuretic hormone secretion (SIADH); one dose/day of 50 to 200 mg. Because of its relatively short half-life, taper slowly.

Three drug–drug combinations are of concern.
1. High levels of one or a combination of strongly serotonergic drugs (best known may be an SSRI + an MAOI) can produce a dangerous **serotonin syndrome** (9): restlessness, tremor and myoclonus, hyperreflexia, diarrhea, hyperactive bowel sounds,

and diaphoresis, leading possibly to severe hypertension, agitated delirium, and death. (Wait 5 weeks to begin an MAOI after stopping fluoxetine; wait 2 to 3 weeks going from an MAOI to fluoxetine.) This is often unrecognized but can be quickly fatal.

2. Fluoxetine increases (sometimes dramatically) blood levels of TCAs, trazodone, maprotiline, carbamazepine, the benzodiazepines, as well as (probably) others, so be careful.

3. L-tryptophan + fluoxetine can produce myoclonic jerks. Finally, early concern was expressed by a few about the possibility that fluoxetine (and other SSRIs) may produce (or worsen) suicidal or aggressive impulses or both; appears to be a "red herring" (but).

Serotonin and norepinephrine reuptake blockers: Drugs with both 5-HT and NE reuptake blocking abilities seem to have a broader spectrum of action: they are generally good anxiolytics as well. These two are at least as effective as the SSRIs for either depression or anxiety.

- **duloxetine** (Cymbalta): Very similar to venlafaxine with primary side effects of constipation, dry mouth, and urinary retention. It seems quite effective with the spectrum of depressions and is likely to be helpful with anxiety disorders and chronic pain. Start dosage at 30 mg/day, and then move to 60 mg (a common steady dose), but consider doses of 90 mg and 120 mg if the response is inadequate. Taper slowly. Looks like a good drug.

- **venlafaxine** (Effexor): This is a "serotonin-like" antidepressant that has NE effects. It has a short half-life (less than 1 day rather than days), few side effects (nausea, sleepiness, dizziness and nervousness, sexual inhibition) and appears safe. Looks like another good one (10). Aim for about 150 mg in divided doses (maximum dose about 375 mg/day), although it also is available in a slow-release form (Effexor XR; maximum dose about 225 mg/day). It appears to be particularly effective for anxious depressions and seems be effective for GAD, social phobia, and chronic pain. *Discontinuation can be difficult.*

Mixed mechanisms of action: Some of these medications are marginally effective, whereas others have gained a central place in the treatment of depression (11) (e.g., bupropion, mirtazapine). Some can be "unpredictably" effective with anxiety disorders, PTSD, and other conditions. Master several of the best, and expect to use them in resistant cases.

- **Alprazolam** (Xanax): This benzodiazepine *may* be antidepressant at higher doses; few side effects except sedation and risk of *addiction*; safe in overdose. (A "second-string" antidepressant.)

- **Amoxapine** (Asendin): This is a metabolite of the antipsychotic loxapine; side effects are similar to those of TCAs; *may* be of particular use in psychotic depressions. Be careful of ODs.
- **Bupropion** (Wellbutrin SR/XL): This is an effective drug with few side effects (no weight gain or sexual side effects) and is safe in overdose; can produce insomnia, tremor, and sweating; may be more likely to produce seizures (particularly at 600 mg/day and higher), so go slowly and avoid patients at risk. Probably one of the better new drugs. It is useful as an adjunct with the SSRIs. Aim for 300 to 450 mg/day in *divided doses* [also available in slow-release (SR) and long-acting (XL) forms]. A second-tier medication for ADHD.
- **Maprotiline** (Ludiomil): Like TCAs, it has less cardiotoxicity in overdose.
- **Mirtazapine** (Remeron): This is a α_2-adrenergic receptor antagonist that thus increases synaptic 5-HT levels and NE release, so it has a peculiar mechanism of action. Weight gain and sedation are problems, but sexual side effects are not. It has rapid onset of action and is effective for anxiety. Begin at 30 mg/day, and aim for 45 mg daily. Looks like a good drug.
- **Nefazodone**: Similar to trazodone, but without the sexual dysfunction; cardiotoxicity is not a problem, and very little anticholinergic and histaminergic activity is seen. Side effects include sedation, dizziness, and headache. Do not use with MAOIs. It has been discontinued under the trade name "Serzone" because of rare severe liver toxicity, but it is still available as a generic. It is effective with severe depression as well as being an anxiolytic (PTSD). Start slowly, and aim for an oral dose of 400 to 600 mg/day.
- **Trazodone** (Desyrel): This is free of anticholinergic and most cardiac effects; produces orthostatic hypotension, sedation (useful if insomnia is a major problem), GI distress, headaches, and (rarely) *priapism*. Start low (e.g., 50 mg) and increase to the 200- to 300-mg range. Is it less effective than others? It is frequently used as a safe hypnotic.

MONOAMINE OXIDASE INHIBITORS (MAOIs)

MAOIs are effective antidepressant/antipanic medications and sometimes work when nothing else will, but because of their side effects, are very rarely the drugs of first choice (Table 23.5). [In addition to the two drugs listed, an additional "classic" MAOI that had been discontinued several years ago has been released again by another company: isocarboxazid (Marplan).]

TABLE 23.5 ■ MAOIs in Common Use (U.S.A.)				
	Anticholinergic	Sedation	Dose (mg/day)	Starting Dose
Phenelzine (Nardil)	1+	1+	30–90	15 mg t.i.d.
Tranylcypromine (Parnate)	1+	1+	20–60	10 mg b.i.d.–t.i.d.

Indications for Use

Recommended for

1. Atypical depression: An MAOI may be the drug of choice for "atypical depressions" (50% to 60% improve) [i.e., depressed (♀:♂=3–4:1) patients with varying degrees of (a) fatigue, anxious affect, rejection sensitivity, irritability, emotional lability, or (b) hyperphagia (often sweets), hypersomnolence, a "leaden feeling" in the limbs, reversed diurnal variation (worse in evening), and hypochondriasis, or both. (Are two types found: anxious and vegetative?) If a TCA or an SSRI is tried unsuccessfully, follow with a trial of an MAOI. ECT often fails with these patients.

Other uses:

- Patients with treatment-resistant major depression (unipolar or bipolar) or dysthymic disorder and for whom ECT is not the obvious next choice.
- Panic disorder with or without agoraphobia (particularly phenelzine; start slowly).
- Others: social phobia; PTSD; "perhaps" bulimia (use carefully in bingers).

Mechanisms of Action

MAOIs block MAO (and other enzymes) throughout the body (e.g., in blood, platelets, gut, CNS). MAO catalyzes the oxidation of such biogenic amines as NE, DA, 5-HT, and the amino acid tyramine. The therapeutic effect of MAOIs is *probably* related to the increase in CNS NE and 5-HT, which results from the ability of MAOI to block oxidation of intracellular catecholamines.

MAO exists in two isoenzymes: MAO-A (in brain, liver, gut, and sympathetic nerves), which acts primarily on 5-HT and NE; and MAO-B (in brain, liver, and platelets), which acts on phenylethylamine and others. They both act on DA and tyramine.

The two available MAOIs (phenelzine, tranylcypromine) also bind irreversibly to, and affect both types of, MAO. Because of the irreversibility, blood levels and drug half-life are of little importance: if you stop the MAOI, you must wait for new MAO to be synthesized (2 weeks) for the drug's effect to disappear.

No new MAOI antidepressants are available in the United States (the newly released effective old one, *isocarboxazid* or Marplan, had been discontinued in 1993), although the **RIMAs** (reversible inhibitors of monoamine oxidase A) are being researched actively, with *moclobemide* looking safe and possibly effective. Other specific MAOIs exist, such as these: *clorgyline* (unavailable) inhibits MAO-A irreversibly; *pargyline* (Eutonyl, an antihypertensive) and *selegiline* (Eldepryl, for Parkinson disease) inhibit MAO-B; and *brofaromine* (unavailable) is another RIMA. Safer, more specific, and effective MAOIs may be coming.

The only recent change (FDA) in the MAOIs is the reappearance of selegiline (an MAOI β blocker) in a 20-, 30-, or 40-mg patch approved for depression (Emsam). Selegiline has been used for years as an antidepressant in pill form (Eldepryl) but without FDA approval. Side effects are few; a rash is common, and hypertensive crises do occur, but less frequently than with other MAOIs. Finally, the serotonin syndrome remains a problem when selegiline is combined with other medications, although it occurs less frequently than with other MAOIs.

Pharmacokinetics

MAOIs are rapidly absorbed and are metabolized into inactive products (in hours) by several means, including acetylation (primarily phenelzine). Some patients may be "rapid acetylators" and require increased oral doses of MAOI. A clinical response usually takes 1 to 4 weeks. An 80% to 90% inhibition of platelet MAO in blood samples seems necessary for clinical effectiveness (research measure).

Side Effects

MAOIs have numerous side effects. However, they lack the range of cardiotoxic effects of the TCAs, although some experts believe that they should be contraindicated in the elderly because of the risk of a potentially fatal hypertensive crisis (see later).

The most common side effects include drowsiness or stimulation (short lived), *insomnia* [10%+ of patients; often with suppression of rapid eye movement (REM) sleep], dizziness, orthostatic *hypotension*, impotence (long-standing), urinary hesitancy, and weight gain (half of patients; mild but chronic). Dry mouth, constipation, and blurred vision are present but less a problem than with TCAs because of minimal anticholinergic effects. MAOIs also can produce restlessness and irritability and can precipitate a manic episode. Up to 5% of patients have mildly elevated SGOT and SGPT; test further if malaise or jaundice develops.

A rare but potentially fatal side effect is the rapid onset of an **hypertensive crisis** (possible cerebrovascular bleeding and death) and hyperpyrexia in response to ingested tyramine (or other pressor amines). The MAO in the gut wall, which usually prevents entrance of large quantities of such ingested amines, is inhibited by MAOIs, and thus a generalized sympathetic effect is allowed when tyramine-containing foods are eaten. The first sign of an impending crisis is usually a sudden, severe occipital or temporal headache [followed/accompanied by sweating, nausea and vomiting, palpitations, restlessness, fever, neck stiffness, photophobia (dilated pupils), and rapidly increasing BP] 20 minutes to 1 hour after eating. Patients (with marked interindividual variation) taking MAOIs should avoid the following foods completely and eat the other foods only in moderation:

- Protein-containing foods that are cultured or spoiled:
    Strong, aged cheeses (e.g., cheddar, blue, camembert, stilton): cottage, ricotta, or cream cheese is OK.
    Pickled or kippered herring; dried, salted fish; snails; shrimp paste.
    Chicken livers (old livers of any kind) or liver paté; any *aged or slightly spoiled meat* (and *sausage, bologna, pepperoni, salami); protein extracts* and *protein dietary supplements.*
    Old yogurt; sour cream; chocolate (large amounts); licorice; *yeast* (except when used in baking).
- Nondistilled alcohol: red or *Chianti* wine (strict moderation); vermouth; beer (particularly *tap/lager*); coffee, tea, and colas.
- *Broad beans* [contain dopamine (e.g., Fava, Italian green, and lima beans)]; *bean curd*; *sauerkraut*; avocados; banana *peels*; soy sauce; soups prepared with bean curd or protein extracts (e.g., *miso soup*).

Treat a crisis with slow administration of phentolamine (Regitine, 5 mg i.v.); 0.25 to 0.5 mg i.m. q4–6 h later, if needed. It usually resolves in a few hours. The responsible patient may carry a 10-mg capsule of nifedipine (Procardia); bite it and place it under the tongue, and then swallow for rapid relief when signs of a crisis appear (good for 3 to 6 hours; *visit an ED*, a risk of overshoot exists).

Drug Interactions

A number of adrenergic and sympathomimetic drugs may also produce serious interactions.

- *Hypertensive crisis:* Can be produced by amphetamines, cocaine, methylphenidate, and anorectics (stimulate NE release from adrenergic neurons), catecholamines (epinephrine, NE), sympathomimetic precursors (dopamine, methyldopa, levodopa), and sympathomimetic amines [ephedrine, phenylephrine, phenylpropanolamine, pseudoephedrine, metaraminol (check ingredients in over-the-counter cold, hay fever, and cough medication)].
- Meperidine (Demerol): Very dangerous combination. In a few patients, severe, immediate hypertension, hyperpyrexia, and sweating *or* hypotension and coma develop. Narcotics may act similarly.
- CNS depression: Potentiated by alcohol, major tranquilizers, and hypnotic–sedatives.
- *Serotonin syndrome* (37) from conflicting antidepressants: Wait 2 weeks after stopping an SSRI, clomipramine, bupropion, nefazodone, or venlafaxine before starting an MAOI, and vice versa. Wait 5 to 6 weeks after stopping fluoxetine (*long* half-life of active metabolite norfluoxetine).

Treatment Principles

- Begin phenelzine, 15 mg p.o., b.i.d. to t.i.d., and increase by 15 mg weekly to 60 to 90 mg/day. Maintain that dosage for 4 weeks before assuming a failure.
- Instruct the patient carefully about the potential side effects and which drugs and foods to avoid. Avoid using MAOIs in patients with pheochromocytoma or severe hypertension, renal disease, or liver disease.
- Maintenance is at acute treatment doses. In some patients, for unknown reasons, both the antidepressant and antiphobic effects become ineffective after 6 months to 1 year of use.
- Allow a 1- to 2-week washout before starting another drug; continue dietary restrictions for 2 weeks as well.
- If insomnia becomes a major problem, give all doses before mid-afternoon.
- Tranylcypromine is related to amphetamine and may have some stimulant properties.
- Do not give large prescriptions to impulsive, potentially suicidal outpatients.

ANTIDEPRESSANT DRUG COMBINATIONS

Combined drug therapy may help a patient for whom trials with single antidepressants have failed. Such treatment is empiric (just about every conceivable combination has been tried by someone at some time): proceed carefully and watch out for side effects (do *not* combine fluoxetine with the MAOIs). Potentially useful combinations include these:

- **Antidepressant** and **antidepressant:** The most common technique.
- **Antidepressant** and **lithium:** Probably the most effective mix for both unipolar and bipolar depression (12); adding lithium to a TCA or an MAOI occasionally may produce a *rapid* (days) improvement. Effective blood level varies from 0.4 to 1.0.
- **Antidepressant** and **antipsychotic:** For psychotic depressions.
- **Antidepressant** and **stimulant:** Used with TCAs, SSRIs, and (carefully) MAOIs; use doses of dextroamphetamine, 5 mg t.i.d. or methylphenidate, 10 mg t.i.d.
- **Antidepressant** and **thyroid:** Occasional patients improve (Did they have a subclinical thyroid dysfunction?). Choose triiodothyronine (T_3; Cytomel), 25 to 50 µg/d; if ineffective, *stop*.
- **SSRI** and **TCA:** Literature is limited; clinical experience is more promising.
- **TCA or SSRIs** and low-dose **buspirone** (10 mg t.i.d.).
- **Lithium or SSRI** and **bupropion:** For patients with rapid-cycling bipolar diseases (13)?
- **Mood stabilizer** and **atypical antipsychotic:** For acute mania.
- **Mood stabilizer** and **antidepressant:** To treat resistant depressed bipolar I; may induce rapid cycling, but bupropion or an SSRI may reduce that risk.
- **Mood stabilizer** and **mood stabilizer:** Usually try standard medication, but also consider using gabapentin or topiramate as one of the choices.

HYPNOTIC AND ANTIANXIETY DRUGS

Drugs Available

Numerous drugs are available for sedation, of which only the benzodiazepines and several new agents (e.g., buspirone, ramelteon) can be recommended. Recognize that venlafaxine XR and perhaps several new antipsychotics may be useful antianxiety agents (Table 23.6).

TABLE 23.6 ■ Sedative-Hypnotic Agents

Drug	Half-life (hr)	Dose (mg/day)
alprazolam (Xanax)	11–14	0.5–4
chlordiazepoxide (Librium)	15–60	15–60
clorazepate (Tranxene)	50–100	15–45
diazepam (Valium)	30–60	5–40
halazepam (Paxipam)	50–100	60–160
lorazepam (Ativan)	10–20	2–6
oxazepam (Serax)	5–10	30–120
prazepam (Centrax)	60–70	20–60
clonazepam (Klonopin)	30–40	1–4
estazolam (ProSom)	10–24	1–2 (HS)
eszopiclone (Lunesta)	6	2–3 (HS)
flurazepam (Dalmane)	50+	15–30 (HS)
quazepam (Doral)	40+	7.5–15 (HS)
ramelteon (Rozerem)	1–2.6	8 (HS)
temazepam (Restoril)	8–18	15–30 (HS)
triazolam (Halcion)	2–3	0.125–0.25 (HS)
zaleplon (Sonata)	1–4	5–20 (HS)
zolpidem (Ambien)	2–3	5–10 (HS)
buspirone (Buspar)	2–3	15–60

Indications for Use

1. Short-term treatment of restlessness and anxiety (e.g., after life crises). They are *sedative at low dosage* and *hypnotic at higher doses*. They have no antipsychotic activity and thus should not be used as the exclusive treatment for psychotic disorders.
2. Generalized anxiety disorder and mild panic symptoms. Panic disorder (alprazolam, clonazepam).
3. Alcohol withdrawal (see Chapter 16); hypnotic–sedative withdrawal; psychosis due to hallucinogens.
4. Various seizure disorders.
5. Muscle relaxant (diazepam).

Mechanisms of Action and Pharmacokinetics

They enhance the inhibitory neurotransmitters (e.g., GABA, glycine), and they have a specific depressant effect on the limbic system. As the dosage increases, generalized CNS depression ensues. Buspirone, conversely, affects dopamine and serotonin receptors.

They are well absorbed orally, are all both water and lipid soluble, and are usually metabolized by the liver but may also be excreted by the kidney. They are slowly and variably absorbed i.m. (faster by p.o. route). Very little hepatic enzyme induction is seen. Peak blood levels usually occur 1 to 4 hours after the oral dose (1 hour for diazepam).

Side Effects

In comparison to other classes of psychoactive drugs, side effects are few.

- The most common problem is CNS depression, manifested by daytime sedation, decreased concentration, and poor coordination in some patients at therapeutic doses. They are very safe drugs, although a massive OD or combination with alcohol or other drugs will produce life-threatening CNS depression.
- Anterograde amnesia can occur after hypnotic-induced sleep with short-acting drugs (e.g., lorazepam, triazolam). Patients may lose memory for events that occurred during the night *or* during the following day.
- Tolerance and physical addiction occur, particularly with short-acting drugs or when taken at high doses for several months. The withdrawal syndrome is usually mild (but may be severe: rebound anxiety, nausea, sweating, hyperalertness, and occasionally seizures) and typically occurs 2 to 14 days after stopping the drug (most rapid with the shorter-acting drugs). Discontinuing alprazolam may be particularly difficult (withdrawal symptoms can include paranoia, marked anxiety and agitation, psychosis, hallucinations, and seizures); go *very* slowly (e.g., decrease 0.5 mg weekly at first, and then 0.25 mg weekly below a total daily dose of 2 mg).
- Untoward but infrequent psychiatric manifestations include exacerbation of schizophrenia and depression.
- *No* autonomic side effects occur.
- Benzodiazepines seem to be safe in pregnancy.

Drug Interactions

- An increased sedative effect is found when combined with CNS depressants (e.g., alcohol). Moreover, the combination with alcohol at times actually may be anxiogenic.
- Disulfiram (Antabuse) and cimetidine impair the metabolism of the long-acting benzodiazepines and thus increase the plasma levels. The shorter-acting drugs appear less affected.

- Food, antacids, and anticholinergic drugs appear to decrease the rate, but not the extent, of drug absorption.

Treatment Principles

- Use the long-acting benzodiazepines (chlordiazepoxide, diazepam, clorazepate) on an hs or b.i.d. schedule. Use a t.i.d. to q.i.d. schedule for the shorter-acting ones (oxazepam, lorazepam).
- Recognize that the longer-acting drugs (and their active metabolites) may accumulate over days or weeks, producing increasing symptoms of sedation, etc. Lorazepam and oxazepam have a simple metabolism and do not accumulate.
- Try to avoid use for longer than 1 to 3 weeks in most patients, either as a sedative or as a hypnotic. Some patients may be able to use them less frequently but long-term on an "as needed" basis, but be alert for those patients prone to abuse. Reevaluate if you find that you have used medications for longer than 2 to 4 months (however, a few patients seem to do well on *low* doses for long periods; not recommended if it can be avoided). Addiction can occur (particularly among alcoholics) but is uncommon.
- Use by p.o. route, if possible.
- Encourage the patient to avoid the simultaneous use of a benzodiazepine and alcohol or another sedative–hypnotic drug.
- Be *very* careful when giving to the elderly; confusion is common. Dosage may need to be 20% or less of the usual young adult dose.
- If the patient has been taking benzodiazepines for several months, stop medications over a 2- to 3-week period (particularly the long-acting drugs).
- The more sedative benzodiazepines and those with shorter half-lives are used primarily as hypnotics, although, in adequate dosage, any drug in this class can be hypnotic. Flurazepam is rapidly absorbed and is useful for sleep-onset problems; temazepam and flurazepam may help frequent awakening. Flurazepam, particularly because of its long-acting metabolite N-desalkylflurazepam (quazepam has the same major active metabolite), accumulates and produces a hangover in a few (often older) patients. Triazolam is very short-acting and does not accumulate but has been associated in a number of patients with "withdrawal-like" symptoms after each dose [e.g., early morning insomnia, irritability, daytime anxiety and dysphoria (and even rare confusion and paranoia)]. It has been "accused" of producing rage attacks in some patients; the issue remains unsettled, but the drug looks suggestive.

Zolpidem (Ambien; rapidly absorbed, short half-life, minimal rebound insomnia or daytime somnolence) is a recent benzodiazepine-like hypnotic that may be an improvement but may have the usual problems of tolerance with extended use and addiction at higher doses. However, addiction occurs less frequently than with the benzodiazepines.

Eszopiclone (Lunesta): Rapidly absorbed, half-life of 4 to 6 hours; patients generally are able to sleep through the night. Tolerance is minimal, and addiction occurs, but even less frequently than with zolpidem. Another benzodiazepine-like hypnotic.

Ramelteon (Rozerem): Just released as of this writing. No evidence of addiction or dependence; works by a unique mechanism; binding the MT receptors of the suprachiasmatic nucleus. The manufacturer claims no tolerance. The question of effectiveness remains to be answered. Potentially a good, safe hypnotic.

Buspirone represents a new class of anxiolytics [a serotonin $(5-HT_{1A})$ agonist]. It has few side effects, produces less sedation and cognitive and psychomotor impairment than the benzodiazepines, is not likely to be abused, but may be less effective as well. It is a reasonable alternative drug, particularly for chronic anxiety states and in the elderly. Begin at 5 mg t.i.d. (5 mg qd in the elderly), and increase over a 10-day period to the average daily dose of 20 to 30 mg, b.i.d. to t.i.d. Unlike the benzodiazepines, expect 2 to 3 weeks before it begins to work. It "may" also augment the antidepressant effects of the SSRIs, decrease agitation in the demented elderly, possibly decrease drinking in alcoholic outpatients, and have a number of additional possible uses.

PSYCHOTROPIC MEDICATION USE DURING PREGNANCY

In general, the absolute risk on the infant of a mother's use of psychotropic medication during pregnancy is low. In most cases (for example, even in the notorious situation of using Li to control mania in the pregnant woman), the treated condition is much safer for the infant. This topic suffers from a general lack of knowledge about the effects of most of the medications, particularly the newer drugs. Most information comes either from animal studies or, after release of a medication, from women discovered to have become pregnant while taking the drug. The most conservative approach is to avoid any medication not proven safe. This is almost certainly unnecessarily cautious. The risk–benefit ratio would suggest that most medications should be used (with care) if needed. No psychotropic medication has been shown to be seriously dangerous to the infant. The "short list" of those medications that generally should be avoided (unless truly needed) includes lithium (due to rare cardiovascular anomalies); fluoxetine (maybe) and paroxetine in the third trimester; valproic acid and carbamazepine in the first trimester because of the 1% to 2% incidence of neural tube defects; diazepam and several other benzodiazepines because of an infrequent oral-cleft defect (clonazepam and lorazepam seem to be OK); and benzodiazepine hypnotics due to decreased intrauterine growth. Interestingly, clozapine seems to be safe.

ELECTROCONVULSIVE THERAPY

In spite of its unjustified notoriety, ECT is legitimate. Although its mechanism of action is unknown, it is effective, painless, and safe (mortality rate less than competing therapies or the untreated state: 0.01% to 0.03% of patients treated; mostly cardiovascular deaths). However, before administration, *always* obtain:

1. Informed consent from a voluntary, competent patient.
2. Informed consent from a relative or guardian of a voluntary, incompetent patient and an independent psychiatric opinion of therapeutic need.
3. Court approval for administration to a resisting, involuntary patient who is a danger to himself or others.

Discuss the risks of amnesia, confusion, and headache with the patient and the family. Also discuss the risks of *not* receiving ECT.

Indications for Use

ECT is a serious procedure; use *only* in those conditions for which it is recommended. It is tempting to give ECT to any patient who is not improving: Do not!

MAJOR AFFECTIVE ILLNESS: Patients with *Major Depression* or *Bipolar disorder, depressed,* respond well to ECT (80% to 90% recover vs. 70%+ treated with antidepressants). Patients with marked vegetative symptoms (e.g., insomnia, constipation, suicidal rumination, obsessions with guilt, anorexia and weight loss, psychomotor retardation) are particularly responsive. ECT is much more effective than antidepressants for psychotically depressed patients (i.e., vegetative symptoms and paranoid or somatic delusions). Give antidepressants a full trial (e.g., imipramine, 200 to 300 mg/day for 4 weeks), and then consider ECT if no improvement is seen. Mania (*Bipolar Disorder, manic*) also responds to ECT: typically used only if lithium carbonate (+ antipsychotic) fails to control the acute phase.

SCHIZOPHRENIC DISORDERS: *Catatonic Schizophrenia* of either the stuporous or the excited type responds well to ECT. Try antipsychotic medication first, but if the condition is life-threatening (e.g., hyperexcited delirium), go quickly to ECT. Occasional acutely psychotic patients (particularly of the schizoaffective type) who do not respond to medication alone may improve if ECT is added, but for most schizophrenics (e.g., chronics), it is of little value.

ECT is the *treatment of choice* for
1. Actively suicidal depressed patients who may not live until antidepressants begin to work.
2. Depressed patients (particularly the elderly) whose medical condition makes administration of antidepressants risky. Patients with both depression and OBS may do better with ECT. ECT *can* be safely performed during pregnancy.
3. Seriously depressed patients who have had an *adequate* trial of antidepressants (60% to 70% recovers with ECT).

Contraindications for Use

No *absolute* contraindications. Always weigh the risk of the procedure against the danger incurred if the patient is untreated. Neurologic disease is not a contraindication. Response improves with age; patients younger than 30 respond more poorly.

■ Very high risk

- Increased intracranial pressure (e.g., brain tumor, CNS infection): ECT briefly increases CSF pressure and risks tentorial herniation. Always check for papilledema before administration.

  Recent MI: ECT frequently causes arrhythmias (vagal arrhythmias producing postictal PVCs and extravagal arrhythmias producing PVCs anytime during the procedure), which can be fatal if there has been recent muscle damage. Wait until enzymes and ECG have stabilized.

■ **Moderate risk:**

- Severe osteoarthritis, osteoporosis, or recent fracture: Prepare thoroughly for treatment (i.e., with muscle relaxants); retinal detachment.
- Cardiovascular disease (e.g., hypertension, angina, aneurysm, arrhythmias): Premedicate carefully; have a cardiologist available.
- Major infections, recent CVA, chronic respiratory difficulty, acute peptic ulcer, pheochromocytoma.

Techniques of Administration

■ **Pre-ECT Medical Workup**

Complete history and physical, concentrating on cardiac and neurologic status, CBC, chemistry, UA, VDRL, chest and spine radiographs, ECG. Get EEG (and/or CT scan) if neurologic results are abnormal.

■ **A Typical Technique**

ECT routines vary: no "one right way" exists. Usually perform in a hospital and with the aid of an anesthesiologist.

1. Prepare the patient with information and psychological support. Have him void and defecate beforehand. NPO after midnight. If markedly anxious, give 5 mg of diazepam i.m. 1 to 2 hours before treatment. Antidepressants, antipsychotics, sedative–hypnotics, and anticonvulsants (among others) should be stopped the day before treatment. Lithium usually should be stopped several days before: risk is organicity.
2. Make patient comfortable. Remove dentures. Hyperextend the back with a pillow.
3. When ready, premedicate with atropine (0.6 to 1.2 mg s.c., i.m., or i.v.). This anticholinergic controls vagal arrhythmias and reduces GI secretions.
4. Provide 90% to 100% oxygen by bag when respirations are not spontaneous.
5. Give sodium *methohexital* (Brevital) (40 to 100 mg i.v., rapidly). This short-acting barbiturate anesthetic is used to produce a light coma.
6. Next quickly give enough of the muscle relaxant *succinylcholine* (Anectine) (30 to 80 mg i.v., rapidly; monitor depth of relaxation by the muscle fasciculations produced) to remove all but very minor evidences of a generalized seizure (e.g., plantarflexion).

7. Once relaxed, place a bite-block in the mouth, and then give electroconvulsive stimulus.

Two methods are common and acceptable today:

Unilateral: One electrode placed in the frontotemporal area, and the other, 7 to 10 cm away in the parietal region, both on the nondominant hemisphere (right side for right-handed persons, 60% R and 40% L for left-handers). Unilateral ECT is commonly used because it produces less postictal confusion and amnesia, but it seems to be less effective than bilateral ECT.

Bilateral: Bifrontotemporal electrode placement. This is the traditional technique; it is effective but produces more side effects (e.g., amnesia, headache).

The effectiveness of either method depends on producing a central generalized seizure (peripheral effects are not necessary) lasting at least 25 seconds. Monitor this with EEG, peripheral EMG, or the tonic/clonic movement of the hand on the same side as the electrode (unilateral), which has been freed of muscle relaxant by a tight cuff applied before the administration of the succinylcholine. If a seizure is not produced, increase the stimulus, and repeat ("missed" or unilateral seizures are usually of little therapeutic value; they occur more frequently with unilateral shock, perhaps accounting for its lesser effectiveness).

8. Monitor patient carefully until stable; usually 15 to 30 minutes of postictal confusion ensues. These patients are at risk for prolonged apnea and a postictal delirium (5 to 10 mg of i.v. diazepam may help).

Complications of ECT

- Amnesia (retrograde and anterograde): Variable; beginning after three to four treatments; lasting weeks to 2 to 3 months (but occasionally much longer); more severe with bilateral placement, increased number of treatments, increased current strength, and prior presence of organicity.
- Headache, muscle aches, nausea.
- Dizziness, confusion: The persistence and severity of the confusion increases with an increasing number of treatments.
- Reserpine and ECT given concurrently have resulted in fatalities.
- Fractures: Rare with good muscle relaxation.
- ECT anesthesia risks:
  Atropine worsens narrow-angle glaucoma.

Succinylcholine's action is prolonged in pseudocholinesterase deficiency states. These conditions (malnutrition, liver disease, chronic renal dialysis, use of echothiophate for glaucoma) can lead to potentially fatal hypotonia.

Procainamide, lidocaine, and quinidine can potentiate succinylcholine.

Methohexital can precipitate an attack of acute intermittent porphyria.

Treatment Principles

1. Usually give one treatment per day, on alternate days.
2. Depressions usually require six to 12 treatments. Mania and catatonia require 10 to 20. Expect to see improved behavior after two to six treatments if it is going to be effective. Allow the clinical response to determine the treatment end point. Be *very cautious* (and seek a second opinion) about exceeding 20 treatments during one period of illness.
3. Maintenance ECT (single treatments every 1 to 3 months during the months or years after recovery) *may* be useful, particularly with elderly depressed patients, but should be used primarily if medication is contraindicated.
4. Maintenance antidepressants, antipsychotics, and lithium (begun after a successful course of ECT) may forestall relapse. Without medication, the relapse rate is high.

PSYCHOSURGERY

Little psychosurgery is currently performed in the United States. Modern psychosurgeons make one of several possible small cuts in the brain (usually in the limbic system), which can improve a variety of psychiatric conditions and which have few side effects (unlike the widely destructive prefrontal lobotomy of the past).

All candidates for surgery must have an intractable and devastating condition unrelieved by any other therapy. Conditions likely to respond include chronic pain with depression and severe depression alone. Improvement occurs in some patients who have severe obsessive–compulsive and anxiety states and in a few schizophrenics. The mechanism for the improvement is uncertain, and a variety of different surgical cuts yield similar results. Despite the lack of theoretic sophistication, for some patients, psychosurgery is a valid "last resort."

REFERENCES

1. Schatzberg AF, Nemeroff CB. *Textbook of psychopharmacology*, 3rd ed. Washington, DC: American Psychiatric Press, 2004.
2. Miyamoto S, Duncan GE, Marx CE, et al. Treatments for schizophrenia: a critical review of pharmacology and mechanisms of action of antipsychotic drugs. *Mol Psychiatry* 2005;10:79–104.
3. Lieberman JA, Stroup TS, McEvoy JP, et al. Effectiveness of antipsychotic drugs in patients with chronic schizophrenia. *N Engl J Med* 2005;353:1209–1223.
4. McGrath PJ, Stewart JW, Fava M, et al. Tranylcypromine versus venlafaxine plus mirtazapine following three failed antidepressant medication trials for depression: a STAR*D report. *Am J Psychiatry* 2006;163:1531–1541.
5. Honer WG, Thornton AE, Chen EYH, et al. Clozapine alone versus clozapine and risperidone with refractory schizophrenia. *N Engl J Med* 2006;354:472–482.
6. Calabrese JR, Kimmel SE, Woyshville MJ, et al. Clozapine for treatment-refractory mania. *Am J Psychiatry* 1996;153:759–764.
7. Faedda GL, Tondo L, Baldessarini RJ. Outcome after rapid vs gradual discontinuation of lithium treatment in bipolar disorders. *Arch Gen Psychiatry* 1993;50:448–455.
8. Dunn RT, Frye MS, Kimbrell TA, et al. The efficacy and use of anticonvulsants in mood disorders. *Clin Neuropharmacol* 1998; 21:215–235.
9. Boyer EW, Shannon M. The serotonin syndrome. *N Engl J Med* 2005;352:1112–1120.
10. Benkert O, Gründer G, Wetzel H. Is there an advantage to venlafaxine in comparison with other antidepressants? *Human Psychopharmacol* 1997;12:53–64.
11. Rush AJ, Trivedi MH, Wisniewski SR, et al. Bupropion-SR, sertraline, or venlafaxine-XR after failure of SSRIs for depression. *N Engl J Med* 2006;354:1231–1242.
12. Nierenberg AA, Fava M, Trivedi MH, et al. A comparison of lithium and T_3 augmentation following two failed medication treatments for depression: a STAR*D report. *Am J Psychiatry* 2006;163:1519–1530.
13. Trivedi MH, Fava M, Wisniewski SR, et al. Medication augmentation after the failure of SSRIs for depression. *N Engl J Med* 2006;354:1243–1252.

Chapter 24

The Elderly Patient

More than 35,000,000 Americans are older than 65: 85% have a chronic illness (usually medical), and 20% to 30% have a psychiatric illness (most common in the very old) (1,2).

EVALUATION OF THE ELDERLY

1. Assess each patient carefully: Mental decline is *not* normal for the aged.
2. Always carefully evaluate physical condition. An impaired physical state can markedly alter the psychiatric evaluation. Make sure the patient can hear and see. Check for deficiency states (iron, folate, vitamins B_{12} and D, calcium, serum proteins).
3. Interview technique: Be respectful, use surname, sit near, speak slowly and clearly, allow time for answers, be friendly and personal, pat and hug, be supportive and issue oriented, ask direct questions if appropriate, keep interview short.
4. Collect history, do mental status: Perhaps in more than one interview.
5. Identify premorbid personality: Defense mechanisms and coping styles (e.g., independent vs. passive–dependent, rigid vs. flexible, use of denial).
6. Assess the major *risk factors:*
   a. Loss: Of spouse, friends, physical health, job, status, independence, etc.
   b. Poverty: Many elderly are poor; some are victims of crime.
   c. Social isolation: Impaired mobility, few friends, etc.
   d. Medications: Particularly steroids, antihypertensives, anticholinergics, L-dopa.
   e. Sensory deprivation: Poor hearing, vision, etc.
   f. Sickness: Chronic illness, chronic pain, forced inactivity, alcohol abuse, etc.
   g. Fears: Of being dependent, of being alone, of being helpless.
7. See family: Assess their strengths, dynamics, support for the patient, hidden agendas.

COMMON PSYCHIATRIC DISORDERS

Delirium (3) (see Chapter 5)

Fluctuating confusion, cognition, and consciousness, of acute onset with lucid intervals; it is common among the elderly and commonly overlooked or mistaken for psychosis or depression (due to agitation or lethargy). May be the primary presentation of:

1. CNS: Cerebral infarction (embolic or thrombotic), transient ischemic attacks (TIAs), neoplasms, infection.
2. Circulation: Myocardial infarction (MI; often without pain), arrhythmia, congestive heart failure (CHF), anemia.
3. Lungs: Pneumonia (without fever or leukocytosis), pulmonary embolism (PE; without chest pain, dyspnea, tachycardia).
4. Medication: Multiple drugs, anticholinergics, benzodiazepines, bupropion, narcotics.
5. Metabolic: Diabetes, liver failure, hyper- or hypothyroidism, electrolyte abnormalities.
6. Psychogenic: Strange surroundings, stress, restraints.
7. Infections: Most kinds, any severe and acute disease.
8. Other: Alcohol abuse, prescription drug misuse, dehydration, fecal impaction, "silent" appendicitis, urinary retention, urinary tract infections (UTIs), eye or ear disease, surgery (e.g., cardiac).

Treat the underlying disease process, if possible. Keep patient in a lighted room and with familiar surroundings and people. Restrain only if absolutely essential. If needed, use small doses of major tranquilizers (e.g., haloperidol, 0.5 to 1.0 mg p.o. or i.m., b.i.d. PRN; quetiapine, 25 mg p.o. b.i.d.). Mild delirium may continue (unnoticed?) for months after the acute episode.

Dementia (see Chapter 6)

Most elderly have unimpaired intellectual functioning. Dementia (30% of those 80 years old) is not "just a result of aging"; it needs an explanation. Dementia often is seen first with agitation, anxiety, depression, somatic complaints, or a combination of these. *Always* do a mental-status examination on elderly patients with these complaints, but remember that it can also be mimicked by depression, serious physical conditions, alcoholism, and malnutrition. Dementia in the elderly frequently occurs with, is confused with, and is made worse by depression or delirium. Treat the depressed and/or agitated demented patient with low-dose atypical neuroleptics (e.g., quetiapine, olanzapine) initially, but consider an early switch to SSRIs, lithium, or anticonvulsants. Marked memory loss may be unrecognized by the patient but is of major concern to the family, who ultimately insist on evaluation and treatment for it. Recent medication includes the cholinergic agonists such as donepezil, rivastigmine, and galantamine; enhance one of these with the possible addition of memantine (a glutamate blocker).

Most patients with a progressive and nonreversible form of dementia can be maintained at home until the late stages of the disease process. The decision to institutionalize depends not only on what facilities are available locally (some may be very good) but also on the realistic strengths and limits of the family. Once the cause and prognosis of the dementia is determined, the physician may most profitably spend his time helping the family draw limits, handle guilt, and adjust.

Depression (see Chapter 4)

Major depression can develop in old age for the first time or be a recurrence of a major affective disorder. In the elderly, it may at times closely mimic a dementia (pseudodementia; although a high percentage of these patients go on to develop a genuine dementia) or be closely related to (caused by?) and share clinical features with a chronic medical illness. It develops in cerebrovascular disease (25%), Alzheimer disease (25%+), and Parkinson disease (50%). Physical symptoms, apathy, or fatigue may dominate the clinical picture. It is common, frequently unrecognized, often has a long course compared with that of a younger person, is potentially fatal (both from physical inanition and from suicide; remember, the highest suicide rate is among elderly men, particularly with alcoholism), and responds well (but usually slowly) to treatment. When in doubt, hospitalize. Treat with psychotherapy and, particularly if severe, with antidepressants (increase slowly; effective final daily oral dose may be as low as 5 mg of escitalopram or 10 mg of fluoxetine). Relapse is common, so consider maintenance antipsychotics (4). Consider a low-dose selective serotonin reuptake inhibitor (SSRI) as an appropriate first-line medication. Electroconvulsive therapy (ECT) may be the therapy of choice in patients with unstable cardiac status or in those patients with very severe and/or psychotic depression (e.g., paranoia, hallucinations).

A less severe depression or depressive equivalent (listlessness, physical complaints, withdrawal) in a patient with long-standing depressive complaints may represent *dysthymic disorder*. Because stress and loss are so common among the elderly, *adjustment disorder with depressed mood* and *bereavement* occur frequently.

Other Disorders

Mania continues in 5%[+] of bipolar patients or as a first event in patients with a history of recurrent depression. Cognitive impairment is common; patients are more often dysphoric; may resemble delirium or schizophrenia. Extreme agitation or manic-like behavior can be caused by organic factors, dementia, schizophrenia, depression, or situational anxiety. Lithium (use low doses; watch for decreased renal clearance; avoid use with antipsychotics; side effects are a problem), anticonvulsants (low-dose valproate or carbamazepine and perhaps lamotrigine), or very low dose and short-term atypical antipsychotics are effective. ECT may be necessary.

Schizophrenia usually has a lifelong history, but approximately 10%[+] have an onset after age 60, perhaps secondary to the stresses of old age. Paranoia is a dominant presentation; occasionally associated intellectual deterioration is found. Treat with support and antipsychotics.

Paranoia or mild suspiciousness among the elderly is very common. Bizarre forms or near-psychotic levels may occur with

1. Early dementia: *Always* check for intellectual loss;
2. Delirium;
3. Vision or hearing problems; may resolve promptly;
4. Social isolation; chronic illness;
5. Drugs (e.g., steroids, antiparkinsonians, hypnotic withdrawal).

Anxiety is common in the elderly, and anxiety disorders are the most common psychiatric problems (5% to 6% of elderly), except for cognitive decline. Phobias lead the list with OCD, panic disorder, and GAD encountered regularly. Treatment of anxiety disorders in the elderly is similar to that of younger adults (5) (see Chapter 8).

DELUSIONAL DISORDER (DSM, p. 323, 297.1) often has an onset late in life (late-life paraphrenia). These patients have fixed paranoid delusions and occasionally auditory hallucinations but not the loose associations, grandiosity, major hallucinations, and autistic thought of paranoid schizophrenics (although the conditions may overlap). Treat with reality-oriented psychotherapy, behavior modification, maintenance antipsychotics, and possibly ECT.

Hypochondriasis

The elderly are frequently ill, and a preoccupation with exaggerated physical complaints and problems may develop. This is particularly common among depressed and/or demented elderly and comorbid with panic disorder and OCD. The physical symptoms may or may not improve with resolution of the depression.

The patient with severe hypochondriasis (5% of elderly), whose life is dominated by ruminations about one or more physical problems, is very difficult to treat. Withdrawal and isolation are frequent. Do not expect a "cure." Develop an ongoing relationship with this patient. Be available. See every 2 to 3 weeks for 10 to 20 minutes. Reassure that the problem may be persistent and incurable but not debilitating or fatal. Recognize that in some cases, symptoms may continue, because to lose them would mean to lose the reason for visiting the physician.

Adjustment Disorders

These are common in old age and are due to the numerous stresses (loss, physical illness, retirement, etc.) encountered. Symptoms include anxiety, depression, agitation, and physical complaints, and most often occur in persons with past adjustment problems. Supportive psychotherapy, attention to concrete problems, and brief use of minor tranquilizers or very-low-dose antipsychotics helps. Grief is common and may mimic a major depression but often has an obvious precipitant, is short-lived with therapy, and does not require antidepressants. *Alcohol abuse* (10% of elderly, mostly men), particularly of recent onset, is also a common response to stress in the elderly, is frequently unrecognized, and carries a high risk for depression and suicide. Treat as an alcoholic: psychosocial interventions, abstinence, naltrexone, etc.

PSYCHOPHARMACOLOGY OF OLD AGE

The elderly usually run higher blood levels (because of decreased hepatic metabolism and renal excretion, reduced plasma albumin and protein binding, and increased fat-to-lean tissue ratios), display increased receptor responsiveness, and thus require more gradual increases and *lower doses* of most psychoactive medication. They are also more susceptible to most side effects (e.g., peripheral and central anticholinergic effects, sedation, hypotension, arrhythmias). They are at risk for bowel obstruction, urinary retention, blood pressure (BP) problems (fainting, stroke), sudden death from fatal arrhythmias, glaucoma crises, delirium, and coma. They also are particularly likely to be taking multiple drugs, to misunderstand and fail to comply with prescribing instruction, and to have symptoms from such polypharmacy. Preferable medications for the elderly include

- **Benzodiazepines:** Second tier for anxiety [use SSRIs, SNRIs (6)] except as initial, short-term (e.g., 2 weeks) treatment for acute symptoms of GAD, panic disorder (clonazepam, alprazolam), and OCD (clonazepam). Oxazepam (10 to 30 mg/day) and lorazepam (0.5 to 3 mg/day) are least likely to accumulate. Long-term use (e.g., longer than 6 weeks) may produce falls, confusion, lethargy, depression, impaired cognition (7), and withdrawal problems. In patients with insomnia, try relaxation or exercise first. If a medication is needed, try (e.g.) temazepam (7.5 to 15 mg hs; limited accumulation).
- **Antidepressants:** Low to normal doses of the SSRIs and other newer antidepressants (bupropion, nefazodone, venlafaxine) have become the drugs of choice for depression, anxious depression, and most anxiety disorders. TCAs and even MAOIs can be used, but secondarily and cautiously (i.e., effective, but many side effects). (Low-dose trazodone is common for insomnia.)
- **Antipsychotics:** Select patients conservatively and intelligently. Use low doses of atypicals (avoid clozapine), but even with them, be guided by patient's side effects. With i.m. medications, consider U-100 insulin syringes to ensure a small dose. Use primarily for psychosis and agitated or delusional dementia or both. (Low-dose quetiapine is common for insomnia.)
- **Lithium:** Effective, but toxicity occurs easily (e.g., delirium, tremor, impaired cognitive function), so keep on a lower maintenance level (e.g., 0.4 to 0.7 mEq/L).
- **Anticonvulsants:** Carbamazepine, valproate, and lamotrigine are useful antimanics and perhaps for the agitated patient, but the typical side effects are common and may occur early.
- **ECT:** Safe, effective, and used for same indications as those in other adults.

GENERAL TREATMENT PRINCIPLES

- Be *supportive*, respectful, sympathetic, and a "good listener." Touch the patient.
- Encourage patients to express themselves (about guilt, loneliness, helplessness) and unburden themselves (e.g., grieve).
- Be directive and reality oriented. Help in a concrete way with

problems (e.g., who to see about rent assistance, calling "Meals-on-Wheels," explanation of Medicare benefits). The quality of the patient's current environment is probably the single most important factor determining recovery and health.

- Strengthen defenses rather than restructure them.
- Encourage self-esteem. Helping patients "review their life" (to see it as complete) can be enormously beneficial. Reminiscence *is* adaptive coping behavior and helps promote self-esteem.
- Encourage continued interests, friendships, socialization, activities, and self-support. Identify those things still done well, and encourage the patients to continue to do them (if they cannot fix the meal, maybe they can still set the table).
- Be an ongoing presence. Be available: frequent, regular, short sessions. Be reachable by telephone.
- Involve and work with the family. Teach them appropriate skills and expectations. Anger, frustrations, and resentment often develop; help the family (and patient) deal with these feelings.
- A psychotherapy group of elderly patients is often very helpful; locate one for the patient.
- Know and use community resources.

REFERENCES

1. Jenike MA. Psychiatric illnesses in the elderly: a review. *J Geriatr Psychiatry Neurol* 1996;9:57–82.
2. Sadavoy J, Lazarus LW, Jarvik LF, et al. *Comprehensive review of geriatric psychiatry*, 2nd ed. Washington, DC: American Psychiatric Press, 1996.
3. Inouye SK. Delirium in older persons. *N Engl J Med* 2006;354:1157–1165.
4. Reynolds CF, Dew MA, Pollock BG, et al. Maintenance treatment of major depression in old age. *N Engl J Med* 2006;354:1130–1138.
5. Sheikh JI, Cassidy EL. Treatment of anxiety disorders in the elderly: issues and strategies. *J Anxiety Disord* 2000;14:173.
6. Katz IR, Reynolds CF, Alexopoulos GS, et al. Venlafaxine ER as a treatment for generalized anxiety disorder in older adults: pooled analysis of five randomized placebo-controlled clinical trials. *J Am Geriatr Soc* 2002;50:18.
7. Paterniti S, Dufouil C, Alperovitch A. Long-term benzodiazepine use and cognitive decline in the elderly: the epidemiology of vascular aging study. *J Clin Psychopharm* 2002;22:285.

Legal Issues

The interface between psychiatry and law is in flux, partly because of recent patient's rights legislation (based on the constitutional assurance that no person shall be deprived of his or her liberty without "due process of law") (1,2). A psychiatrist's dealings with his patients increasingly are constrained by case law and statue. It is essential to learn the limits of your independence in relation to your patients. Laws can differ markedly from state to state and may change with time—become familiar with those laws that apply to your area.

CIVIL LAW

Civil Commitment

All states permit civil commitment to inpatient [and, at times, outpatient (3)] psychiatric care under specific, but differing, criteria. Know your local standards.

1. **Mental Illness:** All states require the presence of a mental illness, but definitions differ. Psychosis usually is included, but personality disorder is not. Drug or alcohol abuse or both may be allowed. Mental illness alone is not sufficient for commitment but requires at least one of the following two additional conditions.
2. **Dangerousness:** To self or others: Most states require that the patient be dangerous but differ in the degree of urgency—an *imminent* danger (e.g., likely to hurt himself in the next 24 hours) versus a relative danger (e.g., physically deteriorating through depressive withdrawal). Dangerousness is the most common reason for commitment in most states. Two major problems with the dangerousness standard are (a) psychiatrists have difficulty accurately predicting future dangerous behavior except in the most obvious cases; and (b) it has been uncertain what level of proof the law requires—states vary widely, from the lowest civil standard of "preponderance of the evidence" (51% certainty) to the most strict criminal standard of "beyond a reasonable doubt"

(95% certainty). This latter issue appears to have been resolved by the U.S. Supreme Court decision (*Addington v Texas*, 1979) causing Federal courts to favor "clear and convincing evidence" (75% certainty).

3. **Disabled and in need of treatment:** Although diminished in degree, most states allow commitment solely on the grounds that a person is significantly handicapped by a mental illness, is unable to provide for his own basic needs (the *parens patriae* provision), and is in need of, and would benefit from, treatment. This is qualified in many states by a requirement proceeding from *Lake v Cameron* (1966) that hospitalization be the "least restrictive" of the treatment options available.

4. Some states now allow commitment of the developmentally disabled, substance users, and mentally disabled minors. Special due-process provisions apply.

Most states also have laws (usually less strict) allowing brief (1 to 14 days) involuntary holds. A growing tendency in the law exists toward "a duty to commit" worrisome patients (*Schuster v Altenberg*, 1988). Committed patients who believe they are being held illegally may obtain a hearing by a *writ of habeas corpus*.

Much recent legislation defining these standards has redressed real past wrongs that occurred when commitment could result merely from a physician's "okay," yet recent controversy has focused on associated losses to the patient and his or her family due to exclusion from treatment because of complex criminal-like commitment proceedings. As fewer patients have been treated involuntarily, some experts have noted a shift of mental patients from the civil to the criminal system (i.e., untreated mental illness *causes* them to break a law they ordinarily would not have broken, and they are then arrested). The extent of this trend remains undetermined.

An additional impact of the changing commitment laws has been to require the release of committed patients much earlier than in the past, resulting in a marked decline in the size of state mental hospitals. An unfortunate effect of this deinstitutionalization has been to release large numbers of marginally functional persons into communities ill equipped to deal with them, with the resultant formation of "psychiatric ghettos" in some large cities.

The Right to Treatment

After the classic Alabama decision of *Wyatt v Stickney* (1972), it has become a general standard (amazingly, it had not been before) that an involuntarily committed person must receive a level of effective treatment adequate to encourage improvement. This concept was challenged, reviewed, and supported in *Youngberg v Romeo* (1982). How to deal with the patient who is unlikely to improve with *any* treatment remains uncertain.

The Right to Refuse Treatment

This is currently one of the most actively contested areas of psychiatric law, and the results of the debate remain uncertain. Involuntary commitment is *not* prima facie evidence that the patient is incompetent to decide what treatment he is to receive. Many "rights-driven" cases recognize a patient's right to refuse treatment by requiring a separate hearing to establish incompetence and attempt to represent the patient's preference before allowing involuntary treatment. Other, "treatment-driven" cases have deferred to professional judgment in allowing involuntary treatment qualified by an appeals process, as in *Rennie v Klein* (1983). As the federal stance on these issues continues to fluctuate, be *very* cautious (and legal) when insisting that a patient receive electroconvulsive therapy (ECT) or medication against his will, even when that patient appears to need it badly. Know your local laws.

Abandonment

Refusing to continue to treat an active and willing (although possibly difficult) patient is to risk the charge of "abandonment." When refusing continued care, always document the reasons (they should be sound, of course), attempt to transfer the patient to another therapist or institution if the patient is willing, make efforts to minimize any risk to the patient (and document), and arrange to care for the patient "in extremis" until the clinical situation has stabilized. Medical cost-containment policies are typically not seen as a legitimate reason for terminating care (thus producing a significant and growing problem in financially strapped, often public, systems).

Competency

Psychiatrists are sometimes asked to assess (the court *decides*) whether a patient is mentally competent to perform *specific* functions (e.g., make a will, handle finances, testify in court). Although a judgment for or against competency depends on the context, rules exist for some of these decisions—the patient must be able to (a) communicate his choices, (b) understand the information involved, (c) grasp the consequences of his decision, and (d) rationally manipulate the information involved (*Appelbaum and Grisso*, 1988). However, to be found incompetent for one task does not necessarily imply incompetence for another (i.e., competency is *task specific*).

CRIMINAL LAW

Competency to Stand Trial

It is held in law that, to receive a fair trial, a person must be able to understand the nature of the charges against him, understand the possible penalties, understand legal issues and procedures, and work with his attorney and participate rationally in his own defense (*Dusky v United States*) (4). If a person cannot do one or more of these, he is "incompetent to stand trial" and usually is transferred to a treatment facility until competency is restored (e.g., medication for a psychosis). Once found competent, the patient is usually returned to court to stand trial. Recently, many states have decided that if a patient's competency cannot be restored in a "reasonable length of time" (e.g., the length of time he probably would serve for the crime charged), that patient must continue treatment in a civil facility if committable or be released. Psychiatrists are most commonly the experts asked to help the court decide on competency (the decision is the court's).

Criminal Responsibility

The "not guilty by reason of insanity" plea is much debated by both the legal and psychiatric professions, yet it continues to be used (infrequently). It is *not* widely abused. Part of the general dissatisfaction with this plea centers on whether psychiatrists (or anyone) can retrospectively determine a patient's mental functioning at the time of a crime. Just as an incompetency decision is concerned with the patient's mental state *at the time of the trial*, a responsibility decision involves the mental state *at the time of the crime*. Also in question are the criteria needed to make that judgment. Several different ones are used in different states:
- *The M'Naughten Rule:* Did the person not *know* the nature of his act and that it was wrong? This is a common test (one third of states).

- *The Irresistible Impulse Test:* Was a person acting under an "irresistible impulse?" This test is considered unsound alone and is typically combined with other tests.
- *The American Law Institute Test* (ALI Test): Does a person have a mental disease or defect such that he "lacks *substantial* capacity either to *appreciate* the criminality of his conduct or to *conform* his conduct to the requirements of the law?" This test adds a "volitional" standard to the "cognitive" standard of the M'Naughten Rule. It is used in approximately one half of the states and in all federal courts.

If one or more of these conditions are met, the patient may be declared "not guilty by reason of insanity" and be freed of responsibility for his crime. If needing treatment at that point, the patient is usually placed in a psychiatric facility until the mental illness remits or until he is no longer believed to be a threat to the community because of mental illness. Such confinement is sometimes longer than the prison confinement sought for the criminal conviction—especially in lesser charges—so the insanity acquittal is not to be seen as "getting away" with crime.

Many states and the U.S. Congress have considered restrictive modifications (or abolition) of the insanity defense in the wake of the public outcry after John Hinckley's "not guilty" verdict in his shooting of President Reagan. The form the insanity defense will take is not clear. Leading possibilities appear to be (a) a return to some form of the M'Naughten Rule by eliminating the "volitional" standard, and (b) a *guilty but mentally ill* verdict [thus a person first would be judged and sentenced criminally, then (ideally but not always) treated in an appropriate, restrictive setting for mental illness].

PERSONAL ISSUES

Malpractice

The risk that a psychiatrist will be successfully sued for malpractice is low but climbing: approximately 20% to 30% of suits against psychiatrists are successful. Most suits involve use of ECT, improper or inadequately informed use of medication, unusual treatments, sexual involvement with patients, successful patient suicide (suit brought by relatives), or "split treatment" involving inadequate communication with another therapist. Although it sounds like a platitude, the best defense *is* a strong and respectful therapeutic alliance with the patient. (Yet even that is uncertain protection, given a recent successful suit by a father arguing that the therapist had induced false memories of abuse by him in his daughter, the patient.) Careful documentation of the therapeutic process, including "risk–benefit notes" in the patient's chart, recording each stage of treatment, will help in defending against many claims. Assessing the risk of suicide or violence in a patient is a particular challenge to the psychiatrist, and a careful record of the risk–benefit assessments he makes in awarding privileges, passes, and discharges is essential.

Confidentiality

Physicians are ethically obligated to maintain patient confidentiality, except when voluntarily waived by the patient. General knowledge by others of details of a patient's psychiatric treatment or even awareness of psychiatric care can be damaging socially and occupationally to a patient. This requirement for confidentiality continues after the patient's death. However, in some cases, the psychiatrist may be liable if he does *not* break privacy [e.g., *Tarasoff v Regents of the University of California* (1976) states that a therapist has a duty to protect a third party threatened harm by the patient]. This is known as the "*Tarasoff* duty" or "duty to warn." When uncertain, seek consultation from a colleague. Finally, utilization review groups and third-party payers are demanding more privileged information. In the courtroom, the patient holds the "testimonial privilege" to prevent the psychiatrist from disclosing confidential information, with exceptions including cases of child abuse reporting and those calling the competency of the patient into question. The Supreme Court ruled in 1996 (*Redmond v Jaffe*) that therapist–patient communications may be withheld from disclosure in Federal courts, but this does not apply in state courts, where most relevant cases occur. Attorney–client privilege, professional ethics codes, and "right of privacy" combine somewhat to protect the physician in maintaining confidentiality in many cases, but comprehensive legal protection is far from complete. Become familiar with your own state's laws, because this is legally uncertain ground.

Informed Consent

Informed consent should be sought from all patients for all treatments, but formal (i.e., written) consent should be obtained for physical procedures (e.g., ECT, medication). The patient should be informed about the reasons for the treatment, its nature, the likelihood of success, the dangers and likelihood of side effects, and any alternative treatments.

A major problem arises if the patient is "incapable of being informed" (e.g., due to retardation, brain damage, psychosis). A guardian may need to be appointed whose duty would be to make the decision for the patient. Even after consent, voluntary treatment can carry legal risks if the patient is later deemed to have been incompetent at the time of informed consent, as in *Zinermon v Burch* (1990). A standard evaluation for competence does not yet exist, so the clinician must take special care in this area.

REFERENCES

1. Rosner R, Ed. *Principles and practice of forensic psychiatry.* 2nd ed. New York: Chapman & Hall, 2003.
2. Simon RI, Gold LH. *The American Psychiatric Publishing textbook of forensic psychiatry.* Washington, DC: American Psychiatric Publishing, 2004.
3. Allen M, Smith VF. Opening Pandora's box: the practical and legal dangers of involuntary outpatient commitment. *Psychiatr Serv* 2001;52:342–346.
4. McGarry AL, Curran WJ, et al. *Competency to stand trial and mental illness.* Rockville, MD: National Institute of Mental Health, 1973.

26 Impulse-control Disorders

Impulse-control disorders (ICD) is an as yet poorly understood grouping of seemingly related conditions, the symptoms of which overlap elements of many other conditions. They seem to have in common an impulse to do something that is innately and ultimately destructive to themselves or others, to feel increasing tension or arousal before acting, to be unable to resist that drive, to feel pleasure or relief during and immediately after the act, and to feel guilty or regretful some time later (depending on their history and what they have done). DSM-IV-TR lists five specific disorders and one general disorder:

Kleptomania
Pyromania
Pathological Gambling
Trichotillomania
Intermittent Explosive Disorder
Impulse-Control Disorder NOS

Most of the disorders that are comorbid with an ICD often have overlapping symptoms with them: OCD, OCPD, depressive disorders, bipolar spectrum disorders, substance abuse, cluster B personality disorders, ADHD, and eating disorders. A genetic basis is suggested by a high incidence in first-degree relatives of conditions such as: depression, bipolar disorders, substance abuse, personality disorders, alcoholism, and pathologic gamblers among the relatives of pathologic gamblers. There is clearly a neurologic basis for much of this behavior, but it is not well understood. Best identified at this point is that, as a group, ICD is related to low levels of CNS serotonin (responsible for impulsivity?) as well as altered activity in the orbitofrontal cortex (1) and the ventromedial prefrontal cortex.

Males seem more common is some disorders, and females in others, but this has not been well separated. The course of the illness takes several forms: (a) a short period of ICD behavior and then remission, (b) waxing and waning periods of ICD behavior and extended problem-free times, and (c) chronic problems with mild waning periods.

KLEPTOMANIA, P. 667, 312.32

These people steal things of little monetary or personal value impulsively and with no preplanning, even though they frequently develop a criminal record for shoplifting. They experience a sudden urge to steal something, often surprising themselves, and that urge accompanied by increasing tension becomes overpowering, only to be relieved by shoplifting something. They may feel remorseful later and either give the object away or try to return it to the store. A few patients have amnesia for their theft, and another subgroup "don't even think about it" and do it by habit (2). In severe cases, they may become homebound because of fear of exposure to places where they might steal. The female-to-male ratio is 2–3:1; the "typical" patient is a married woman in her 30s; and approximately 5%+ of all shoplifters have kleptomania.

These patients have marked comorbidity, with mood (high rate of attempted suicide) and substance disorders particularly common, as well as anxiety disorders, eating disorders, and other ICDs. Although OCD is not common, hoarding is (3). Treatment is of unproven effectiveness, but consists of a variety of behavioral techniques as well as occasionally effective SSRIs, valproate, lithium, and naltrexone (4).

PYROMANIA, P. 669, 312.33

Individuals with pyromania usually are entranced by fires, become aroused at the thought of setting them, may make detailed preparations for starting a fire, want to watch the results of their efforts (e.g., may become firefighters), and experience pleasure and satisfaction from having created a major fire. They often give little thought to the loss of property or life or both that may result. Pyromania is a subset of, but is not, simple arson; arsonists set fire(s) for understandable, usually concrete, often self-aggrandizing reasons. To meet criteria for pyromania, a person must be responsible for multiple fires.

Men make up the vast majority of pyromaniacs (85%+). This is a chronic condition with a variable course: some people set fires only occasionally, whereas others seldom stop thinking about, and planning for, a fire. Depression is very common among these individuals, as are alcoholism and other ICDs. Treatment is almost nonexistent, although a recent educational approach shows promise (5).

PATHOLOGIC GAMBLING, P. 671, 312.31

Gambling is a common entertainment (70% of the general population), but approximately 1% to 2% of the U.S. population will either rapidly (early 20s) or more slowly (by their 30s or 40s) develop a preoccupation and even obsession with gambling, to the point that it may ruin their lives (pathologic gambling). These individuals are more likely to be male (2:1), to have major depression at some time (50%), alcoholism or some other drug abuse (60%), bipolar disorder, ADHD, some other ICD, and/or a cluster B personality disorder, and to have a family history of major depression, alcoholism, and pathologic gambling.

Pathologic gamblers differ from other gamblers by their daily preoccupation with thoughts of gambling, an inability to stop wagering even when they are deeply in debt and have to obtain money by unacceptable or even illicit means, an inability to stop *chasing* their losses, an ability to convince themselves that they will eventually "catch up," even when common sense and past experience argues otherwise, and a "need" to gamble for excitement and a craving for "action" (and they keep needing to raise the stakes to keep getting that sense of excitement). They possess many characteristics of an addiction, including an inability to cut back, irritability and dysphoria when they do stop gambling, a sense of tension driving them to gamble, a sense of pleasure and relief of depressive feelings when they start gambling again, and increasingly living a life of lies as they get deeper in debt and have to get money any way they can, all the while allowing their personal relationships, employment, and good name to fall apart. They differ from professional gamblers because they cannot stop at previously decided loss limits. The course tends to be lifelong, until they no longer have, or can get, the money to gamble. Treatment is difficult; these gamblers have a high level of denial, optimism, and even manic-like confidence. Moreover, chronic drug or alcohol use worsens their judgment and tendency to gamble.

Similar to alcoholics, compliance with treatment is very poor, and group therapy seems to be the only psychotherapy of real use (Gamblers Anonymous), and even there, the dropout rate is very high. Some medications show promise. The SSRIs display mixed results with a slight tendency in the direction of effectiveness. Mood stabilizers (specifically lithium and valproate) have been shown to be moderately effective in a few limited studies. Kim et al. (6), in a small naltrexone study, found improvement in 75% of pathologic gamblers (opioid antagonists can block the pleasure of addictive behavior), a result that needs further study.

TRICHOTILLOMANIA, P. 674, 312.39

Although a mild, self-limited form of trichotillomania exists in childhood, the serious variety of this disorder typically begins during adolescence and may last a lifetime. Like the other ICDs, the patient (predominantly females) develops a sense of tension and may covertly pull out individual or small groups of hair over a period of minutes to an hour or more. This releases the tension and may even produce a sense of pleasure briefly but usually leaves the person with profound self-regret and a worsened self-image. Hair is usually pulled from the crown of the head or the eyebrows. Make no mistake, this is a serious and debilitating chronic illness that often starts in the teens and may last a lifetime. Perhaps the oddest complication is the formation of *trichobezoars* (or hair balls, because approximately one third of individuals eat the hair), which can result in intestinal obstruction.

Unlike other ICDs, it is common for these patients to be comorbid with OCD, OCPD, and tics. Treatment with medication remains at the case-study level with SSRIs, clonazepam, and perhaps naltrexone being of some use. Conversely, cognitive–behavioral therapy has shown promise (7).

INTERMITTENT EXPLOSIVE DISORDER, P. 663, 312.34

After a period of growing tension and feelings of aggressiveness, these individuals (80% males) will attack someone either verbally or physically, break nearby objects, and perhaps actually seriously hurt someone for no, or very little, reason. Their aggressiveness is far more extreme than warranted by circumstances. Low central serotonin levels is the most constant biologic finding. A major problem with the diagnosis is that this condition is unusual, whereas many other causes of episodic violence are comparatively common (e.g., antisocial personality disorder, psychosis, mania, ADHD, substance intoxication, borderline personality disorder). Treatment with medication is far from developed;

numerous drugs are used from time to time, including mood stabilizers, antipsychotics, and antidepressants, but as yet, no magic bullet exists.

IMPULSE-CONTROL DISORDER NOT OTHERWISE SPECIFIED, P. 677, 312.30

This is a growing group of conditions that may or may not end up being classified as ICDs. Among their number are very poorly defined phenomena such as binge-eating disorder, sexual addictions, Internet addiction, pornography addiction, and compulsive shopping. Even whether these deserve the label of disorders remains to be seen.

REFERENCES

1. Winstanley CA, Theobald DE, Cardinal RN, et al. Contrasting roles of basolateral amygdala and orbitofrontal cortex in impulsive choice. *J Neurosci* 2004;24:4718–4722.
2. Grant JE. Dissociative symptoms in kleptomania. *Psychol Rep* 2004;94:77–82.
3. Grant JE, Kim SW. Clinical characteristics and associated psychopathology of 22 patients with kleptomania. *Compr Psychiatry* 2002;43:378–384.
4. Grant JE, Kim SW. An open label study of naltrexone in the treatment of kleptomania. *J Clin Psychiatry* 2002;63:349–356.
5. Franklin GA, Pucci PS, Arbabi S, et al. Decreased juvenile arson and firesetting recidivism after implementation of a multidisciplinary prevention program. *J Trauma* 2002;53:260–266.
6. Kim SW, Grant JE, Adson DE, et al. Double-blind naltrexone and placebo comparison study in the treatment of pathological gambling. *Biol Psychiatry* 2001;49:914–921.
7. Ninan PT, Rothbaum BO, Marsteller FA, et al. A placebo-controlled trial of cognitive-behavioral therapy and clomipramine in trichotillomania. *J Clin Psychiatry* 2000;61:47–50.

Index

Note: Page numbers followed by a *t* denote tables.

A

AA. *See* Alcoholics Anonymous
Abandonment, 269
Abilify (aripiprazole), 216t, 226
Abstraction, selective, 211
Abstractive thinking, 10–11
  testing for, 10
Acamprosate (Campral), 152
Accident proneness, 124
Acute brain syndrome. *See* Delirium
Acute confusional state. *See* Delirium
Acute intermittent porphyria, 135
Acute psychosis, 23
Acute stress disorder (ASD), 88
Adapinx (doxepin), 235t, 236, 238
ADD. *See* Attention-deficit disorder
Addington v Texas, 268
Addison disease, 134
ADHD. *See* Attention-deficit/hyperactivity disorder
Adjustment disorder(s)
  with anxiety, 81
  with depressed mood, 44, 263
  in elderly patients, 264
  with mixed anxiety and depressed mood, 44
Adolescents, use of antidepressants in, 234
Adoption studies, of schizophrenia, 29
Adrenal corticosteroids, psychiatric symptoms of, 127
α-Adrenergic blocking symptoms, 220
Adult antisocial behavior, 198
Affect, 9
  blunted or flat, 25
  inappropriate, 25
  labile, 25

Affective disorders, form of thought in, 10
Affective spectrum disorder (ASD), 93
Age/aging
  dementia and normal, 68
  mental retardation and, 203
Aggression
  intermittent explosive disorder, 277–278
  lithium for, 227
Agonist maintenance, 157
Agoraphobia, 83–84
  panic disorder with, 85
  tricyclic antidepressants for, 236
  without history of panic disorder, 85
Agranulocytosis, 221, 224, 225, 233
Akathisia, 219
Akineton (biperiden), 128, 220t
Alcohol. *See also* Alcoholic(s); Alcoholism (alcohol dependence)
  abuse of, 142, 264
  alcohol-withdrawal syndromes, 146–147
  in elderly patients, 264
  insomnia and, 188
  intoxication, 145–146
  intoxication syndromes, 145–146
  treatment of withdrawal, 149–150, 250
  tricyclic antidepressants and, 239
Alcoholic cerebellar degeneration, 147
Alcoholic coma, 145
Alcoholic convulsions, 146
Alcoholic hallucinosis, 31
Alcoholic paranoia, 146

Alcoholic(s)
  biological markers of, 144
  clinical markers of, 143–144
  screening tests, 144
  types of, 143
Alcoholics Anonymous (AA), 152, 212
Alcohol-induced persisting amnestic
    disorder (Korsakoff syndrome),
    93, 137, 138, 148
Alcohol-induced persisting dementia,
    148
Alcohol-induced psychotic disorder,
    with hallucinations, 146–147
Alcohol intoxication, 145–146
Alcoholism (alcohol dependence),
    142–143, 264
  classification of, 142–143
  complications of chronic, 147–149
  depression and, 46, 51
  risk of violence and, 76, 77
  suicide risk and, 74
  treatment of, 151–152
Alcohol withdrawal, 146
  treatment of, 149–150, 250
Alcohol-withdrawal delirium, 17, 147
Alcohol-withdrawal syndromes,
    146–147
  alcohol withdrawal, with
    perceptual disturbance, 146
Aldomet (methyldopa), 128, 231,
    239, 248
Alertness, 8
Alogia, 24
Alprazolam (Xanax), 160, 235t,
    243–244
  half-life/dose, 250t
  for panic disorder, 83–84
  side effects of, 251
  use in elderly patient, 265
  withdrawal from, 163
Alzheimer disease, 17, 65–66, 204
  early-onset, 65
  late-onset, 65
  mild cognitive impairment, 66
Amantadine (Symmetrel), 171, 220t
Ambien (zolpidem), 160, 161, 188,
    191, 250t, 253
American Law Institute Test (ALI
    Test), 271
Aminophylline
  insomnia and, 189
  lithium and, 231

Amitriptyline (Elavil, Endep), 122,
    235t, 236, 237, 239
Amnesia, 93–95
  dissociative, 94
  dissociative fugue, 94
  evaluation of, 18
  transient global, 94
Amnestic disorder, sedative,
    hypnotic, or anxiolytic-
    induced, 164
Amnestic syndrome due to general
    medical condition, 60
Amobarbital (Amytal), 17, 160
Amoxapine (Asendin), 235t, 244
Amphetamine dependence, 170
Amphetamine-induced psychotic
    disorder, with delusions, 170
Amphetamine intoxication, 170
Amphetamine intoxication delirium,
    170
Amphetamine psychosis, 29
Amphetamines, 169–171
  abuse of, 170
  impotence and, 178
  insomnia and, 189
  MAOIs and, 248
  tricyclic antidepressants and, 239
Amphetamine withdrawal, 170–171
Amytal (amobarbital), 17, 160
Amytal interview, 17–18, 68, 109
Amytal (sodium amobarbital) test,
    17–18, 68, 109
Anabolic steroids, abuse of, 173–174
Anafranil (clomipramine), 83, 91,
    124, 179, 180, 206, 222, 235t,
    236, 241, 248
Androgens, psychiatric symptoms of,
    127
Anectine (succinylcholine), 231,
    256, 258
Anemia
  as cause of depression, 49
  pernicious, 135
Anorectics, MAOIs and, 248
Anorexia nervosa, 120
Antabuse (disulfiram), 151, 171,
    239, 251
Antacids, interaction with traditional
    antipsychotics, 221
Antianxiety drugs. See Hypnotic and
    antianxiety drugs
Antiarrhythmias, 128

Antibiotics, psychiatric symptoms of, 129–130
Anticholinergic psychosis, 128
Anticholinergics, psychiatric symptoms of, 127–128
Anticipatory anxiety, 83, 85
Anticipatory grief, 98
Anticonvulsants
   for depression, 53
   psychiatric symptoms of, 126
   use in elderly patients, 265
Antidepressant drugs, 234–241, 235t
   children and adolescents and, 234
   combinations of, 249
   for delusional disorder, 37
   for depression, 53
   elderly patients and, 265
   monoamine oxidase inhibitors, 234, 235t, 244–248
   SNRIs, 234, 235t, 241, 243–244
   SSRIs, 234, 235t, 241–244
   tricyclic antidepressants, 234, 235t, 236–241
Antihistamines, 127
Antihypertensives, 128
Anti-inflammatory agents, psychiatric symptoms of, 127
Antimalarials, 130
Antineoplastics, 130
Antiparkinsonism drugs, 128, 220, 220t
Antipsychotics, 215–226
   antidepressant drugs and, 249
   atypical, 215, 216t, 223–226
      mood stabilizers and, 249
   in elderly patient, 265
   traditional, 215–223, 216t
Antisocial personality disorder, 77, 197–198
   alcoholism and, 143
   amnesia and, 94
   dissociative disorders and, 93
   EEG of, 17
   somatization disorder and, 111
Antispasmodics, 128
Anxiety
   amnesia and, 94
   anticipatory, 83, 85
   chronic illness and, 104
   defined, 81
   in dying patient, 102
   in elderly patient, 263

impotence and, 178
   infections and, 135
   insomnia and, 188
   medical diseases presenting, 132t
   rebound, 163
   tests for, 14
Anxiety disorders, 81–92
   acute anxiety-panic attacks, 82–84
   acute stress disorder, 88
   alcoholism and, 143
   anxiety disorder due to general medical condition, 88–89
   anxiety with obsessions and compulsions, 90–91
   anxiety with specific fears: phobic disorders, 84–86
   chronic, mild anxiety, 81
   chronic, moderately severe anxiety, 82
   defined, 81
   generalized. See Generalized anxiety disorder
   pain and, 111
   posttraumatic stress disorder, 86–88
   substance-induced anxiety disorder, 89–90
Anxiolytic abuse, 162
Anxiolytic intoxication, 161–162
Anxiolytic withdrawal, 163
Anxious, fearful personality disorders, 195, 200–201
   attention-deficit/hyperactivity disorder, 200–201
   avoidant personality disorder, 200
   dependent personality disorder, 200
   obsessive-compulsive personality disorder, 200
Aphasia, 9
   dementia and, 68
Appearance, 7–8
Aricept (donepezil), 60, 70, 262
Aripiprazole (Abilify), 216t, 226
Arrhythmias, 119
Artane (trihexyphenidyl), 128, 220t
ASD. See Acute stress disorder; Affective spectrum disorder
Asendin (amoxapine), 235t, 244
Asperger syndrome, 196
Assessment, 4–19
   amytal interview, 17–18
   brain imaging, 16–17

Assessment *(contd.)*
  components of, 4
  electroencephalogram, 15–16
  mental status examination, 4, 7–13
  psychiatric history, 4, 5–7
  psychological tests, 4, 13–15
  purposes of, 4
  of suicide risk, 73–74
Associations, loosening of, 10, 23
Astasia-abasia, 108
Asthma
  anxiety disorder and, 89
  bronchial, 119
Atenolol, for phobias, 86
Ativan (lorazepam), 60, 69, 78, 150,
    160, 163, 219, 232, 250t, 251,
    252, 254, 265
Atomoxetine, for ADHD, 201
Atropine, 128, 256, 257
Attention, 8
  disturbed, 57
Attention deficit, 57
Attention-deficit disorder (ADD),
    201
Attention-deficit/hyperactivity
    disorder (ADHD), 200–201
  antisocial personality disorder and,
    198
  impulse-control disorders and, 274
  in partial remission, 201
Attitude toward examiner, 8
Atypical antipsychotics, 31, 223–226
Atypical depression, 41
Auditory hallucinations, 11, 24
Autistic disorder, 21
Automatic thoughts, 211–212
Aversion therapy, 211
Avoidant personality disorder, 85,
    200
Axis I disorders, 2, 195
Axis II disorders, 2
Axis III disorders, 2
Axis IV disorders, 2
Axis V disorders, 2

B
Barbiturates, 160, 239
Beck Depression Inventory, 14, 42
Behavior
  disturbance of, 25
  general, 8
Behavioral medicine, 118

Behavior modification, 33, 210
Behavior therapy, 210–211
  group, 212
Beliefs, core, 211
Benadryl (diphenhydramine), 127,
    220t
Bender-Gestalt test, 14, 64, 195
Benign prostate hyperplasia, tricyclic
    antidepressants and, 238
Benzodiazepine-like drugs, 160
Benzodiazepines. *See also* Hypnotic
    and antianxiety drugs
  for acute stress disorder, 88
  for alcohol intoxication, 146
  for alcohol withdrawal, 149–150
  for amphetamine abuse, 171
  for delirium, 60
  as drugs of abuse, 160, 161
  in elderly patient, 265
  for hallucinogen abuse, 166
  for insomnia associated with
    narcolepsy, 192
  for mania, 232
  for panic disorder, 83
  for PTSD, 87
  for schizophrenia, 31
  for violent patient, 79
Benztropine (Cogentin), 128, 220t
Bereavement, 43, 98–99, 263
β-blockers, 128
  for anxiety disorder, 82
  for delirium, 150
  for panic disorder, 84
  for phobias, 86
Bethanechol, for dry mouth, 218
Bethanidine, 239
Binge-eating disorder, 278
Biochemistry, of schizophrenia, 29
Biological causes, of mental
    retardation, 204–205
Biologic therapy
  antidepressants. *See* Antidepressant
    drugs
  antipsychotics. *See* Antipsychotics
  electroconvulsive therapy, 254–258
  hypnotic and antianxiety, 249–253
  monoamine oxidase inhibitors,
    244–248
  mood stabilizers. *See* Mood
    stabilizers
  psychiatric symptoms of
    nonpsychiatric, 126–130

psychosurgery, 258
psychotropic medication use
  during pregnancy, 253–254
Biology, of schizophrenia, 28–29
Biperiden (Akineton), 128, 220t
Bipolar depression (bipolar disorder,
  depressed), 47
  carbamazepine for, 233
  electroconvulsive therapy for,
    254–255
  with psychotic features, 45
  treatment for, 53, 233
Bipolar disorders, 21, 47–48
  Bipolar I Disorder (manic-
    depression), 40, 45, 47, 48
  Bipolar II Disorder, 45, 48
  Bipolar II Disorder: Hypomania,
    40
  depressed. *See* Bipolar depression
    (bipolar disorder, depressed)
  impulse-control disorders and, 274
  lamotrigine for, 233
  mania, 47
    electroconvulsive therapy for,
      255
    lithium for, 227
  mixed, 48
  not otherwise specified, 50
  with rapid cycling, 48
  tricyclic antidepressants for, 236
Birth and early development, 6
Birth trauma, mental retardation
  and, 205
Bizarre confused delusions, 24
Blackouts, 142
Blindness, conversion, 108–109
Blocking, 10, 23
Blood, lithium effects on, 229
Blunted affect, 25
Blurred vision, as side effect, 218
Body dysmorphic disorder, 113
Borderline intellectual functioning,
  205
Borderline personality disorder,
  198–199
  dissociative disorders and, 93
  distinguishing from depression,
    51
  distinguishing from mania, 51
  somatization disorder and, 111
BPRS. *See* Brief Psychiatric Rating
  Scale

Brain changes, in schizophrenia,
  28–29
Brain imaging, 16–17
  functional techniques, 16–17
  structural techniques, 16
Brain trauma
  dementia and, 67
  mental retardation and, 205
Brain tumors, dementia and, 67
Breathing-related sleep disorder,
  192–193
Brevital (methohexital), 256
Brief Psychiatric Rating Scale
  (BPRS), 14
Brief psychotherapy, 208–209
Brief psychotic disorder, 34–35
Briquet syndrome. *See* Somatization
  disorder
Brofaromine, 246
Bromide, 129
Bronchial asthma, 119
Bulimia nervosa, 120–121, 245
Buprenex (buprenorphine), 157
Buprenorphine (Buprenex), 157
Bupropion (Wellbutrin), 244
  for ADHD, 201
  for cocaine withdrawal, 171
  for depression, 243
  dose, 235t
  in elderly patient, 265
  for female orgasmic disorder,
    180
  for hypoactive sexual disorder,
    181
  lithium and, 249
  for nicotine withdrawal, 173
  serotonin syndrome and, 248
  SSRIs and, 249
Buspar (buspirone), 79, 82, 87, 152,
  249, 250, 253
Buspirone (Buspar), 249, 253
  for alcoholism, 152
  for anxiety disorder, 82
  half-life/dose, 250t
  for PTSD, 87
  SSRIs and, 249
  tricyclic antidepressants and, 249
  for violent patients, 79
Butabarbital (Butisol), 160
Butalbital (Fiorinal), 160
Butisol (butabarbital), 160
Butyrophenones, 216t

C
Caffeine, insomnia and, 189
Calcium-channel blockers, 128
Calculations, intellectual functioning
     assessment and, 13
Campral (acamprosate), 152
Cannabis, 165, 168–169
Cannabis abuse, 169
Cannabis dependence, 169
Cannabis-induced psychotic disorder,
     with delusions, 168–169
Cannabis intoxication, 168
Carbamazepine (Tegretol), 233
   for alcohol withdrawal, 149, 150
   for bipolar depression, 53
   contraindication during pregnancy,
        254
   in elderly patients, 265
   interaction with clozapine, 225
   for mania, 54, 232, 263
   for panic disorder, 84
   for prophylaxis of mania/
        depression, 232
   psychiatric symptoms of, 126
   for PTSD, 87
   tricyclic antidepressants and, 239
   for violent patients, 79
Carbidopa/levodopa, for restless legs
     syndrome, 190
Carcinoma, pancreatic, 49, 135–136
Cardiac drugs, 128
Cardiac glycosides, 128
Cardiovascular disease
   psychiatric symptoms of, 133
   psychosomatic contribution to,
        118–119
Cataplexy, 191, 192
Catapres (clonidine), 87, 128, 140,
     150, 160
Catatonia, 60
Catatonic disorder due to general
     medical condition, 60–61
Catatonic excitement, 26
Catatonic negativism, 26
Catatonic posturing, 26
Catatonic rigidity, 26
Catatonic schizophrenia, 18, 68, 255
Catatonic stupor, 26
Catecholamines, 129, 248
CBT. See Cognitive-behavioral
     therapy
Celexa (citalopram), 235t, 241

Central anticholinergic syndrome,
     218–219
Central pontine myelinolysis, 147
Central sleep apnea, 192
Centrax (prazepam), 160, 250t
CFS. See Chronic fatigue syndrome
Childhood, history of, 6
Children, use of antidepressants in,
     234
Chloral hydrate, 161
Chlordiazepoxide (Librium), 160
   for delirium, 150
   half-life/dose, 250t
   for sedative withdrawal, 164
   treatment principles for, 252
Chlorpheniramine (Teldrin), 127
Chlorpromazine (Thorazine), 216t
   for acute psychosis, 222
   lithium and, 231
   pharmacokinetics of, 217
   for side effects of traditional
        antipsychotics, 221
Cholestatic jaundice, 220–221
Chronically ill patient, 103–104
Chronic depression, 41
Chronic drug addiction, 154–155
Chronic fatigue syndrome (CFS),
     124
Chronic obstructive pulmonary
     disease (COPD), 136
Chronic pain, psychosomatic
     contribution to, 122–123
Cialis (tadalafil), 179
Cimetidine, 239, 251
Cinnarizine, 128
Circadian rhythm sleep disorder,
     189
Circumstantiality, 9
Citalopram (Celexa), 235t, 241
Civil commitment, 267–268
Civil law
   abandonment, 269
   civil commitment, 267–268
   competency, 269–270
   right to refuse treatment, 269
   right to treatment, 268–269
Clanging, in disturbance of thought
     form, 23
Clinical disorders, 2
Clinical presentation
   of mood disorders, 41–43
   of schizophrenia, 22–25

Clomipramine (Anafranil), 241
  for acute psychosis, 222
  dose, 235t
  male orgasmic disorder and, 180
  for obsessive-compulsive disorder,
    91, 236
  for panic disorder, 83
  for premature ejaculation, 179
  for self-mutilation, 206
  serotonin syndrome and, 248
  for trichotillomania, 124
Clonazepam (Klonopin), 160
  for delirium, 60
  in elderly patient, 265
  half-life/dose, 250t
  for nocturnal myoclonus, 189
  for obsessive-compulsive disorder,
    91
  for panic disorder, 83
  pregnancy and, 254
  for prophylaxis of
    mania/depression, 232
  for schizophrenia, 31
  for sedative withdrawal, 164
  for Tourette disorder, 140
  for trichotillomania, 277
Clonidine (Catapres), 128
  for delirium, 150
  for opiate withdrawal, 160
  for PTSD, 87
  for Tourette disorder, 140
Clorazepate (Tranxene), 160, 250t,
    252
Clorgyline, 246
Clozapine (Clozaril), 216t, 225, 265
  for schizophrenia, 31, 224
  for violent patient, 79
Clozaril (cozapine), 31, 79, 216t,
    224, 225, 265
Cluster B personality disorders,
    impulse-control disorders and,
    274
Cluster headaches, lithium for, 227
CNS disease, undetected, 106
CNS infection, psychiatric symptoms
    of, 139
Cocaine, 169, 171, 189, 248
Cocaine abuse, 170
Cocaine intoxication, 170
Codeine, 122, 155
Cogentin (benztropine), 128, 220t
Cognex (tacrine), 70

Cognitive-behavioral therapy (CBT),
    210–212
  behavior therapy, 210–211
  cognitive therapy, 211–212
  for depression, 52
  for hypochondriasis, 113
  for panic disorder, 84
  for phobias, 86
  for PTSD, 87
  for somatization disorder, 111
  for trichotillomania, 277
Cognitive disorders
  amnestic syndrome due to general
    medical condition, 60
  catatonic disorder due to general
    medical condition, 60–61
  delirium, 56–60
  personality change due to general
    medical condition, 61
  substance-induced persisting
    amnestic disorder, 60
Cognitive restructuring, 86
Cognitive theory, depression and, 51
Cognitive therapy, 211–212
COLD, anxiety disorder and, 89
Command hallucinations, 24
Competency (civil), 269–270
Competency to stand trial, 270
Compliance, traditional
    antipsychotics and, 223
Compulsions, 90. *See also* Obsessive-
    compulsive disorder
Compulsive shopping, 278
Computed tomography (CT), 16
Concentrate, 8
Concreteness, in disturbance of
    thought form, 23
Conditioned insomnia, 188
Conduct disorder, 93, 197
Confidentiality, 272
Confusion, medical diseases
    presenting, 132t
Congestive heart failure, 67, 119
Consanguinity studies, of
    schizophrenia, 29
Consciousness
  clouding of, 57
  state of, 8
Consent, informed, 272–273
Constructional ability, 12, 64
Continuous positive airway pressure
    (CPAP), 193

Conversion blindness, 108–109
Conversion disorder, 106–109
  diagnosis of, 107–109
  differential diagnosis of, 109
  evaluation of, 18
  treatment of, 109
Conversion paralysis, 108
Conversion seizures, 107–108
Conversion sensory changes, 108
Conversion unconsciousness, 108
Convulsions, alcoholic, 146
COPD. *See* Chronic obstructive
    pulmonary disease
Core beliefs, 211
Coronary artery disease, 118–119
Cortical dementia, 62
Cortisone, 127
Covert sensitization, 211
CPAP. *See* Continuous positive
    airway pressure
Crack cocaine, 169, 171
"Crack lung," 171
Creutzfeldt-Jakob disease, dementia
    and, 66
Cri-du-chat syndrome, 204
Criminal law, 270–271
Criminal responsibility, 270–271
Crohn disease, 120
CT. *See* Computed tomography
Cushing disease, 89
Cushing syndrome, 49, 67, 134
1-Cyclohexyl-1-phenyl-3-(1-
    piperidyl)propan-1-ol
    hydrochloride (Tremin),
    128
Cyclopentolate, 128
Cycloserine, 130
Cyclothymic disorder, 40, 41, 45
Cymbalta (duloxetine), 235t, 243
Cyproheptadine, for PTSD, 87
Cyproterone acetate, for paraphilia,
    182

D
Dalmane (flurazepam), 160, 250t,
    252
Darvon (propoxyphene), 122, 155
Dangerousness, civil commitment
    and, 267–268
Date-rape drug, 164–165
Deferred diagnosis, 1
Delayed grief, 99

Delirium, 11, 56–60, 68, 150
  with agitation or psychotic
      features, 59–60
  alcohol-withdrawal, 60, 147
  anticholinergic, 60
  dementia *vs.*, 59
  diagnosis of, 57–58
  differential diagnosis of, 58–59
  as drug side effect, 219
  due to general medical condition,
      56
  due to multiple etiologies, 56
  EEG of, 17
  in elderly patients, 261
  etiology of, 58–59
  organic psychoses and, 21
  postcardiotomy, 133
  sedative, hypnotic, or anxiolytic
      withdrawal and, 60, 163
  substance intoxication or
      withdrawal and, 56
  synonyms of, 56
  treatment of, 59–60, 219
Delirium tremens (DTs), 17, 147
Delusional disorder, 35–37, 263
Delusions, 10
  bizarre confused, 24
  grandiose, 24
  of influence, 24
  in major depression, 45
  persecutory, 24
  of reference, 24
  of thought broadcasting, 24
  of thought insertion, 24
Dementia, 56, 62–71
  alcohol-induced persisting, 148
  alcoholism and, 143
  of Alzheimer type, 17, 65–66
  cortical, 62
  delirium *vs.*, 59
  diagnosing, 62–64
  differential diagnosis of, 68
  distinguishing from depression, 51
  due to other general medical
      conditions, 66–68
  in elderly patients, 261–262
  HIV-associated, 67
  laboratory examination for, 64
  Lewy body, 65–66
  major types of, 65–66
  physical examination for, 64
  psychological testing for, 64

retardation *vs.*, 203
subcortical, 62
substance-induced persisting, 68
treatment of, 69–70
vascular, 66
Demerol (meperidine), 122, 155,
158t, 248
Depakene (valproic acid), 79, 233,
254
Depakote (divalproex sodium), 149,
150, 152, 199
Dependent personality disorder, 200
Dependent retarded, 204
Depersonalization disorder, 96
Depersonalizations, 24
Depo-Provera (medroxyprogesterone
acetate), 182
Depression, 40, 44. *See also* Bipolar
depression; Mood disorders
amnesia and, 94
atypical, 41, 245
MAOIs for, 245
brain imaging in, 16
cardiovascular disease and, 133
chronic, 41
cognitive-behavioral therapy for,
210
cognitive therapy for, 212
dementia and, 63
differential diagnosis of, 50–51
dissociative disorders and, 93
due to general medical condition,
49
in dying patient, 102
in elderly patient, 262–263
electroconvulsive therapy for,
254–255
general presentation of, 8
impotence and, 178
impulse-control disorders and, 274
infections and, 135
insomnia and, 188
interpersonal therapy and, 209
lithium prophylaxis of, 232
major, 45–47
major depressive disorder, 21
masked, 41
medical diseases presenting, 132t
obsessive-compulsive disorder and,
90
pain and, 111
panic disorder and, 83
postpartum, 46, 236
postpsychotic, 28
poststroke, 139
pseudodementia and, 68
seasonal affective disorder, 46
substance-induced, 50
symptoms of, 42t
tests for, 14
treatment of, 52–53, 215, 236,
245
tricyclic antidepressants for, 236
unipolar, 227
Depressive disorder NOS, 50, 134
Depressive spectrum disorders, 46
Derealizations, 24
Desensitization, systematic, 211
Designer drugs, 166
Desipramine (Norpramin), 239
action mechanism of, 236
for ADHD, 201
for cocaine withdrawal, 171
dose, 235t
for panic disorder, 83
pharmacokinetics of, 237
for Tourette disorder, 140
Desoxyn, methedrine
(methamphetamine), 169
Desyrel (trazodone), 69, 191, 235t,
244, 265
Dexamethasone, 127
Dexamethasone suppression test
(DST-positive test), 47
Dexedrine (dextroamphetamine),
169, 192, 201
Dextroamphetamine (Dexedrine),
169, 192, 201
Diabetes mellitus, 122
psychiatric symptoms of, 134
Diacetylmorphine, 155
Diagnoses, psychiatric. *See*
Psychiatric diagnoses
*Diagnostic and Statistical Manual of
Mental Disorders* (DSM-IV-TR),
1–2
assessment and, 4
mood disorders, 40–41
Dialectical behavior therapy, 199
Diazepam (Valium), 160
for alcohol intoxication, 145
for alcohol withdrawal, 150
for amphetamine abuse, 171
for chronic pain, 122

Diazepam (Valium) *(contd.)*
  contraindication during pregnancy, 254
  half-life/dose, 250t
  for hallucinogen abuse, 167
  for PCP abuse, 167
  pre-electroconvulsive therapy, 256
  for schizophrenia, 31
  for sedative withdrawal, 164
  for somnambulism, 190
  treatment principles for, 252
  for tremulousness, 150
  for unresolved grief, 100
Dibenzoxazepines, 216t
Dicumarol, tricyclic antidepressants and, 239
DID. *See* Dissociative identity disorder
Differential diagnosis
  of conversion disorder, 109
  of delirium, 58–59
  of dementia, 68
  of mood disorders, 50–51
  of obsessive-compulsive disorder, 90–91
  of schizophrenia, 31
Digitalis, 128
Digit recall, 8
Digit repetition test, 12
Digit span, 8
Dihydroindolones, 216t
Dilaudid (hydromorphone), 155
Dimenhydrinate (Dramamine), 127
Dimethoxymethylamphetamine (DOM), 165
Dimethyltryptamine (DMT), 165
Diphenhydramine (Benadryl), 127, 220t
Diphenyl butylpiperidines, 216t
Diphenylhydantoin, for alcohol withdrawal, 150
Disabled and in need of treatment, civil commitment and, 268
Disorientation, delirium and, 57
Dissociative amnesia, 94
Dissociative disorders, 93–97
  amnesia, 93–95
  depersonalization disorder, 96
  dissociative identity disorder, 95–96
Dissociative fugue, 94

Dissociative identity disorder (DID), 95–96
Distorted grief, 99
Disturbance of behavior, 25
Disturbance of emotions, 25
Disturbance of perception, 24
Disturbance of thought content, 24
Disturbance of thought form, in schizophrenia, 23–24
Disulfiram (Antabuse)
  for alcoholism, 151
  for cocaine withdrawal, 171
  sedatives and, 251
Diuretics, 128, 231
Divalproex sodium (Depakote)
  for alcoholism, 152
  for alcohol withdrawal, 149, 150
  for borderline personality disorder, 199
Donepezil (Aricept), 60, 70, 262
Dopamine hypothesis, 29, 217
Doral (quazepam), 160, 250t, 252
Doriden (glutethimide), 161
Down syndrome, 204
Doxepin (Sinequan, Adapin), 235t, 236, 238
Doxycycline, 239
Dramamine (dimenhydrinate), 127
Dramatic, emotional, and erratic personality disorders, 195, 197–199
  antisocial personality disorder, 197–198
  borderline personality disorder, 198–199
  histrionic personality disorder, 199
  narcissistic personality disorder, 199
Draw-a-Person Test, 14
Dreaming, 187
Droperidol, for violent patient, 78
Drug abuse, 154–175
  defined, 154
  distinguishing from depression, 51
  impulse-control disorders and, 274
  patterns of, 154
  violence and, 77
Drug addiction
  chronic, 154–155
  iatrogenic, 154
Drug dependence, 154

Drug interactions
  lithium, 231
  monoamine oxidase inhibitors, 248
  sedative-hypnotic drugs, 251–252
  traditional antipsychotics, 221
  tricyclic antidepressants, 239
Drugs. *See* Biologic therapy
Drugs of abuse
  anabolic steroids, 173–174
  designer drugs, 166
  hallucinogens, 165–169
  inhalants, 172–173
  nicotine, 173
  opioids, 155–160
  sedative-hypnotics, 160–165
  stimulants, 169–172
Drug use, schizophrenia and chronic, 31
Dry mouth, as side effect, 218
DST. *See* Dynamic system test
DTs. *See* Delirium tremens
Duloxetine (Cymbalta), 235t, 243
Duodenal ulcer, anxiety disorder and, 89
Dusky v United States, 270
"Duty to warn," 272
Dying patient, 101–103
  normal responses, 101–102
  treatment of, 102–103
Dynamic system test (DST), 68
Dyspareunia, 177, 180–181
Dyssomnia NOS, 189–190
Dyssomnias, 186
Dysthymic disorder, 40, 41, 44, 236, 263

E
Eating disorders
  cognitive-behavioral therapy for, 210
  impulse-control disorders and, 274
Echolalia, 23, 60–61
Echopraxia, 61
ECT. *See* Electroconvulsive therapy
"Educable," 203
Education
  in interpersonal therapy, 209
  as part of personal history, 6
EEG. *See* Electroencephalogram
Effexor (venlafaxine), 84, 124, 235t, 243, 248, 249, 265
Ego-alien symptoms, 81

Ego-dystonic symptoms, 81
Ejaculation
  premature, 179
  retrograde, 180
Elavil (amitriptyline), 122, 235t, 236, 237, 239
Eldepryl (selegiline), 235t, 246
Elderly patient, 260–266
  adjustment disorder in, 264
  anxiety in, 263
  common psychiatric disorders in, 261–264
  delirium in, 56, 261
  delusional disorder in, 263
  dementia in, 261–262
  depression in, 262–263
  evaluation of, 260
  hypochondriasis in, 264
  mania in, 263
  paranoia in, 263
  psychopharmacology of, 264–265
  schizophrenia in, 263
  treatment principles for, 265–266
Electroconvulsive therapy (ECT), 254–258
  administration techniques, 256–257
  complications of, 257–258
  contraindications for use, 255–256
  for depression, 53, 262
  in elderly patient, 265
  indications for use, 254–255
  for pseudodementia, 68
  right to refuse, 269
  for schizophrenia, 31
  treatment principles for, 258
  for violent patient, 79
Electroencephalogram (EEG), 15–16, 58
Electrolyte imbalances, 49, 67
Emotions
  disturbance of, 25
  expressed, 30
Encephalitis, 139
Encounter therapy, 212
Endep (amitriptyline), 122, 235t, 236, 237, 239
Endocrine disorders
  as cause of depression, 49
  psychiatric symptoms of, 133–134
  psychosomatic contribution to, 122
Endorphins, 118

Enuresis, tricyclic antidepressants for, 236
Environmental problems, psychiatric classification and, 2
Ephedrine, 189, 248
Epidemiology, of suicidal patient, 72
Epilepsy
  dementia and, 67
  EEG of, 17
  as physical cause of psychogenic illness, 106
  psychiatric symptoms of, 140
Epinephrine, 239
EPs. *See* Evoked potentials
Equanil (meprobamate), 161
Erythroblastosis fetalis, 205
Escitalopram (Lexapro), 235t, 241–242, 262
EST, 212
Estazolam (ProSom), 160, 250t
Estrogens
  impotence and, 178
  psychiatric symptoms of, 127
Eszopiclone (Lunesta), 160, 250t, 253
Ethacrynic acid, 128, 231
Ethchlorvynol (Placidyl), 161
Ethinamate (Valmid), 161
Ethyl alcohol, impotence and, 178
Etiology of delirium, 58–59
Eutonyl (pargyline), 246
Evaluation, of elderly patient, 260
Evasiveness, 10
Evoked potentials (EPs), 18
Excitement phase, of sexual response, 176
Exelon (rivastigmine), 70, 262
Exercise, for depression, 53
Exhibitionism, 182–183
Exogenous thyroid, psychiatric symptoms of, 127
Explosive disorder, 21
Explosive outbursts, lithium for, 227
Exposure, for obsessive-compulsive disorder, 91
Expressed emotion, 30
Extrapyramidal symptoms, 219
  treatment of, 220–221
Eye movement, rapid synchronous, 187

F
Factitious disorder, 110
  with predominantly physical signs and symptoms, 114
  with predominantly psychological signs and symptoms, 21
False memory, 18
False memory syndrome, 94
Family history, 7
  suicide risk and, 74
Family of dying patient, 103
Family processes, in schizophrenia, 30
Family psychiatric history, 7
Family studies, of depression, 46
Family therapy, 213
  for schizophrenia, 33
Fear, 81
Female orgasmic disorder, 180
Female sexual arousal disorder, 179
Fetal alcohol syndrome, 148–149, 205
Fetishism, 183
Fibromyalgia, 121–122
Fiorinal (butalbital), 160
Flat affect, 25
Flight of ideas, 9–10
Flooding, 86, 211
Flunarizine, 128
Fluoxetine (Prozac), 242, 243
  for borderline personality disorder, 199
  for bulimia nervosa, 121
  for cataplexy, 192
  contraindication during pregnancy, 254
  for depression, 262
  dose, 235t
  for premenstrual syndrome, 134
  serotonin syndrome and, 248
  for trichotillomania, 124
  for violent patient, 79
Fluphenazine (Prolixin), 216t, 222, 223
Flurazepam (Dalmane), 160, 250t, 252
Fluvoxamine (Luvox), 235t, 242
Folie à deux, 37
Foods, MAOIs interactions with, 247
Formal thought disorder, 23
Formication, 163
Form of thought, 9–10

Fragile X syndrome, 204
Frontal lobe syndrome, 76, 137
Frotteurism, 183
Fructose intolerance, 204
Fugues, evaluation of, 18
Functional MRI (fMRI), 16, 17
Fund of knowledge, 12–13
Furosemide, 128, 231

G
Gabapentin (Neurontin), 86, 234
GAD. *See* Generalized anxiety disorder
GAF. *See* Global Assessment of Functioning Scale
Gain
  primary, 106
  secondary, 107
Gait ataxia, 66
Galactosemia, 204
Galantamine (Razadyne), 70, 262
Gamblers Anonymous, 276
Gambling, pathological, 198, 276–277
GAS. *See* Global Assessment Scale
Gastrointestinal disorders, psychosomatic contribution to, 120–121
Gastrointestinal side effects, of lithium, 230
Gender differences
  gender identity disorder and, 183
  paraphilia and, 182
Gender identity disorder, 183–184
General behavior, 8
Generalized anxiety disorder (GAD), 82
  cognitive therapy for, 212
  distinguishing from depression, 51
  in elderly patient, 263
  venlafaxine for, 243
General presentation of patient, 7–8
Genetics
  of Alzheimer disease, 65
  of antisocial personality disorder, 197
  of bipolar disorder, 48
  of mental retardation, 204
  of schizophrenia, 29–30, 30t
Genitourinary disorders, psychosomatic contribution to, 122

Geodon (ziprasidone), 59, 78, 140, 216t, 226
Gestalt therapy, 212
GHB (γ-hydroxybutyrate), 164–165
Global Assessment of Functioning Scale (GAF), 2
Global Assessment Scale (GAS), 14
Glutethimide (Doriden), 161
Grandiose delusions, 24
Grief, 43, 98–101
  anticipatory, 98
  chronic illness and, 103–104
  delayed, 99
  distorted, 99
  of family of dying patient, 103
  interpersonal therapy and, 210
  normal, 98–99
  prolonged, 99
  treatment of, 100–101
  unresolved, 99–100
Group therapy, 212–213
  for alcoholism, 152
  for cocaine addiction, 171
  for drug abuse, 155
  for schizophrenia, 33
Guanethidine (Ismelin), 128, 239
Guidance-inspirational groups, 212
Guilty but mentally ill, 271

H
Halazepam (Paxipam), 160, 250t
Halcion (triazolam), 160, 163, 250t, 251, 252
Haldol (haloperidol), 54, 59–60, 69, 78, 79, 140, 146, 150, 167, 171, 215, 216t, 217, 222, 223, 231, 232
Hallucinations
  alcohol-induced psychotic disorder, with, 146–147
  auditory, 11, 24
  command, 24
  hypnagogic, 191–192
  tactile, 11
  visual, 11
Hallucinogen abuse, 166
Hallucinogen-induced mood disorder, 166
Hallucinogen-induced psychotic disorder, with delusions, 166
Hallucinogen intoxication, 166

Hallucinogen persisting perception
disorder, 166
Hallucinogens
as drugs of abuse, 165–169
cannabis, 168–169
drugs involved, 165
LSD, 165–167
MDMA, 168
mescaline, 165–167
phencyclidine, 167
insomnia and, 189
Haloperidol (Haldol), 216t
for alcohol intoxication, 146
for amphetamine abuse, 171
for delirium, 59–60, 150
for dementia, 69
for hallucinogen abuse, 167
lithium and, 231
for mania, 54, 232
for PCP abuse, 167
pharmacokinetics of, 217
for Tourette syndrome, 140, 215
use of, 222, 223
for violent patient, 78, 79
Halstead and Reitan Batteries, 64
Hamilton Anxiety Rating Scale, 14
Hamilton Depression Rating Scale,
14, 42
Hartnup disease, 204
Hay fever, 119
Headaches
cluster, 227
migraine, 119
tension, 121
Head trauma, psychiatric symptoms,
49, 139
Heart, lithium effects on, 230
Hematologic disease, psychosocial
stressors and, 124
Hematoma, subdural, 67
Hepatolenticular degeneration
(Wilson disease), 31, 49, 67,
135, 204
Heroin, 155, 156, 158t
Heroin addiction, 156–157
Herpes simplex encephalitis, 67
Heterosexual pedophilia, 182
Histrionic patients, general
presentation of, 8
Histrionic personality disorder, 199
distinguishing from depression, 51
somatization disorder and, 111

HIV/AIDS, psychiatric symptoms of,
139–140
HIV-associated dementia, 67
Homatropine, 128
Homeostasis, 118
Homosexuality, 184
Homosexual pedophilia, 182
Hopelessness, 73
Hormones
for gender identity disorder, 184
psychiatric symptoms of, 127
Huntington chorea
dementia and, 66
depression and, 49
differentiating from schizophrenia,
31
mental retardation and, 204
psychiatric symptoms, 138
Hydrocodone (Lortab), 155
Hydromorphone (Dilaudid), 155
Hyperadrenalism (Cushing
syndrome), 49, 67, 134
Hyperalertness, 8
Hyperparathyroidism
depression and, 49
lithium use and, 230
as physical cause of psychogenic
illness, 106
psychiatric symptoms of, 133
Hypersomnia, 186, 191–193
narcolepsy, 191–192
primary, 191–193
related to another mental disorder,
191
sleep apnea, 192–193
Hypertension, 119
Hypertensive crisis, 247, 248
Hyperthyroidism
anxiety disorder and, 89
dementia and, 67
depression and, 49
as physical cause of psychogenic
illness, 106
psychiatric symptoms of, 133
stress and, 122
Hyperventilation syndrome, 119
Hypnagogic hallucinations, 191–192
Hypnopompic, 192
Hypnotic abuse, 162
Hypnotic and antianxiety drugs,
249–253
drug interactions, 251–252

drugs available, 249, 250t
as drugs of abuse, 160–165
  clinical syndromes, 161–163
  GHB, 164–165
  tolerance test, 163–164
  withdrawal symptoms, 163
indications for use, 250
for insomnia, 190–191
insomnia and, 189
mechanisms of actions, 250–251
pharmacokinetics of, 250–251
side effects of, 251
treatment principles for, 252–253
Hypnotic intoxication, 161–162
Hypnotic withdrawal, 163
Hypoactive sexual desire disorder, 181
Hypoadrenalism (Addison disease),
  psychiatric symptoms of, 134
Hypochondriasis, 112–113
in elderly patient, 264
Hypoglycemia
anxiety and, 89
mental retardation and, 204
as physical cause of psychogenic
  illness, 106
psychiatric symptoms of, 129, 134
Hypomania, 45, 188
Hypoparathyroidism
depression and, 49
psychiatric symptoms of, 134
Hypotension, 119
Hypothyroidism
dementia and, 67
depression and, 49
mental retardation and, 204
as physical cause of psychogenic
  illness, 106
psychiatric symptoms of, 133
Hysterical phenomena, evaluation of,
  18

I

Iatrogenic addiction, 154
ICD. *See* Impulse-control disorders
Identification of patient, 5
Illusions, 11, 24
Imaginal exposure, 91
Imipramine (Tofranil)
action mechanism of, 236
for cataplexy, 192
dose, 235t
for panic disorder, 83

pharmacokinetics of, 237
for PTSD, 87
for somnambulism, 190
treatment principles for, 239–240
Implosion, 86, 211
Implosive therapy, 211
Impotence, 177–181
causes of, 178
primary, 177
secondary, 178
selective, 178
Impulse-control disorders (ICD),
  274–278
impulse-control disorder not
  otherwise specified, 278
intermittent explosive disorder,
  277–278
kleptomania, 275
pathological gambling, 276–277
pyromania, 275
trichotillomania, 277
Inappropriate affect, 25
Incoherence, delirium and, 57
Incontinence, 66
Inderal (propranolol), 79, 84, 86, 87,
  128, 206, 219
Individual therapy, 207–212
cognitive-behavioral therapy,
  210–212
interpersonal therapy, 209–210
psychoanalytic psychotherapy,
  208–209
supportive therapy, 207–208
Indomethacin, lithium and, 231
Infections
as cause of depression, 49
as cause of mania, 49
CNS, 139
dementia and, 67
psychiatric symptoms of, 133–134
Information collection, in
  interpersonal therapy, 209
Informed consent, 272–273
INH. *See* Isoniazid
Inhalant intoxication, 172
Inhalants, as drugs of abuse, 172–173
Inhibition, reciprocal, 211
Insight, 10
lack of, 24
Insomnia, 186, 187–191
conditioned, 188
delirium and, 57

Insomnia *(contd.)*
  primary, 187–190
  pseudo-, 187
  psychophysiologic, 188
  related to another mental disorder,
    188
  situational, 188
  sleeping-pill, 189
  treatment of, 190–191
Insulin, 129
Intellectual functioning, 12–13
Intellectual impairment, dementia
    and, 63
Intelligence, abstractive thinking and,
    11
Intercourse, pain with, 180–181
Intermediate memory, 11, 12
Intermittent explosive disorder, 77,
    277–278
Internet addiction, 278
Interpersonal exploration groups,
    212
Interpersonal role disputes, 209–210
Interpersonal style, patient's, 4
Interpersonal therapy (ITP),
    209–210
Intoxication syndromes, 145–146
Intracranial tumors, psychiatric
    symptoms, 138–139
Irresistible impulse test, 271
Irritable bowel syndrome, 120, 136
Ismelin (guanethidine), 128, 239
Isocarboxazid (Marplan), 235t, 244,
    245, 246
Isoniazid (INH), 130
Isoproterenol, tricyclic
    antidepressants and, 239
ITP. *See* Interpersonal therapy

J
Jaundice, cholestatic, 220–221
"Jittery babies," 171
Judgment
  assessing, 11
  dementia and compromised, 63

Kx
K complexes, 186
Kemadrin (procyclidine), 128, 220t
Ketamine (Ketalar), 165
Ketalar (ketamine), 165

Kidney, lithium effects on, 229
Kleine-Levin syndrome, 193
Kleptomania, 198, 275
Klinefelter syndrome, 204
Klonopin (clonazepam), 31, 60, 83,
    91, 140, 160, 164, 189, 232,
    250t, 254, 265, 277
Kluver-Bucy syndrome, 137
Knowledge, fund of, 12–13
Korsakoff syndrome, 93, 137, 138,
    148

L
LAAM (levo-a-acetylmethadol), 157
La belle indifference, 107
Labile affect, 25
Laboratory examination, dementia
    and, 64
Laboratory screening evaluation, 4
Lack of insight, in schizophrenia, 24
Lake v Cameron, 268
Lamictal (lamotrigine), 53, 54, 87,
    233–234, 263, 265
Lamotrigine (Lamictal), 233–234
  for bipolar depression, 53
  for mania, 54, 263
  for PTSD, 87
  use in elderly patient, 265
Language, deficiency in, 9
  dementia and, 63
Lead, mental retardation and
    exposure to, 205
Learning theory, 210
Legal issues in psychiatry, 267–273
  abandonment, 269
  civil commitment, 267–268
  competency, 269–270
  competency to stand trial, 270
  confidentiality, 272
  criminal law, 270–271
  criminal responsibility, 270–271
  informed consent, 272–273
  malpractice, 271–272
  right to refuse treatment, 269
  right to treatment, 268–269
Lethargy, 8
Leukocytosis, 229
Levitra (vardenafil), 179
Levodopa, 129, 248
Lewy body dementia, 65–66
Lexapro (escitalopram), 235t,
    241–242, 262

Librium (chlordiazepoxide), 150,
160, 164, 250t, 252
Lidocaine, 128, 258
Limbic system, 138
Lithium carbonate, 227–232
for alcoholism, 152
antidepressant drugs and, 249
for borderline personality disorder,
199
bupropion and, 249
contraindication during pregnancy,
254
for dementia, 262
for depression, 53, 234
drug interactions, 231
in elderly patient, 265
indications for use, 227
for insomnia with mania, 188
for kleptomania, 275
for mania, 54, 263
mechanisms of action, 227
for pathological gambling, 276
pharmacokinetics of, 228
for PTSD, 87
for schizoaffective disorder, 35
for schizophrenia, 31
for self-abuse/aggression, 206
side effects of, 219, 228–230
traditional antipsychotics used
with, 215
treatment principles for, 231–232
for violent patient, 79
Lithium-induced dysphoria, 228
Locus coerulus cell receptors, opioids
and, 156
Loosening of associations, 10, 23
Lorazepam (Ativan), 160, 163
for akathisia, 219
for delirium, 60
for dementia, 69
in elderly patient, 265
half-life/dose, 250t
for mania, 232
pregnancy and, 254
side effects of, 251
treatment principles for, 252
for tremulousness, 150
for violent patient, 78
Lortab (hydrocodone), 155
Low back pain, 122
Loxapine (Loxitane), 216t
Loxitane (loxapine), 216t

LSD, 165–167
L-Tryptophan, fluoxetine and, 243
Ludiomil (maprotiline), 235t, 244
Luminal (phenobarbital), 126, 160,
164
Lunesta (eszopiclone), 160, 250t, 253
Luria test, 64
Luvox (fluvoxamine), 235t, 242
Lyme disease meningitis, 139

M
MacAndrew Scale, 144
Magnesium sulfate, for alcohol
withdrawal, 150
Magnetic resonance imaging (MRI),
16
Magnification, 211
Mainstreaming, 205
Maintenance treatment, of opioid
addiction, 157
Major depression, 45–47. *See also*
Depression
with psychotic features, 45
recurrent, 46
single episode, 46
Major depressive disorder, 21, 40, 45
Male erectile dysfunction, 177–179
Male orgasmic disorder, 180
Malignant disease, psychosocial
stressors and, 124
Malingering, 21, 109, 110, 113
Malnutrition, dementia and, 67
Malpractice, 271–272
Mania, 40, 47. *See also* Bipolar
disorders; Mood disorders
carbamazepine for, 233
due to general medical condition,
49
in elderly patient, 263
insomnia and, 188
lithium for, 227, 231–232
lithium prophylaxis of, 232
maintenance treatment of, 232
substance-induced, 50
symptoms of, 42, 43t
treatment of, 54
unipolar, 48
violence and, 77
Manic patients, speech of, 9
MAOIs. *See* Monoamine oxidase
inhibitors
Maprotiline (Ludiomil), 235t, 244

Marathon therapy, 212
Marchiafava-Bignami disease, 147
Marijuana, 165, 168–169
Marital therapy, 213
Marplan (isocarboxazid), 235t, 244, 245, 246
Marriage, as part of personal history, 6
Masked depressions, 41
MDD. *See* Multiplex developmental disorder
MDMA (ecstasy), 165, 168
Medical complications of chronic alcoholism, 147
Medical disease, psychiatric presentations of, 131–136, 132t
Medical history, 7
Medications. *See* Biologic therapy; Drugs of abuse
Medroxyprogesterone acetate (Depo-Provera), 182
Melancholia, 41
Melatonin, 186, 189
Mellaril (thioridazine), 216t
Memantine (Namenda), 70, 262
Memory
  assessing, 11–12
  delirium and impairment in, 57
  false *vs.* repressed, 18
  intermediate, 11, 12
  lithium effects on, 230
  loss of
    in dementia, 63
    medical diseases presenting, 132t
  remote, 11, 12
  short-term, 11, 12
Ménière disease, 89
Meningitis, 139
  Lyme disease, 139
Mental illness, civil commitment and, 267
Mental retardation, 203–206
  causes of, 204–205
  classification of, 203–204
  mild, 203
  moderate, 203
  profound, 204
  prognosis for, 205–206
  severe, 204
  severity unspecified, 204
  treatment of, 205–206

Mental status examination, 4, 7–13
  attention, 8
  form of thought, 9–10
  general presentation, 7–8
  intellectual functioning, 12–13
  judgment, 11
  memory, 11–12
  mood and affect, 9
  orientation, 9
  perceptions, 11
  speech, 9
  state of consciousness, 8
  thought content, 10–11
Meperidine (Demerol), 122, 155, 158t, 248
Meprobamate (Equanil), 161
Mercury, mental retardation and, 205
Mescaline, 165–167
Mesoridazine (Serentil), 216t
Metabolic disorders
  dementia and, 67
  mental retardation and, 204
Metabolic encephalopathy. *See* Delirium
Metachromatic leukodystrophy, 31
Metaraminol, MAOIs and, 248
Methadone, 155, 157, 158t, 159–160
Methamphetamine (Desoxyn, Methedrine), 169
Methandienone, 173
Meth mouth, 170
Methohexital (Brevital), 256
Methyldopa (Aldomet), 128, 231, 239, 248
3,4-Methylenedioxyamphetamine (MDA), 165
Methylphenidate (Ritalin), 169
  for ADHD, 201
  insomnia and, 189
  MAOIs and, 248
  for sleep attacks, 192
  tricyclic antidepressants and, 239
Methyprylon (Noludar), 161
Migraine, 119
Mild cognitive impairment, 66
Mild mental retardation, 203
Milieu therapy, 213
Mini-Mental State Examination (MMSE), 14, 64
Minnesota Multiphasic Personality Inventory (MMPI), 13–14, 106, 195

Mirtazapine (Remeron), 235t, 243, 244
Misperceptions, 11
Mitral valve prolapse, 136
Mitral valve prolapse syndrome, 88
Mixed sleep apnea, 193
MMPI. *See* Minnesota Multiphasic Personality Inventory
MMSE. *See* Mini-Mental State Examination
M'Naughten rule, 270, 271
Moban (molindone), 216t
Moclobemide, 246
Modafinil (Provigil), 192, 201
Moderate mental retardation, 203
Molindone (Moban), 216t
Monoamine oxidase inhibitors (MAOIs), 234, 235t, 244–248, 245t
  for anxiety disorder, 82
  for depression, 53
  drug interactions, 248
  indications for use, 245
  male orgasmic disorder and, 180
  mechanisms of action, 51, 245–246
  for panic disorder, 84
  pharmacokinetics of, 246
  side effects of, 246–247
  SSRIs and, 242–243
  treatment principles for, 248
  tricyclic antidepressants and, 240
Monophobias, 85–86
Mood, 9
  changes in, in dementia, 63
  normal processes of, 43–44
Mood disorders, 40–54
  alcoholism and, 143
  classification of, 40–41
  clinical presentation of, 41–43
  differential diagnosis of, 50–51
  due to general medical condition, 48–49
  hallucinogen-induced, 166
  major, 45–48
  minor, 44–45
  normal mood processes of, 43–44
  not otherwise specified, 50
  PCP-induced, 167
  psychobiologic theories of, 51–52
  substance-induced, 49–50
  suicide risk and, 74

  treatment of depression, 52–53
  treatment of mania, 54
Mood stabilizers, 227–234
  antidepressant drugs and, 249
  atypical antipsychotics and, 249
  carbamazepine, 233
  combined with other mood stabilizers, 249
  gabapentin, 234
  lamotrigine, 233–234
  lithium carbonate, 227–232
  oxcarbazepine, 234
  for pathological gambling, 276
  topiramate, 234
  valproic acid, 233
Morphine, 155
MRI. *See* Magnetic resonance imaging
Multiaxial classification, 2
Multiple personality disorder. *See* Dissociative identity disorder
Multiple sclerosis, 31, 49, 67, 106
  psychiatric symptoms of, 138
Multiplex developmental disorder (MDD), 111
  body dysmorphic disorder and, 113
Mu receptors, 156
Musculoskeletal disorders, psychosomatic contribution to, 121–122
Mute patients, evaluation of, 18
Mutism, 26, 60
Myasthenia gravis, 106
Myxedema madness, 127, 133

N
Nadolol, for violent patient, 79
Nalidixic acid, 129
Naloxone (Narcan), for opioid overdose, 158–159
Naltrexone (nefazodone), 244
Naltrexone (ReVia)
  for alcoholism, 152
  for kleptomania, 275
  for opioid withdrawal, 160
  for pathological gambling, 276–277
  for trichotillomania, 277
Namenda (memantine), 70, 262
Nandrolone, 173
Narcan (naloxone), for opioid overdose, 158–159

Narcissistic personality disorder, 199
Narcoanalysis, 17
Narcolepsy, 191–192
Narcoleptic tetrad, 191
Nardil (phenelzine), 84, 235t, 245t, 246, 248
Navane (thiothixene), 216t, 217
Nefazodone (Serzone), 244
  dose, 235t
  serotonin syndrome and, 248
  use in elderly patient, 265
Negative reinforcement, 211
Negative symptoms, 27
Nembutal (pentobarbital), 17, 160, 164
Neologisms, 23
Neostigmine, for dry mouth, 218
Neuroendocrine system, disease production and, 118
Neurofibromatosis, 204
Neuroleptic malignant syndrome (NMS), 221
Neurologic complications of chronic alcoholism, 147–148
Neurologic diseases, psychiatric presentation of, 137–141
Neurologic side effects of lithium, 229
Neuromuscular side effects of lithium, 229
Neurontin (gabapentin), 86, 234
Newborns
  of crack mothers, 171
  opioid addiction in, 159
New Haven-Boston Collaborative Depression Project, 209
Nicotine
  as drug of abuse, 173
  insomnia and, 189
Nicotine dependence, 173
Nicotine replacement therapy, 173
Nicotine withdrawal, 173
Nifedipine (Procardia), 128, 247
Nightmares, 190
Night terrors, 190
Nitrofurantoin, 129
NMS. See Neuroleptic malignant syndrome
Nocturnal myoclonus, 189
Nocturnal penile tumescence (NPT), 178
Noludar (methyprylon), 161

Nonsteroidal anti-inflammatory drugs (NSAIDs), psychiatric symptoms of, 127
Nonverbal communication, patient's, 4
Norepinephrine, depression and, 51–52
Normal-pressure hydrocephalus, dementia and, 66
Norpramin (desipramine), 83, 140, 171, 201, 235t, 236, 237, 239
Nortriptyline (Pamelor), 173, 235t, 236, 237, 238, 239
Not Otherwise Specified (NOS), 1
NPT. See Nocturnal penile tumescence
NREM sleep, 186
Nupercaine ointment, 179
Nutrition, as cause of depression, 49

O
Obesity, psychosomatic contribution to, 120
OBS. See Organic brain syndrome
Obsessions, 10, 90
Obsessive-compulsive disorder (OCD), 90–91
  body dysmorphic disorder and, 113
  cognitive-behavioral therapy for, 210
  distinguishing from depression, 51
  in elderly patient, 263
  impulse-control disorders and, 274
  schizophrenia and, 30
  temporal lobes and, 137
  trichotillomania and, 277
  tricyclic antidepressants for, 236
Obsessive-compulsive personality disorder (OCPD), 200
  impulse-control disorders and, 274
  trichotillomania and, 277
Obsessive-compulsive spectrum disorders, 91
Obstructive sleep apnea, 192–193
Occipital lobe lesions, 138
Occupational history, 6
OCD. See Obsessive-compulsive disorder
OCPD. See Obsessive-compulsive personality disorder
Odd eccentric personality disorders, 195, 196–197
  paranoid personality disorder, 196

schizoid personality disorder, 196
schizotypal personality disorder,
   196–197
Olanzapine (Zyprexa), 216t, 226
   for borderline personality disorder,
      199
   for delirium, 59
   for dementia, 262
   for Tourette disorder, 140
   for violent patient, 78
Operant conditioning, 211
Ophthalmic drops, 128
Opioid intoxication, 158–159, 158t
Opioids, 155–160
   abuse of, 156–157
   dependence on, 156–157
   drugs involved, 155
   opioid intoxication, 158–159, 158t
   opioid withdrawal, 159–160, 159t
   overdose of, 158–159
   treatment of addicts, 157
Opium, 155
Orap (pimozide), 140, 216t
Organic brain syndrome (OBS), 135,
   198, 220
Organicity, test of, 14
Organic psychoses, psychotic
   disorders *vs.*, 21
Orgasm, 176
   female orgasmic disorder, 180
   male orgasmic disorder, 180
Orientation, 9
   dementia and loss of, 63
Ornade (phenylpropanolamine),
   127, 248
Overdose, of opioids, 158–159
Overgeneralization, 211
Overinclusiveness, 23
Oxandrolone, 173
Oxazepam (Serax), 160
   for dementia, 69
   half-life/dose, 250t
   treatment principles for, 252
   for tremulousness, 150
   use in elderly patient, 265
Oxcarbazepine (Trileptal), 234
Oxycodone (Percodan), 122, 155

P
Pain
   chronic, 122–123
   low back, 122
      tricyclic antidepressants for
         chronic, 236
Pain disorder, 111–112
Pamelor (nortriptyline), 173, 235t,
   236, 237, 238, 239
Pancreatic carcinoma, 135–136
   mood disorder and, 49
Panic attacks, 21, 82–84, 85
Panic disorder
   with agoraphobia, 83–84, 85
   cognitive therapy for, 212
   in elderly patient, 263
   MAOIs for, 245
   somatization disorder and, 111
   suicide risk and, 74
   treatment of, 236, 245, 250
   tricyclic antidepressants for, 236
   without agoraphobia, 82–83
Panic states, evaluation of acute,
   18
Paralysis
   conversion, 108
   sleep, 192
Paranoia
   alcoholic, 146
   delusional disorder and, 36
   dementia and, 63
   in elderly patient, 263
   general presentation of, 8
Paranoid personality disorder, 196
Paraphilia, 181–183
   exhibitionism, 182–183
   pedophilia, 182
Parasomnias, 186, 190
Parens patriae provision, 268
Paresis, 31
   general, 139
Pargyline (Eutonyl), 246
Parietal lobe lesions, 137–138
Parkinson disease
   dementia and, 66
   depression and, 49
   psychiatric symptoms of, 138
Parkinsonism-dementia complex of
   Guam, 67
Parkinson-like syndrome, 219
Paroxetine (Paxil), 134, 179, 235t
Partial sleep deprivation, for
   depression, 52–53
Partner relational problem, 98
Pathological gambling, 198,
   276–277

Patient. *See also* Elderly patient; Suicidal patient; Violent patient
  general presentation of, 7–8
  identification of, 5
Pavor nocturnus, 190
Paxil (paroxetine), 134, 179, 235t
Paxipam (halazepam), 160, 250t
PCP (phencyclidine) intoxication, 167
PCP. *See under* Phencyclidine
Pedophilia, 182
Pellagra, 49, 135
Pentazocine (Talwin), 122, 155
Pentobarbital (Nembutal), 17, 160, 164
Pentobarbital (perphenazine), 216t
Pentothal (thiopental), 17
Peptic ulcer, 120
Perceptions, 11
Perceptual disturbances, delirium and, 57
Percodan (oxycodone), 122, 155
Pergolide, 189–190
Periodic limb movement of sleep, 189
Pernicious anemia, 135
Perphenazine (Trilafon), 216t
Persecutory delusions, 24
Perseveration, 10
Person, orientation and, 9
Personal history, 6–7
Personality
  changes in, in dementia, 63
  defined, 195
Personality change due to general medical condition, 61
Personality change due to general medical condition, disinhibited type, 78
Personality disorders, 2, 195–202
  antisocial, 197–198
  anxious, fearful, 195, 200–201
  attention-deficit/hyperactivity, 200–201
  avoidant, 200
  borderline, 198–199
  defined, 195
  dependent, 200
  dramatic, emotional, and erratic, 195, 197–199
  heroin addiction and, 156
  histrionic, 199
  narcissistic, 199
  obsessive-compulsive, 200
  odd eccentric, 195, 196–197
  paranoid, 196
  psychotic disorders and, 21
  risk of violence and, 77
  schizoid, 196
  schizotypal, 196–197
Personalization, 211
Pervasive developmental disorder NOS, 21
PET. *See* Positron emission tomography
Pharmacokinetics
  of lithium, 228
  of monoamine oxidase inhibitors, 246
  of sedative-hypnotic drugs, 250–251
  of traditional antipsychotics, 217
  of tricyclic antidepressants, 237
Phenacemide, psychiatric symptoms of, 126
Phencyclidine (PCP), 165, 167
Phencyclidine (PCP) abuse, 167
Phencyclidine (PCP) dependence, 167
Phencyclidine (PCP)-induced mood disorder, 167
Phencyclidine (PCP)-induced psychotic disorder, with delusions, 167
Phencyclidine (PCP) intoxication, 167
Phenelzine (Nardil), 84, 235t, 245t, 246, 248
Phenergan (promethazine), 127
Phenmetrazine (Preludin), 169
Phenobarbital (Luminal), 126, 160, 164
Phenothiazines, 216t
Phentolamine, 247
Phenylbutazone, lithium and, 231
Phenylephrine, 239, 248
Phenylketonuria (PKU), 204
Phenylpropanolamine (Ornade), 127, 248
Phenytoin, 126, 239
Pheochromocytoma, 89, 134
Phobias, 10
  defined, 84
  in elderly patient, 263
Phobic avoidance, 85
Phobic disorders, 84–86
Physical disorders, 2

Physical examination, 4, 64
Physical illness
  conditions mimicking, 105–115
  undetected, 105–106
Physical symptoms, simulation of,
    113–114
Physical therapies, for depression,
    53
Physiological mechanisms of disease
    production, 117–118
Physostigmine, 60, 218, 219
Pickwickian syndrome, 193
Pimozide (Orap), 140, 216t
Pindolol, 79, 91
PKU. See Phenylketonuria
Place, orientation and, 9
Placidyl (ethchlorvynol), 161
Plateau phase, of sexual response, 176
Polyarteritis nodosa, 106
Polysomnography, 186
Polythetic diagnosis, 1
Pornography addiction, 278
Porphyria
  acute intermittent, 135
  anxiety disorder and, 89
  differentiating from schizophrenia,
    31
  as physical cause of psychogenic
    illness, 106
Positive reinforcement, 211
Positive symptoms, 27
Positron emission tomography
    (PET), 17
Postcardiotomy delirium, 133
Postconcussion syndrome, 106
Postpartum depression, 46, 236
Postpsychotic depression, 28
Poststroke depression, 139
Posttraumatic stress disorder
    (PTSD), 86–88
  amnesia and, 94
  brain imaging in, 16
  dissociative disorders and, 93
  MAOIs for, 245
  tricyclic antidepressants for, 236
  violence and, 77
Poverty of speech, 24
Poverty of speech content, 24
Pramipexole, for restless legs
    syndrome, 189
Prazepam (Centrax), 160, 250t
Prednisone, 127

Pregnancy
  lithium use in, 230
  psychotropic medication use
    during, 253–254
  tricyclic antidepressant use during,
    238
Preludin (phenmetrazine), 169
Premature ejaculation, 179
Premenstrual dysphoric disorder,
    134
Premenstrual syndrome
  depression and, 49
  psychiatric symptoms of, 134
Premorbid personality, 6
Prepsychotic personality, 23
Primary gain, 106
Primary hypersomnia, 191–193
Primary impotence, 177
Primidone, psychiatric symptoms of,
    126
Prion, 66
Pro-Banthine (propantheline), 128
Procainamide, 128, 258
Procardia (nifedipine), 128, 247
Process schizophrenia, 27
Procyclidine (Kemadrin), 128, 220t
Prodromal phase, of schizophrenia,
    23
Prodromal symptoms, 58
Profound mental retardation, 204
Progesterones, psychiatric symptoms
    of, 127
Prognosis, for schizophrenia, 27–28
Progressive dementia, 66
Progressive supranuclear palsy, 67
Projective test, 14
Prolapse of the mitral valve, 136
Prolixin (fluphenazine), 216t, 222,
    223
Prolonged grief, 99
Promethazine (Phenergan), 127
Propantheline (Pro-Banthine), 128
Propoxyphene (Darvon), 122, 155
Propranolol (Inderal), 128
  for akathisia, 219
  for panic disorder, 84
  for phobias, 86
  for PTSD, 87
  for self-abuse/aggression, 206
  for violent patient, 79
ProSom (estazolam), 160, 250t
Protriptyline (Vivactil), 235t, 236

Proverbs, testing for abstractive
  ability and, 10
Provigil (modafinil), 192, 201
Provisional diagnosis, 1
Prozac (fluoxetine), 79, 121, 124,
  134, 192, 199, 235t, 242, 243,
  248, 254, 262
Pseudodementia, 17, 45, 68
Pseudodepression, 51
Pseudoephedrine, MAOIs and, 248
Pseudoinsomnia, 187
Pseudotumor cerebri, 127
Psilocybin, 165
Psychiatric classification, 1–3
  DMS-IV, 1–2
  multiaxial classification, 2
Psychiatric complications of chronic
  alcoholism, 148
Psychiatric diagnoses, 1–3
  deferred, 1
  not otherwise specified, 1
  provisional, 1
  reliability of, 2
  specifiers, 1
  subtypes, 1
  validity of, 2
Psychiatric evaluation. *See* Assessment
Psychiatric history, 4, 5–7
  chief complaint, 5
  family history, 7
  medical history, 7
  past psychiatric illness, 6
  patient identification, 5
  personal history, 6–7
  present illness, 5–6
Psychiatric symptoms, 131–132,
  132t
Psychoanalysis, 208
Psychoanalytically oriented therapy,
  212
Psychoanalytic theory, depression
  and, 51
Psychoanalytic therapy, 208–209
Psychobiologic theories, of mood
  disorders, 51–52
Psychodrama, 212
Psychogenic pain disorder,
  conversion disorder and, 109
Psychological factors affecting
  medical condition, 116
Psychological mechanisms of disease
  production, 116–117

Psychological tests, 4, 13–15. *See also*
  individual tests
  for dementia, 64
  for personality disorders, 195
Psychological therapies, for
  depression, 52–53
Psychomotor activity, delirium and
  altered, 57
Psychopharmacology, of old age,
  264–265
Psychophysiologic insomnia, 188
Psychosexual disorders, 176–185
  gender identity disorders, 183–184
  paraphilia, 181–183
  psychosexual dysfunction,
    176–181
Psychosexual dysfunction, 176–181
  dyspareunia, 180–181
  female orgasmic disorder, 180
  female sexual arousal disorder, 179
  hypoactive sexual desire disorder,
    181
  male erectile disorder, 177–179
  male orgasmic disorder, 180
  premature ejaculation, 179
  sexual aversion disorder, 181
  vaginismus, 181
Psychosis
  acute, 23
    insomnia and, 188
    treatment of, 222
  defined, 20
Psychosocial problems, 2
Psychosocial treatment methods, for
  schizophrenia, 32–34
Psychosomatic disorders, 116–125
  accident proneness, 124
  cardiovascular, 118–119
  chronic fatigue syndrome, 124
  chronic pain, 122–123
  endocrine, 122
  gastrointestinal, 120–121
  genitourinary, 122
  hematologic, 124
  malignant disease, 124
  mechanisms of disease production,
    116–118
  musculoskeletal, 121–122
  respiratory, 119
  seizures, 124
  skin, 123–124
Psychosurgery, 91, 258

Psychotherapies, 207–214
  cognitive-behavioral therapy, 210–212
  family therapy, 213
  group therapy, 212–213
  individual therapy, 207–212
  interpersonal therapy, 209–210
  marital therapy, 213
  milieu therapy, 213
  psychoanalytic psychotherapy, 208–209
  supportive therapy, 207–208
Psychotherapy
  brief, 208–209
  for PTSD, 87
Psychotic disorders, 20–39
  brief psychotic disorder, 20, 34–35
  delusional (paranoid) disorder, 20, 35–37
  differential diagnosis of, 20–21
  due to general medical condition, 37
  not otherwise specified, 38
  psychotic disorder due to general medical condition, 20, 37
  psychotic disorder NOS, 20, 38
  schizoaffective disorder, 20, 35
  schizophrenia. See Schizophrenia
  schizophreniform disorder, 34
  shared psychotic disorder, 20, 37
  substance-induced psychotic disorder, 20, 37–38
Psychotic-hysterical symptoms, medical diseases presenting, 132t
Psychotic states, evaluation of, 18
PTSD. See Posttraumatic stress disorder
Pyromania, 198, 275

Q
Quazepam (Doral), 160, 250t, 252
Quetiapine (Seroquel), 216t, 226
  for delirium, 59
  for dementia, 69, 262
  use in elderly patient, 265
Quinidine, 128, 258

R
Rabbit syndrome, 219
Rage attacks, 21

Ramelteon (Rozerem), 249, 250t, 253
Random Letter Test, 8, 57
Rauwolfia alkaloids, 128
Raynaud disease, 119
Razadyne (galantamine), 70, 262
Reactive schizophrenia, 27
Rebound anxiety, 163
Reciprocal inhibition, 211
Recreational use, of drugs, 154
Redmond v Jaffe, 272
Regional enteritis, 120
Reinforcement, positive and negative, 211
Relaxation therapy, 119
Reliability, of psychiatric diagnoses, 2
Remeron (mirtazapine), 235t, 243, 244
Remote memory, 11, 12
Rennie v Klein, 269
Repressed memory, 18
Reserpine, 128
Residual phase, of schizophrenia, 22
Resolution phase, of sexual response, 176
Respiratory disorders, psychosomatic contribution to, 119
Restoril (temazepam), 160, 188, 250t, 252, 265
Restless legs syndrome, 189
Restlessness, 8
Retinitis pigmentosa, 221
Retrograde ejaculation, 180
ReVia (naltrexone), 152, 160, 275, 276–277
Rheumatoid arthritis, 106, 121
Right to refuse treatment, 269
Right to treatment, 268–269
RIMAs (reversible inhibitors of monoamine oxidase), 246
Risk factors
  for suicide, 73–74
  for violence, 76
Risperdal (risperidone), 59, 69, 79, 140, 180, 196, 206, 216t, 226
Risperidone (Risperdal), 216t, 226
  for delirium, 59
  for dementia, 69
  male orgasmic disorder and, 180
  for paranoid personality disorder, 196

Risperidone (Risperdal) *(contd.)*
  for psychiatric syndromes in
      mentally retarded patients, 206
  for Tourette disorder, 140
  for violent patient, 79
Ritalin (methylphenidate), 169, 189,
      192, 201, 239, 248
Rivastigmine (Exelon), 70, 262
Roid rage, 173
Role disputes, interpersonal,
      209–210
Role transitions, 210
Rorschach test, 14, 195
Rozerem (ramelteon), 249, 250t,
      253
Rubella, maternal, 205

S
SAAST (Self-Administered
      Alcoholic Screening Test), 144
SAD. *See* Seasonal affective disorder
Sadness, 43
SADS. *See* Schedule for Affective
      Disorders and Schizophrenia
Salicylates, psychiatric symptoms of,
      127
Salvinorin A, 165
SBE. *See* Subacute bacterial
      endocarditis
Schedule for Affective Disorders and
      Schizophrenia (SADS), 14
Schizoaffective disorder, 35
  distinguishing from depression, 50
  distinguishing from mania, 51
  distinguishing from schizophrenia,
      31
Schizoid personality disorder, 196
Schizophrenia, 22–34
  alcoholism and, 143
  antisocial personality disorder and,
      198
  atypical antipsychotics for, 223
  biochemistry of, 29
  biology of, 28–29
  brain imaging in, 16
  catatonic, 18, 26, 68, 255
  classification of, 20, 26–27
  clinical presentation, 22–25
  differential diagnosis of, 31
  disorganized type, 26
  disturbance of behavior in, 25
  disturbance of emotions in, 25

disturbance of perception in, 24
disturbance of thought content in,
      24
disturbance of thought form in,
      23–24
in elderly patient, 263
family processes in, 30
form of thought in, 10
general presentation of, 8
genetics of, 29–30, 30t
impotence and, 178
lifetime risk of developing, 30t
paranoid personality disorder and,
      196
paranoid type, 26, 170
perceptions in, 11
process, 27
prodromal phase of, 23
prognosis, 27–28
reactive, 27
residual phase of, 22
residual type, 27
schizoid personality disorder and,
      196
suicide risk and, 74
treatment of, 31–34, 215
tricyclic antidepressants and, 239
undifferentiated type, 27
violence and, 77
Schizophrenia spectrum disorders,
      30
Schizophrenic disorders
  distinguishing from depression, 50
  distinguishing from mania, 51
  electroconvulsive therapy for, 255
Schizophreniform disorder, 34
Schizotypal personality disorder,
      196–197
School phobia, tricyclic
      antidepressants for, 236
Schuster v Altenberg, 268
Seasonal affective disorder (SAD),
      46
Secobarbital (Seconal), 160
Seconal (secobarbital), 160
Secondary amines, 236
Secondary gain, 107
Secondary impotence, 178
Sedation, as side effect of traditional
      antipsychotics, 218
Sedative, hypnotic, or anxiolytic
      dependence, 162

Sedative, hypnotic, or anxiolytic-induced persisting amnestic disorder, 164
Sedative, hypnotic, or anxiolytic withdrawal delirium, 163
Sedative abuse, 162
Sedative-hypnotics. *See* Hypnotic and antianxiety drugs
Sedative intoxication, 161–162
Sedative withdrawal, 163
Seizures, 124
    conversion, 107–108
    temporal lobe, 140
Selective abstraction, 211
Selective impotence, 178
Selective serotonin reuptake inhibitor (SSRI) discontinuation syndrome, 242
Selective serotonin reuptake inhibitors (SSRIs), 234, 235t, 241–244
    for anxiety disorder, 82
    for borderline personality disorder, 199
    for dementia, 69, 262
    for depression, 53, 262
    for heart patients with depression, 133
    impotence and, 178
    for insomnia with depression, 188
    interaction with traditional antipsychotics, 221
    for kleptomania, 275
    male orgasmic disorder and, 180
    MAOIs and, 242–243
    for night terrors, 190
    for phobias, 86
    for premature ejaculation, 179
    for premenstrual syndrome, 134
    for PTSD, 87
    for somnambulism, 190
    for trichotillomania, 277
    tricyclic antidepressants and, 249
Selegiline (Eldepryl), 235t, 246
Self-medication, 154–155
Self-mutilation, 206
Sensitization, covert, 211
Sensorimotor polyneuropathy, 147
Sensory changes, conversion, 108
Serax (oxazepam), 69, 150, 160, 250t, 252, 265
Serentil (mesoridazine), 216t

Seroquel (quetiapine), 216t, 226
Serotonin, depression and, 51
Serotonin-norepinephrine reuptake inhibitors (SNRIs), 234, 235t, 241, 243–244
Serotonin syndrome, 242–243, 248
Sertraline (Zoloft), 134, 179, 235t, 242
Serzone (nefazodone), 235t, 244, 248, 265
Severe mental retardation, 204
Sex therapy, 177
Sexual addition, 278
Sexual aversion disorder, 181
Sexual deviation, 181–183
Sexual disorder not otherwise specified, 184
Sexual dysfunction due to general medical condition, 178
Sexual history, 6
Sexual masochism, 183
Sexual response cycle, 176
Sexual sadism, 183
Shared psychotic disorder, 37
Short-term memory, 11, 12
Side effects
    of lithium, 228–230
    of monoamine oxidase inhibitors, 246–247
    of sedative-hypnotic drugs, 251
    of traditional antipsychotics, 217–221, 218t
    of tricyclic antidepressants, 237–239
Sildenafil (Viagra), 179
Similarities, testing for abstractive ability and, 10
Simulation of physical symptoms, 113–114
Sinequan (doxepin), 235t, 236, 238
Single-photon emission CT (SPECT), 16, 17
Situation, orientation and, 9
Situational insomnia, 188
Skin disorders
    psychosocial stressors and, 123–124
    psychosomatic contribution to, 123–124
SLE. *See* Systemic lupus erythematosus
Sleep, normal, 186–187
    NREM sleep, 186
    REM sleep, 187

Sleep apnea, 192–193
  central, 192
  mixed, 193
  obstructive, 192–193
Sleep attacks, 191, 192
Sleep cycle disruption, 189
Sleep disorders
  breathing-related, 192–193
  circadian rhythm, 189
  due to general medical condition,
      hypersomnia type, 193
  due to general medical condition,
      insomnia type, 188
  substance-induced, 188–189
Sleep disturbances, 186–194
  hypersomnia, 186, 191–193
  insomnia, 186, 187–191
  narcolepsy, 191–192
  sleep apnea, 192–193
Sleep hygiene, 190
Sleeping-pill insomnia, 189
Sleep paralysis, 192
Sleep spindles, 186
Sleep-state misperception syndrome,
    187
Sleep terror disorder, 190
Sleep-wake alteration, 57
Sleepwalking, 190
Sleepwalking disorder, 190
SNRIs. *See* Serotonin-norepinephrine
    reuptake inhibitors
Social causes, of mental retardation,
    205
Social history, 6
Social phobia, 85, 243, 245
Social situation, current, 7
Social skills training, 86
  for schizophrenia, 33
Sodium amobarbital (Amytal) test,
    17–18, 68, 109
Somatization disorder, 93, 110–111
  conversion disorder and, 109
Somatoform disorders, 106–109
  conversion disorder, 106–109
  not otherwise specified, 111
  undifferentiated, 111
Somnambulism, 94, 190
Sonata (zaleplon), 191, 250t
Spasmodic torticollis, 121
Specifiers, of psychiatric disorders, 1
SPECT. *See* Single-photon emission
    CT

Speech
  assessment of, 9
  poverty of, 24
Spinocerebellar degenerations, 67
Spironolactone, lithium and, 231
SSPE. *See* Subacute sclerosing
    panendocarditis
SSRIs. *See* Selective serotonin
    reuptake inhibitors
Staff, of dying patient, 103
State of consciousness, 8
State-Trait Anxiety Scale, 14
Stelazine (trifluoperazine), 216t
Stevens-Johnson syndrome, 233
Stimulants
  antidepressant drugs and, 249
  as drugs of abuse, 169–172
    clinical syndromes, 170–171
    drugs involved, 169
    treatment for, 171–172
Stress
  depression and, 41, 46
  disease production and, 116–118
Stroke
  mood disorder and, 49
  poststroke depression, 139
  psychiatric symptoms of, 139
Sturge-Weber syndrome, 204
Subacute bacterial endocarditis
    (SBE), 67
Subacute sclerosing panendocarditis
    (SSPE), 67
Subcortical dementia, 62
Subdural hematoma, 67
Substance-induced anxiety disorder,
    89–90
Substance-induced mood disorder,
    49–50
Substance-induced persisting
    amnestic disorder, 60, 93–94
Substance-induced psychotic
    disorder, 37–38
Substance-induced sexual
    dysfunction, 178
Substance-induced sleep disorder,
    188–189
Substance-inducing persisting
    dementia, 68
Subtypes, of psychiatric disorders, 1
Succinylcholine (Anectine)
  ECT and, 256, 258
  lithium and, 231

Sudden sniffing death syndrome, 172
Suicidal patient, 72–76
  assessing suicidal risk, 73–74
  epidemiology of, 72
  identifying potentially, 72–73
  initiating treatment, 74–75
  treatment principles for, 75–76
Supportive therapy, 207–208
Symmetrel (amantadine), 171, 220t
Surmontil (trimipramine), 235t
Sympathomimetics, 129
Symptoms, 5
  negative, 27
  positive, 27
  prodromal, 58
  psychiatric, 131–132, 132t
Syphilis, 106, 205
Systematic desensitization, 86, 211
Systemic lupus erythematosus (SLE),
    31, 67, 106
  psychiatric symptoms of, 135

T
TA. *See* Transactional analysis
Tacrine (Cognex), 70
Tactile hallucinations, 11
Tadalafil (Cialis), 179
Talwin (pentazocine), 122, 155
Tarasoff duty, 272
*Tarasoff v Regents of the University of
    California*, 272
Tardive dyskinesia, 219–220
TAT. *See* Thematic Apperception
    Test
TBI. *See* Traumatic brain injury
TCAs. *See* Tricyclic antidepressants
TCP. *See* Thiocyclidine
Tegretol (carbamazepine), 53, 54,
    79, 84, 87, 126, 149, 150, 225,
    232, 233, 239, 254, 263, 265
Teldrin (chlorpheniramine), 127
Temazepam (Restoril), 160
  in elderly patient, 265
  half-life/dose, 250t
  for insomnia, 188
  treatment principles for, 252
Temporal lobe epilepsy, 17, 31
Temporal lobe lesions, 137
Temporal lobe seizures, 140
Tension headaches, 121
Tertiary amines, 236
Testimonial privilege, 272

Testosterone
  as drug of abuse, 173–174
  for hypoactive sexual disorder, 181
Tetracyclines, 129, 231
TGA. *See* Transient global amnesia
Thalidomide, 205
THC (delta-9-tetrahydrocannabinol),
    165
Thematic Apperception Test (TAT),
    14
Therapeutic alliance, assessment and,
    4
Therapeutic milieus, 32–33
Thiamine, for alcohol withdrawal,
    150
Thiazides, 128, 231
Thiocyclidine (TCP), 165
Thiopental (Pentothal), 17
Thioridazine (Mellaril), 216t
  for borderline personality disorder,
    199
  impotence and, 178
  male orgasmic disorder and, 180
Thiothixene (Navane), 216t, 217
Thioxanthenes, 216t
Thorazine (chlorpromazine), 216t
Thought content, 10–11
Thought(s)
  automatic, 211–212
  disturbance of thought content,
    24
  disturbance of thought form,
    23–24
  form of, 9–10
Thought stopping, 91
Thyroid. *See also* Hyperthyroidism;
    Hypothyroidism
  antidepressant drugs and, 249
  lithium effects on, 230
Tics, trichotillomania and, 277
Time, orientation and, 9
Tofranil (imipramine), 83, 87, 190,
    192, 235t, 236, 237, 239–240
Token economy, 211
Tolbutamide, 129
Tolerance test, 163–164
Topiramate (Topomax), 53, 152,
    234
Topomax (topiramate), 53, 152,
    234
Tourette syndrome, 90, 140, 215
Toxic psychosis. *See* Delirium

Toxoplasmosis, 205
Traditional antipsychotics, 215–223,
  216t
  drug interactions, 221
  indications for use, 215–216
  mechanisms of action, 217
  pharmacokinetics of, 217
  side effects of, 217–221, 218t
  treatment principles for, 222–223
"Trainable," 203
Transactional analysis (TA), 212
Transient global amnesia (TGA),
  94
Transsexuals, 183
Transvestic fetishism, 183
Tranxene (clorazepate), 160, 250t,
  252
Tranylcypromine (Parnate), 235t,
  245t, 246, 248
Traumatic brain injury (TBI), 67
Trazodone (Desyrel), 244
  for dementia, 69
  dose, 235t
  for insomnia, 191
  use in elderly patient, 265
Treatment, 5
  of alcoholism, 151–152
  of alcohol withdrawal, 149–150
  for amphetamine abuse, 171–172
  of chronic pain, 122–123
  of conversion disorder, 109
  of delirium, 59–60
  of delusional disorder, 36–37
  of dementia, 69–70
  of depression, 52–53
  of dissociative identity disorder,
    95–96
  of drug abuse, 155
  of dying patient, 102–103
  of insomnia, 190–191
  of mania, 54
  of narcolepsy, 192
  of obsessive-compulsive disorder,
    91
  of opioid addiction, 157
  of phobias, 86
  right to, 268–269
  right to refuse, 269
  of schizophrenia, 31–34
  of somatization disorder, 111
  of suicide, 74–76
  of unresolved grief, 100–101

using monoamine oxidase
    inhibitors, 248
  using sedative-hypnotic drugs,
    252–253
  using tricyclic antidepressants,
    239–241
Tremin (1-cyclohexyl-1-phenyl-3-(1-
    piperidyl)propan-1-ol
    hydrochloride), 128
Tremulousness, 150
Triamterene, 231
Triazolam (Halcion), 160, 163, 250t,
    251, 252
Trichobezoars, 277
Trichotillomania, 124, 277
Tricyclic antidepressants (TCAs),
    234, 235t, 236–241
  for anxiety disorder, 82
  for depression, 53
  drug interactions, 239
  impotence and, 178
  indications for use, 236
  interaction with traditional
    antipsychotics, 221
  lithium and, 231
  mechanisms of action, 236–237
  for panic disorder, 83
  pharmacokinetics of, 237
  for PTSD, 87
  side effects of, 219, 237–239
  SSRIs and, 249
  treatment principles for, 239–241
Trifluoperazine (Stelazine), 216t
Trihexyphenidyl (Artane), 128, 220t
Trilafon (perphenazine), 216t
Trileptal (oxcarbazepine), 234
Trimipramine (Surmontil), 235t
Tuberculosis, 106, 119
Tuberous sclerosis, 204
Tumors
  as cause of depression, 49
  as cause of mania, 49
  dementia and brain, 67
  intracranial, 138–139
Turner syndrome, 204
Twin studies
  of depression, 46
  of schizophrenia, 29

U
Ulcer, peptic, 120
Ulcerative colitis, 89, 120

Unconsciousness, conversion, 108
Undifferentiated somatoform
    disorder, 111
Unipolar depression, 227
Unipolar mania, 48
Unresolved grief, 99–100
Urecholine, 218

V
Vaginismus, 181
Validity, of psychiatric diagnoses, 2
Valium (diazepam), 31, 100, 122,
    145, 150, 160, 164, 167, 171,
    190, 250t, 252, 254, 256
Valmid (ethinamate), 161
Valproate
    for alcohol withdrawal, 149
    for depression, 53
    in elderly patient, 265
    for kleptomania, 275
    for mania, 54, 263
    for panic disorder, 84
    for pathological gambling, 276
    for prophylaxis of
        mania/depression, 232
    for PTSD, 87
Valproic acid (Depakene), 233
    contraindication during pregnancy,
        254
    for violent patients, 79
Vardenafil (Levitra), 179
Vascular dementia, 66
Venlafaxine (Effexor), 243, 249
    dose, 235t
    for panic disorder, 84
    serotonin syndrome and, 248
    for trichotillomania, 124
    use in elderly patient, 265
Venlafaxine XR, 82
Verapamil, 128
Viagra (sildenafil), 179
Violent patient, 76–80
    evaluating threats of violence, 78
    individual predictors of, 76
    management of, 78–79

    mental disorders with associated
        violent behavior, 77
    ongoing care of, 79–80
    patterns of violence, 77–78
Visual hallucinations, 11
Vivactil (protriptyline), 235t, 236
Vivitrol, for alcoholism, 152
Von Recklinghausen disease, 204
Voyeurism, 183

W
WAIS. *See* Wechsler Adult
    Intelligence Scale
Waking, 186
Watson-Schwartz Test, 89
Wechsler Adult Intelligence Scale
    (WAIS), 13, 64, 195
Wellbutrin (bupropion), 244
Wernicke encephalopathy, 148
Wilson disease, 31, 49, 67, 135, 204
Writ of habeus corpus, 268
Wyatt v Stickney, 268

X
Xanax (alprazolam), 160, 235t,
    243–244

Y
Youngberg v Romeo, 269

Z
Zaleplon (Sonata), 191, 250t
Zinermon v Burch, 273
Ziprasidone (Geodon), 216t, 226
    for delirium, 59
    for Tourette disorder, 140
    for violent patient, 78
Zoloft, (sertraline), 134, 179, 235t,
    242
Zolpidem (Ambien), 160, 161
    half-life/dose, 250t
    for insomnia, 188, 191
    treatment principles for, 253
Zyprexa (olanzapine), 59, 78, 140,
    199, 216t, 226, 262